Data quality in
longitudinal research

European Network on Longitudinal Studies on Individual Development

Chairman: David Magnusson

Coordination Committee Members: Paul Baltes, Paul Casaer, Alex Kalverboer, Jostein Mykletun, Anik de Ribaupierre, Michael Rutter, Fini Schulsinger, and Martti Takala

The European Science Foundation (ESF) is an association of 50 research councils and scientific academies in 18 European countries. The member organizations represent all scientific disciplines – in natural sciences, in medical and biosciences, in social sciences and in humanities. One of its main modes of operation is establishing scientific networks.

In this frame the European Network on Longitudinal Studies on Individual Development (ENLS) was established. By organizing a series of workshops on substantive and methodological topics, the network has brought together several hundred scientists from very different fields – criminology, developmental biology, epidemiology, pediatrics, psychiatrics, psychology, sociology, statistics, and others – all actively involved in longitudinal research. By distributing fellowships to young researchers and twinning grants to researchers for planning common projects, and by the development and administration of an inventory covering all major longitudinal projects in Europe, longitudinal research has been further supported and stimulated.

Michael Rutter, ed., Studies of psychosocial risk: The power of longitudinal data

Anik de Ribaupierre, ed., Transition mechanisms in child development: The longitudinal perspective

Data quality in longitudinal research

O.18
MAG

Edited by
DAVID MAGNUSSON
and
LARS R. BERGMAN

Department of Psychology
University of Stockholm

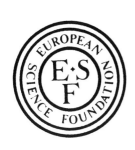

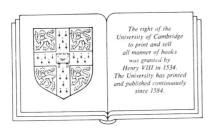

The right of the
University of Cambridge
to print and sell
all manner of books
was granted by
Henry VIII in 1534.
The University has printed
and published continuously
since 1584.

CAMBRIDGE UNIVERSITY PRESS

Cambridge
New York   Port Chester   Melbourne   Sydney

Published by the Press Syndicate of the University of Cambridge
The Pitt Building, Trumpington Street, Cambridge CB2 1RP
40 West 20th Street, New York, NY 10011, USA
10 Stamford Road, Oakleigh, Melbourne 3166, Australia

First published 1990

Printed in the United States of America

Library of Congress Cataloging-in-Publication Data

Data quality in longitudinal research / edited by David Magnusson and
Lars R. Bergman.
    p.   cm.
   ISBN 0-521-38091-X
   1. Medicine – Psychology – Sociology – Research – Quality control. 2. Medicine –
Psychology – Sociology – Longitudinal studies. I. Magnusson, David. II. Bergman,
Lars R.
R850.D37   1990
610'.72–dc20

                        89-34500
                           CIP

British Library Cataloguing in Publication Data

Data quality in longitudinal research.
1. Longitudinal studies
I. Magnusson, David II. Bergman, Lars R.
001. 4'2

ISBN 0-521-38091-X hard covers

Contents

Foreword

This text is the third in a series of volumes, emanating from the workshops organized by the European Network on Longitudinal Studies on Individual Development (ENLS) within the framework of the European Science Foundation.

The effective study of individual development in its biological, psychological, and social aspects involves many difficult problems with respect to substantive theories, methodologies for treatment of data, and research strategy. These aspects of developmental research have been analyzed in a large number of publications. Substantive theories on cognitive, moral, social, and biological development have been discussed extensively, and highly sophisticated models and methods for data treatment have been presented. During recent years, the necessity of a longitudinal research strategy for the study of individual development has been demonstrated. However, a basic requirement for effective empirical research on individual development, that is, the quality of the data expected to cover the structures and processes involved in individual development, on which the models and methods for data treatment are applied, has not drawn the attention it deserves from developmental researchers. No theory, no matter how functional and relevant it may be to the question under consideration, can be effectively studied in empirical research if data used to reflect the structures and processes involved do not meet certain requirements with respect to reliability, validity, and representativeness. And no methods for data treatment, however technically sophisticated they may be, can save data that do not meet these requirements. An explicit analysis of the quality of the data collected and used for the elucidation of the problem should be a main element of the planning and implementation of any developmental research project. This claim is particularly crucial for the planning and implementation of longitudinal research with reference to the long-term consequences of deficient planning and bad implementation, which cannot be remedied later.

A primary aim of this volume is to emphasize the importance of this claim and to draw the attention of researchers involved in longitudinal research to this aspect of the total research process. It is my conviction and that of my colleagues in the Network's Coordination Committee that by taking the claim seriously, longitudinal research will be in a much better position to contribute solid knowledge concerning the biological, psychological, and social factors that are involved in the life courses of individuals.

David Magnusson
Chairman of the ENLS Coordination Committee

Preface

In December 1987 the third workshop organized by the European Science Foundation Network on Longitudinal Studies on Individual Development was held at Rönneberga, Stockholm. The volume presented here contains the papers discussed at the workshop, revised on the basis of the comments and suggestions made, and a selection of the discussants' contributions.

The book is organized into three parts, preceded by an introductory chapter written by the editors. The introductory chapter discusses some general aspects of the central topic of the volume. Although it does not attempt to summarize the major points of the following chapters, we have profited from the other papers and have attempted to refer to them in the appropriate places.

The organization of the chapters emanating from the workshop is not necessarily self-evident. Because many of the papers discuss problems and issues that are appropriate to all parts of this book, the papers could have been organized in several ways. The organization we selected was as follows:

I. Data quality issues in different areas
II. Drop out and attrition
III. Design, methods, and data quality

Part I contains chapters on data quality within the areas of psychiatry, epidemiology, pediatrics, alcohol research, and research on antisocial behavior. The two chapters comprising Part II deal with minimizing drop-out rate and with estimating, and, where possible, correcting for, the effect of drop-out bias. Part III contains six chapters on issues of research design and strategy in relation to data quality. Topics such as types of data, age and cohort effects, implementing a longitudinal research program, and archiving longitudinal data are addressed.

We would like to express our gratitude to the participants of the symposium. Their scientific knowledge led to very fruitful and constructive discussions during the workshop. We are also thankful to Michael Rutter, who read and commented on the introductory chapter.

We wish to thank Bertil Törestad and Luki Hagen-Norberg for their invaluable contribution to the planning of the workshop and to the publication of this volume, and Sigrid Gustafson, who carefully checked the English of some of the chapters in this volume.

David Magnusson
Lars R. Bergman

Contributors to this volume

Jens B. Asendorpf, M.D.
MPI for Psychological Research
Munich

Lars R. Bergman, Ph.D.
Department of Psychology
University of Stockholm

Anne Colby, Ph.D.
Henry A. Murray Research Center, Radcliffe
  College
Cambridge, Massachusetts

Gunnar Eklund, Ph.D.
Department of Cancer Epidemiology
Karolinska Hospital, Stockholm

David P. Farrington, Ph.D.
Institute of Criminology, University of
  Cambridge
Cambridge

Ken Fogelman, M.D.
Institute of Criminology, University of
  Cambridge
Cambridge

John Fox, Ph.D.
Social Statistics Research Unit
City University, London

Bernard Gallagher, Ph.D.
Institute of Criminology, University of
  Cambridge
Cambridge

Johannes Huinink, M.D.
MPI for Human Development and Education
Berlin

Carl-Gunnar Janson, Ph.D.
Department of Sociology
University of Stockholm

David Magnusson, Ph.D.
Department of Psychology
University of Stockholm

Karl-Ulrich Mayer, M.D.
MPI for Human Development and Education
Berlin

Lynda Morley, Ph.D.
Institute of Criminology, University of
  Cambridge
Cambridge

Michael Murphy, M.D.
London School of Economics and Political Science
University of London

Erin Phelps, M.D.
Henry A. Murray Research Center, Radcliffe
  College
Cambridge, Massachusetts

Andrew Pickles, M.D.
MRC Child Psychiatry Unit
Institute of Psychiatry, London

Georg Rudinger, Ph.D.
Department of Psychology, Methodology and
  Statistics
University of Bonn

Michael Rutter, Ph.D.
MRC Child Psychiatric Unit
Institute of Psychiatry, London

Fini Schulsinger, Ph.D.
Psykologisk Institut, Psykiatrisk Afdelning
Kommunehospitalet, Copenhagen

Raymond J. St. Ledger, Ph.D.
Institute of Criminology, University of
*   Cambridge*
Cambridge

Franz E. Weinert, Ph.D.
MPI for Psychological Research
Munich

Donald J. West, M.D.
Institute of Criminology, University of
*   Cambridge*
Cambridge

Phillip Karl Wood, Ph.D.
Department of Individual and Family Studies
Pennsylvania State University
State College, Pennsylvania

Ambros Uchtenhagen, M.D.
Sozialpsychiatrischer Dienst der Psychiatrischen
*   Universitätsklinik Zürich*
Zurich

Rolf Zetterström, Ph.D.
Department of Pediatrics, Karolinska Institute
St. Göran's Children's Hospital, Stockholm

1 General issues about data quality in longitudinal research

LARS R. BERGMAN AND DAVID MAGNUSSON

Introduction

Longitudinal research is the lifeblood of the study of individual development. It has been pointed out many times that the most important questions concerning individual development can be answered only by applying a longitudinal design whereby the same individuals are followed through time (e.g., Magnusson, 1988; Mednick, Harway, & Finello, 1984; Rutter, 1981). However, no research can go beyond the quality of the basic data that are used, and this volume deals with the important topic of data quality in longitudinal research.

This introductory chapter discusses certain important general aspects of data quality as a background to the later chapters, which contain more detailed and specific expositions within different areas. Certain basic facts regarding, for instance, sampling, reliability, and validity are reiterated. Though these issues are important, they are too often neglected in empirical research.

Validity issues

Hypothetical and nonhypothetical variables

A fundamental prerequisite for the use of a certain type of data is that data are valid, that is, that they reflect the aspect of individual characteristics that they are expected to reflect and not something else. As long as we deal with basic somatic data – data for height, weight, pulse rate, blood pressure, for example – the validity of the data does not cause any serious problems in most cases. Data for these aspects have the following characteristics that are of importance for the application of most traditional measurement models and methods for data treatment:

1. These variables can be unequivocally defined and operationalized with enough precision for most purposes. This precision in definition implies, among other things, that the data for such variables directly reflect the individual characteristic in which we are interested. For practical purposes, such data can be interpreted straightforwardly without the use of a theory that explicates the nature of the phenomena or posits intervening variables.

1

2. Data reflect interindividual differences in *quantity* for a certain variable, without confounding quantitative differences with qualitative differences. Data for height refer to the same quality independent of the quantitative level that is measured.

3. Data for such variables retain their qualitative meaning across age levels. Height has the same quality at the age of 8, at the age of 18, and at the age of 70. This property makes data for various ages comparable and is a prerequisite for longitudinal studies of single variables.

Thus, when the issue under consideration can be elucidated by data of the kind just discussed the situation offers no major problems in the application of traditional models and methods for treatment of data, as long as other conditions, for example, representativeness, are met. In the following we will call such measures "direct measures."

The situation is quite different and much more troublesome when our interest is in what are usually designated "hypothetical constructs," that is, variables that are derived abstractions, the operationalization of which is not clear-cut but must be chosen by the researcher. Such hypothetical constructs – social class, intelligence, aggressiveness, hyperactivity, attachment, independence, anxiety, mobility, and many, many others – are very common and very central in developmental research, both when the interest is in normal development, such as in the areas of cognition and social development, and when it is in the developmental background of adult problems like health problems, criminal behavior, and alcohol abuse. Here it is very important to distinguish between the theoretical construct level and the operationalized level where the data exist. (For a discussion of hypothetical constructs the reader is referred to Marx, 1951, among others). In the following, data for operationalized hypothetical constructs will be designated "indirect measures." In chapter 2, Rutter and Pickles have drawn attention to the central role of such factors in psychiatric research and to the importance of considering the special properties of "hypothetical constructs" that are similar to what they call "latent variables" in that field.

Indirect measures. For the application of a measurement model using indirect measures of hypothetical constructs it is imperative to consider the fact that such constructs or variables do not have the properties that were summarized above for nonhypothetical variables. In contrast to what is valid for nonhypothetical variables, the following holds for variables that can be characterized as hypothetical constructs:

1. Hypothetical constructs are fuzzy; they are not unequivocally delineated and thus are not unequivocally defined theoretically in a manner that leads to one and only one measurement method. A variable on a hypothetical level is assumed to reflect a certain aspect of the total functioning of an individual. What will be studied (i.e., the indirect measure) is then determined by the properties of the method that is introduced for the collection of data, that is, by the way in which the construct is operationalized.

2. Indirect measures often cannot be assumed to reflect only quantitative differences; rather, such measures are frequently confounded because they may also reflect related qualitative differences. For example, a low aggressiveness score may reflect not only less of the same kind/quality of aggressiveness than does a high aggressiveness score. Rather, an indirect measure of the hypothetical construct "aggressiveness" may well reflect both quantitative and qualitative differences at various levels, and the two cannot always be separated from one another.

3. Indirect measures that are assumed to assess the same hypothetical construct at various age levels may reflect qualitatively different hypothetical constructs even if they are measured by the same instrument (e.g., Wohlwill, 1980). The constructs may differ both with respect to their very nature and meaning per se and with respect to the role they play in the total functioning of the individual.

Implications for the use of indirect measures

The foregoing discussion concerning the characteristics of hypothetical constructs and the properties of their indirect measures leads to specific consequences for the use of such data:

1. One obvious implication of the characteristic features of indirect measures is the necessity of seriously investigating the validity of the measures used in each case, because they have only an indirect relation to the theoretical construct they are assumed to indicate. The validity cannot be established once and for all. For each specific purpose it is crucial that the validity of the data used be estimated in one way or another. This can be done by the use of external criteria (*predictive* and *concurrent* validity), by the analysis of the content of the instrument (*content* validity), or by the study of how well the instrument functions in accordance with theoretical expectations (*construct* validity). (Cf. Magnusson, 1967; Nunnally, 1978)

2. As emphasized above, what determines the actual aspect of individual functioning or of the environment, covered by a certain theoretical definition of a hypothetical construct, is determined by the kinds of indirect measures used, that is, how it is operationalized. Maintaining strict definitions of hypothetical constructs in terms of operationalization was early stressed as a means to avoid confusion in the interpretation of results of empirical research. (Cf. the early definition of intelligence as "what is measured by a certain test".) In the extreme case this demand led to operationalism, pure operationalization without a solid basis in theory, a movement which has been strongly criticized. However, there are strong reasons to emphasize this need again. The lack of adherence to operational definitions has caused much confusion in the interpretation of the vast amount of empirical research in such important areas as social class, stress and anxiety, intelligence, and others.

In the beginning of this century much energy was expended in discussions regarding what intelligence really is. Of course, intelligence "isn't"; it does not exist as a unity, the boundaries of which can be delimited once and for all. It is a hypothetical construct aimed at assessing a certain chosen aspect of the total functioning of an organism. What is actually assessed by a certain measure of this aspect of individual functioning is, of course, defined by the properties of the instrument used for data collection.

An operational definition of a hypothetical construct, one that reflects a sound, substantive theory, enables us to interpret and discuss empirical results in a more meaningful way. It also provides a solid basis for theorizing about the character of the structures and processes under consideration, and their role in the total functioning of an individual.

3. A special problem in longitudinal studies concerns the measurement and analysis of change, an area in which it is particularly important to be clear in the formulation of relevant concepts and their nature. The conceptualization of change and stability is discussed by Asendorpf and Weinert in chapter 10.

4. In their chapter in this volume, Rutter and Pickles (chapter 2) draw attention to the importance of employing theory to underlie the empirical study of hypothetical constructs. The application of any method to data collection/scaling and data treatment/statistical analysis must rely on an appropriate measurement model. Such a model should include an assumption, based on theory, regarding the manner in which the aspect of individual functioning that is expressed in the definition of the hypothetical construct is reflected in the various types of data that can be used.

Very commonly, linear regression models are applied to the treatment of data used in the study of the relations among variables. This implies, among other things, the assumption that there is a monotonic (often linear) relation between individuals' positions on a dimension for the latent hypothetical construct and the overt behavior that is reflected in data (Figure 1.1A).

The effectiveness of the study then relies on the validity of that assumption. If, for example, the hypothetical construct under study is aggressiveness as a latent disposition, and the question is how well data for overt aggression reflect individuals' positions on the dimension for latent aggressiveness, a competing measurement model could be advocated from a psychodynamic point of view (see Figure 1.1B). According to such a model, for low to medium latent aggressiveness there is a monotonic positive relation, such that the more aggressive a person is, the more overt aggression he or she will show. However, when the latent aggressiveness becomes very strong, the aggressive impulses are repressed and overt aggression is inhibited. The stronger the aggressive impulses, the stronger the defense mechanisms, and the relation between hypothetical latent aggressiveness and overt aggression will take the form shown in Figure 1.1B. The example serves to demonstrate the necessity of being aware of which measurement model, with its explicit or implicit assumptions about the underlying hypothetical construct and its role in the functioning of the total individual, appropriately reflects the researcher's theoretical position. It is crucial to base the choice of methods for data collection and of procedure for data treatment on a proper measurement model.

The possibility of different individuals having a different functional relationship between the value in the observed indicator and the position with regard to a latent

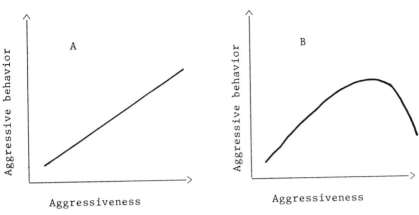

Figure 1.1. The assumed function of actual aggressive behavior on latent aggressiveness for (A) the trait measurement model and (B) the psychodynamic measurement model. From Magnusson (1976).

disposition must also be taken seriously, especially with regard to attitude measurement (Saris, 1988). Such differences can invalidate ordinary statistical procedures and Saris points to the importance of providing fixed reference points in opinion measurement in order to reduce differences in response functions.

Aspects of data

Different types of data

Many types of data may be used in a longitudinal framework, and Rudinger and Wood give an overview of this issue in chapter 9 (see also Coombs, 1964, for a general discussion of types of data). Most of the data used in empirical, developmental research take the form of numbers assigned to the phenomena under consideration. Nevertheless, it is sometimes possible and suitable to use more qualitative information, which is not normally used in quantitative analyses. In chapter 11 Schulsinger discusses a possible way of using such data for case-wise analyses. Here, however, to serve as a background to the discussion of measurement errors, we give a brief presentation of different types of data, classified according to the data collection method.

There are, of course, many ways of classifying data and, without claiming that a complete classification is presented, we just state that the following data collection methods are frequently used:

1. Data collection from records (e.g., school records, criminal records);
2. Laboratory procedures and procedures yielding direct measures (e.g., the measurement of length, weight, determination of hormone levels from blood samples);
3. Inventories (e.g., a questionnaire about work conditions and attitudes to work);

4. Tests (e.g., an intelligence test in which there are a number of standardized questions that can be answered right or wrong).
5. Direct observations (e.g., of children in play situations leading to simple counts of the number of times a certain behavior is displayed or to more global ratings of the behavior);
6. Interviews (e.g., a psychiatric interview that often includes ratings or a standardized interview about working conditions).

Obviously, these categories sometimes overlap, and it is possible to carry out one kind of data collection in conjunction with another (e.g., giving an inventory as a handout during an interview). It should also be pointed out that the subjective methods are more controllable now than they were previously because video recording can be used to document interviews and observation situations. Depending on what construct regarding which the collection method is supposed to yield data, direct or indirect measures can be produced by all classes of data collection methods; but in practice, methods 3 – 6 are more frequently used in generating indirect measures.

State and trait data

The appropriate type of data for analysis and description of individual functioning in a certain study depends primarily on the characteristics of the problem under study. Thus, it is important to clarify whether the problem is to be considered as individual momentary functioning at a certain occasion in a certain situation, that is, as an individual *state,* or if it is individual functioning in terms of general dispositions to react in a certain way, that is, in terms of *traits.* Each of these two types of problems requires its specific type of data. The first type of problem requires situation-specific data, and the second type requires nonsituation-specific data. Situation-specific data for aggressive behavior, for example, collected in a certain situation at a certain occasion reflect the individual's momentary state(s) and can be used for the study of the relation between momentary state(s) and specific situational factors, as is done in laboratory research and for the study of the relation between various momentary states in that type of situation. Data for aggressiveness aggregated across situations, that is, nonsituation-specific data, on the other hand, can be used for the analysis of individual differences with respect to general dispositions to react with aggressiveness. But such data aggregated across situations cannot, for example, be used for analyses of cross-situational variation in individual behavior. This statement is obvious and may even seem trivial. However, negligence in considering the point made here is one reason why much of the last decade's discussion over personality consistency has become more of a semantic quarrel than a scientific debate (Magnusson, 1988).

Aggregation of data

The above discussion regarding (a) the fuzziness of hypothetical constructs and the connected problems in their operationalization and in the interpretation of data that reflect them and (b) the importance of maintaining the distinction between situation-specific and nonsituation-specific data can be discussed from the viewpoint of data aggregation.

For the study of individual functioning we can distinguish three types of aggregation of data:

1. Across situations
2. Across subvariables
3. Across time

Aggregations of these types are very common in developmental research. They often occur in conjunction. For example, ratings of personality traits in children, say hyperactivity, made by teachers are usually based on observations in various types of situations across time and may reflect a trait at a high level of generality.

A fundamental requirement for any study of individual functioning is that the data used for analysis be appropriate with respect to the level of the structures and processes involved (Magnusson, 1988). The level of the structures and processes that are reflected in data depends on if, how, and to what extent data are aggregated in one of the ways described above. For the choice of the appropriate data for the elucidation of a specific problem, it is thus fundamental to know the properties of aggregated data.

Aggregation across situations. Aggregation of data across situations yields nonsituation-specific data. A nonsituation-specific datum is usually obtained in one of two ways. The first way is by summing or averaging situation-specific data covering a range of situations. The second and the most common type of aggregation takes place when raters who have observed the ratees across situations express their generalizations directly in nonsituation-specific data. This type of aggregation is concealed in the answers to questions in traditional inventories ("Do you often . . . ?"), in which respondents aggregate observations about themselves across situations that they usually choose themselves. This type of aggregation also occurs in nonsituation-specific ratings of, for example, social behavior, in which situation-specific observations are aggregated by an observer to arrive directly at an aggregated nonsituation-specific datum. Moreover, in order to ensure high reliability in observational data, ratings are often aggregated across raters. Ratings from several observers are thus aggregated twice: First, the individual observer has aggregated observations across situations, the properties of which are seldom known and controlled, and, second, such aggregated ratings from several observers have been aggregated again.

Aggregation of observations across situations implies that situation-specific information is lost and, consequently, that the analysis of such data will reflect structures and processes at a nonsituation-specific level. Thus, nonsituation-specific data are not representative of, nor do they reflect, individual responses in a specific situation. Most of the common methods for data collection in developmental research, like ratings based on direct observation, interviews, and inventories, often yield nonsituation-specific data with the characteristics just described.

Aggregation, reliability, internal consistency, and homogeneity

A fundamental requirement for the use of a certain method for data collection is that it yields data that are replicable. That is, if we measure the same characteristic twice for a certain individual under similar conditions, the results should be the same. The extent to which a method for data collection meets this requirement is expressed in terms of its *reliability*. Empirically, the reliability of a method for data collection is usually expressed in a reliability coefficient.

Under the general heading of reliability a series of various methods are covered: methods for the calculation of test–retest coefficients, coefficient alpha (Kuder-Richardson's 20 and 21), split-half coefficients, and so forth. Each of these coefficients for estimating the reliability in a certain type of data has its own properties. It is essential that the researcher be aware of these characteristics in order to arrive at the correct interpretation of a certain type of reliability coefficient. General presentations and discussions of the various methods for estimation of reliability are given elsewhere (see, e.g., Magnusson, 1967; Nunnally, 1978). Here only two main points will be made: one referring to the interpretation of what is usually designated "internal consistency coefficients"; the other concerning the interpretation of "homogeneous factors."

The interpretation of internal consistency. It should be observed that a reliability coefficient is assumed to reflect the extent to which a certain measure of a certain variable is replicable. This fact must be remembered when reliability coefficients of any composite measure, for example, test scores and sums of ratings, are interpreted. Coefficients such as the common KR 20 and KR 21 are often incorrectly interpreted as reflecting the internal consistency or homogeneity of the composite measure. This misunderstanding is easily made, given the use of the term *internal consistency coefficient* for some types of reliability coefficients (e.g., KR 21); although, as a matter of fact, the size of such a coefficient is not only dependent upon and reflective of the intercorrelations among the parts on which a composite measure is based. It is also dependent on the number of parts making up the composite measure, the reliability of which is being estimated. Thus, an instrument consisting of many items may have a very high KR 21 reliability, although the intercorrelations among the items are very low. For instance, the average coefficient for the intercorrelations among single items in a 40-item questionnaire with an estimated KR 21 of 0.88 is only 0.15, and the average intercorrelation among six raters whose summarized ratings yield a reliability coefficient of 0.80 can be estimated to be only 0.40.

Agreement among raters does not mean high validity. Ratings made by competent observers are powerful and very useful data in developmental research (Cairns & Green, 1979; Magnusson, 1988; Scarr, 1981). As is the case for other types of data, reliability of ratings aggregated across raters is most often estimated by some sort of reliability coefficient. As emphasized above, the size of such coefficients depends upon the degree of agreement among the observers and upon the number of observers. Interpreted correctly, such coefficients are useful. However, high reliability coefficients for composite ratings are sometimes also interpreted as indicating high validity of the ratings, that is, the extent to which they stand for what they are assumed to reflect. This incorrect interpretation is especially easy to make when the raters are experts in their field. It has, nevertheless, been demonstrated empirically that high agreement among raters, even among highly competent experts, can primarily reflect a common bias dominating the field (Nystedt & Magnusson, 1973). Thus, the validity of ratings, even those made by experts, must be confirmed, as is the case for other types of data.

Aggregation and homogeneity. Aggregating data to enable the researcher to work with more reliable measures is a common feature of research on individual functioning. This aggregation is often done without considering that the degree to which data are aggregated across subvariables and across situations determines the level of individual structures and processes that will be reflected in the aggregated data. The frequent use of factor analysis in order to arrive at more reliable data in terms of what is misleadingly called "homogeneous factors" offers a good example. From a purely statistical point of view it is possible to show that factors that are regarded as homogeneous when obtained by factor analysis actually may yield factor scores containing subvariables with very low intercorrelations. Methodologically, this fact emphasizes the need for caution in the interpretation of factors and for a careful consideration of the measurement model for the factors and how it explains the intercorrelations among factors at the aggregated level. With respect to the interpretation of the contents of a factor, it is essential to keep in mind that aggregation of scores from subvariables belonging to a homogeneous factor may conceal important individual differences in specific aspects of the domain covered by the factor.

A striking example of this issue is given by Magnusson (1988). In a factor analysis of teachers' ratings of schoolchildren's behavior, a main factor emerged with the highest loadings for two variables: aggressiveness and motor restlessness. The intercorrelation between these two variables was .66. In spite of this result, both these variables were included separately in a study of the relation between manifest behavior and physiological activity/reactivity in terms of adrenaline excretion. Both variables were found to be significantly negatively related to adrenaline excretion in two independent situations. However, partial regression analyses showed that with motor restlessness partialed out, the original correlation between aggressiveness and adrenaline excretion totally disappeared. On the other hand, when ratings of aggressiveness were partialed out from the relation between motor restlessness and adrenaline excretion, the relation was still significant. Thus, there were differences in the relation of aggression and of motor restlessness to adrenalin excretion that were of theoretical importance. This result clearly demonstrates the danger in working at the factor level for the sole purpose of obtaining the more statistically reliable data aggregation may provide. It is as if a meteorologist always would prefer to aggregate data for various aspects of the weather across the days of a whole season, because that kind of data are more reliable and would be more stable across years than are data for single days. If, in the above study, aggressiveness and motor restlessness had been viewed as measuring the same homogeneous factor, and the sum of the scores for these two variables had been used in the analyses instead of the separate variables, the above reported results would not have been found.

Aspects of sampling

The sampling aspects in longitudinal settings have many facets; here the interrelated topics of sample representativeness, sample size, and sample attrition are briefly discussed.

Sample representativeness

An obvious, important prerequisite for effective longitudinal research is that the sample studied be reasonably representative of the population to which one wishes to make inferences; otherwise, one should refrain from conducting the study. However, representativeness is a relative and a multidimensional concept. Very rarely is it possible to obtain a strictly random sample of the exact population to which one wants to generalize.

With random samples there is also a representativeness problem if the samples are small, because a sample by chance can deviate from the population in important aspects. However, this situation can be modeled and ordinary inferential statistics applied. The importance of the sample size in this situation will be discussed in the next section, "Sample size." Often the sample under consideration is not a strictly random sample for the following two reasons:

1. Practical considerations frequently lead to using nonrandom sampling procedures (e.g., enrolling in a longitudinal study all children born at a certain hospital during a two-month period).

2. Full information is not obtained for all persons in the initial sample; a drop out occurs influencing the size of the effective sample. In longitudinal studies this problem of sample attrition can be troublesome (see the section "Sample attrition").

The degree of sample representativeness should be judged by comparing the effective sample with (a) the initial sample and (b) the population, using whatever

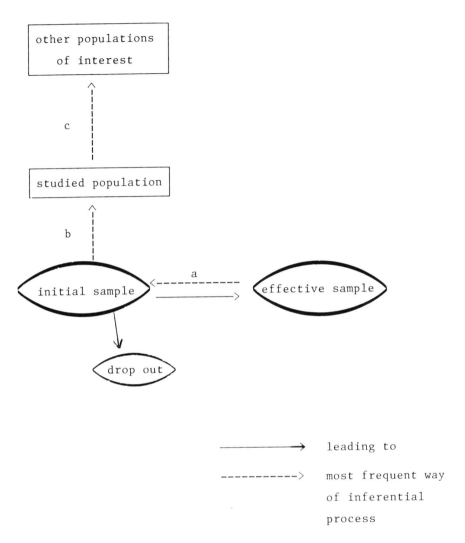

Figure 1.2. The inferential process.

information is available. This corresponds to studying the arrows *a* and *b* in Figure 1.2.

It is also important that a detailed description of the sampling procedure be given to aid the reader in judging the quality of the sample. Considering the nonrandom nature of most samples that are studied, it is surprising to note the strong importance that sometimes is given to the results of significance tests for which the assumptions are not even remotely fulfilled.

With regard to the *population* the sample is drawn from, one usually has to compromise and use a sample from a reasonably accessible population that one judges to be relevant but not exactly what one would like to have. For instance, one might use a sample of children from a certain urban community ("studied population" in Figure 1.2) to investigate a specific research question instead of sampling children from all urban communities in the country, the population the researcher judges as ideal in that situation ("other populations" in Figure 1.2). In the nonideal case, one must assume that there is a reasonably strong similarity between the two populations in relevant aspects, thus implying the generalizability represented by arrow *c* in Figure 1.2.

However, a careful description of the population under study, as well as a discussion of the similarities and differences between it and other, more general populations, is quite frequently missing in publications. It should not be left to the reader to make this kind of difficult judgment without the necessary information's being furnished by the author (see Bergman, 1972). The importance of a careful description of the population under study and of a discussion of its similarity and dissimilarity in relevant aspects to other populations of interest has been emphasized before. Such information is particularly important when the interest is in comparing cohorts that vary in different aspects. The comparison can also be simpler for a longitudinal study than for a cross-sectional study, because the former contains data from many ages, thereby increasing the chances of finding a good comparison population for at least one of the ages.

Sample size

Obviously, other things being equal, it is better to have a large sample than a small sample. However, especially in a longitudinal setting it might not be possible to obtain a large sample. There is also a trade-off between a larger sample with less in-depth information collected and fewer resources for reducing the drop out, and so forth, versus a smaller sample of a higher quality.

An important aspect of sample size is its relation to the standard error of measurement. Let us assume that a random sample can be obtained. To illustrate the size of random fluctuations in a rather frequent empirical case, Figure 1.3 was constructed. It shows how much one can expect the obtained percentage to vary for different sample sizes when the percentage in the population is 30. The upper and lower limits contain 95% of the observed percentages.

Two basic conclusions can be drawn from Figure 1.3. First, it is seen that for very small samples the size of the variation in the obtained percentages can be expected to be so large that the percentage estimate is almost useless. For instance, for $n = 10$ the obtained percentage can, in 95% of the cases, be expected to vary between 2 and 58% when the population percentage is 30%. (The size of this interval varies not only with the sample size and confidence level but also with the population percentage.) Second, the law of diminishing returns can also be seen, because a large increase

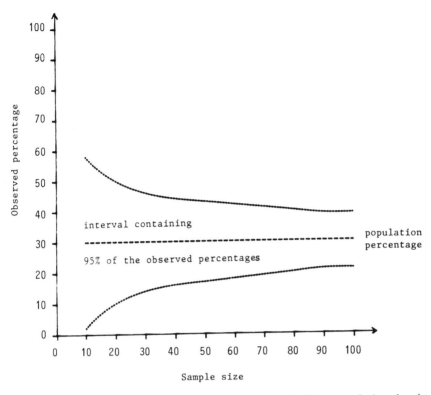

Figure 1.3. Interval of expected variation of the sample percentage for different sample sizes when the population percentage is 30%.

in an already large sample is necessary to decrease appreciably the range of the expected variation of the obtained percentage. Figure 1.3 shows that the important groups on which percentage calculations are to be based must not be too small, with an absolute minimum of 20–50, depending on the kind of inferences one wants to make. It is informative for researchers to envision, in the planning of a project, the most important analyses to be made and to consider how large the standard errors, power, and so forth, will be for the sample size they have in mind.

For the study of most aspects of individual development, longitudinal data are necessary, and they cannot be replaced by cross-sectional data. However, it should also be pointed out that even if one has a problem that in principle can be answered by a cross-sectional design (such as comparing the mean of some variable between ages), a longitudinal design or a mixed design can sometimes be more efficient. For instance, when studying the difference between means from two ages, the relative precision of a longitudinal design as compared to a cross-sectional design of the same sample size is 2.0 when the measures correlate 0.5. This means that to obtain the same precision when using a cross-sectional design, a sample is needed that is twice as large as that needed when using a longitudinal design. For higher correlations the difference is even larger. This is discussed more fully in Goldstein (1979).

Sample attrition

Sample attrition can be a serious problem when performing a longitudinal study, because even with a moderate drop out at each point in time the number of subjects with incomplete data will accumulate. The seriousness of the drop out will depend not only on its relative size but also on the characteristics of the drop out and on the problem under study. For instance, children with severe adjustment problems tend to be overrepresented in the drop out (Cox, Rutter, Yule, & Quinton, 1977; see also chapter 7 in this book); and it is obvious that in a longitudinal study of adjustment problems it is very important to achieve a low drop out rate. This point is also made by Zetterström in chapter 4 when discussing the study of problem families. Otherwise, the conclusion may be seriously undermined by the fact that the majority of children with severe problems in the population are lost from the study. However, in some settings the values on the main variables are not very different between the sample and the drop out because drop out is normally influenced by many different factors (cf. Bergman, Hanve, & Rapp, 1978, for a discussion of this). Thus, the effects of drop out on the results must be judged separately for each specific study with reference to its characteristic features.

In the above, it has implicitly been assumed that a lower drop out is preferable to a higher drop out. This is a natural assumption to make but not as unproblematic as it sounds. The main concern about the drop out from a statistical viewpoint is that, if biased, it leads to the effective sample's no longer being representative of the population. However, in some cases it might be that the cases creating the bias are, for instance, persons with severe adjustment problems who will end up in the drop out regardless of whether a more or less ambitious policy for drop-out reduction is followed. What is gained by more persistent fieldwork in such a case is only data from persons whose absence would not have created bias in the first place. Thus, in some cases the gain of a drop out reduction might not be as large as one would believe.

Of course, the most important recommendation with regard to sample attrition is to minimize it. For instance, in chapter 7 Farrington, Gallagher, Morley, St. Ledger, and West have shown how, by an extreme effort, the drop out can be reduced to a very low level; another example of this is given by Cairns, Cairns, and Neckerman (1987). The main factor behind their remarkable success in reducing the drop out appears to be persistent fieldwork utilizing a variety of methods for tracing and securing cooperation. In Cairns et al.'s study there had also been continuous contact with the subjects, but this was not the case in Farrington et al.'s study.

In chapter 8 Murphy raises the ethical problem of a possible intrusion of privacy if the fieldwork is too intense. However, this issue must be balanced against the ethical demand for conducting research that reaches valid conclusions about important phenomena. Of course, it is the responsibility of the researcher to point out to the subject that participation is voluntary, but once this is done it is the responsibility of the researcher to try to convince potential respondents to participate and to make a real effort to trace them. If the research performed is not important enough to outweigh the possible small intrusion of privacy that might result from efficient fieldwork, it should not be performed at all.

A longitudinal study not only tends to have drop out problems; it also offers possibilities for estimating the effects of the drop out and even for correcting for it. For instance, if a drop out occurs in a later wave of a longitudinal study, information is often available for a majority of the drop out from earlier waves. This information can be used for comparing the drop out and the respondents, and in this way a good basis is obtained for estimating the possible bias created by the drop out.

Denote with D_k the drop out group at time k. In certain situations, information from other points in time can be used for estimating the values for the key variables at time k for D_k (e.g., by using regression analysis). The mean of D_k can then be compared to that of the respondents (or the mean of the respondents compared with the mean of the whole sample), and in this way very direct information is obtained about the bias of the drop out in the investigation variables. Depending on the type of analysis being performed in the study, the results may even be corrected for the effect of the drop out (Bergman, 1972). The feasibility of this approach depends mainly on the following three factors:

1. The availability of good predictors from other points in time of the key variables at time k;
2. The feasibility of the assumption that similar relationships between predictors and key variables hold for the group with complete data and for D_k;
3. The information obtained by this approach, which usually is in terms of estimated means for D_k, must be relevant for the issue at hand. (For example, if the purpose is to build a structural equation model at time k, the information is rather indirect for judging the effects of the drop out on the results of such an analysis.)

The above discussion has centered around handling the situation when *all* information is missing for certain subjects at one or more points in time. Partial drop out of some types of data for certain individuals at a specific point in time can also create problems. Often multivariate analyses are performed on longitudinal data where the analyses formally require complete information for a substantial number of variables from several points in time. Even a very moderate drop out rate for each variable can then create serious problems, because the rate tends to be rather additive when complete data are demanded, sometimes resulting in a prohibitive drop out rate.

Various ways have been followed to "solve" this problem:

1. When a correlation matrix is the basis for the multivariate analysis, each correlation is calculated for all subjects having the necessary data for the specific correlation. For instance, in SPSSX (1986) this procedure is called "pairwise dele-

tion." Thus, the sample for which the correlations have been calculated varies across cells in the correlation matrix.

2. The overall mean for the variable is imputed for cases having a missing datum for this variable.

3. A regression analytic method, like the one described above, is used for the imputation (see also Dalenius, 1962; Gleason & Staelin, 1975).

4. A twin method is used; that is, for a subject with incomplete data a twin with complete data is searched for, and the twin's value(s) in the missing variable(s) is imputed (see, e.g., Bergman & El-Khouri, 1986, who applied this method within the context of pattern analysis).

It should also be pointed out that item 1 above is a kind of imputation and, in our opinion, often not a very sound one. Which method is preferable is, of course, specific to the particular study, but a careful use of imputed values is often preferable to accepting a heavy drop out due to incomplete data. Two conditions must then be met: values should only be imputed for subjects with almost complete data, and the resulting data file containing the imputed values must not be considered as a permanent data file but only as a temporary file for a specific analysis.

Errors of measurement

Errors of measurement are ubiquitous in longitudinal research, as in almost all other scientific endeavors involving measurement. For instance, Eklund in chapter 3 discusses the possible errors introduced by using a datum referring to one point in time as representative of the conditions during a long period of time. The importance of considering errors of measurement in relation to theory and not as an isolated phenomenon is emphasized by Rudinger and Wood in chapter 9 and by Rutter and Pickles in chapter 2. The main point is that there should be a simultaneous consideration of (1) the theory regarding the substantive phenomena under study, the hypothetical constructs evolving from the theory, and their relation to the observables, and (2) how the errors of measurement operate in influencing the observables and their relations to the latent variables.

In the research endeavor this should be expressed in the general design of the study, in the choice of relevant indicators and careful measurement procedures, and in the choice of appropriate statistical models for handling and estimating errors.

It has repeatedly been emphasized that errors can be conceptualized differently with reference to the characteristics of the study under consideration. The proper conceptualization of possible errors is vital both for the design of the study and the data to be collected and for the choice of appropriate statistical models for analyzing the data (Bergman, 1988; Cronbach, Gleser, Nanda, & Rajaratnam, 1972). In a longitudinal study, the issue of errors of measurement is complicated by the fact that a time dimension is introduced; for instance, the use of the same instrument at two different points in time may create a systematic retest effect. However, it cannot generally be stated that errors of measurement should be a more serious problem in a longitudinal

effects of errors of measurement. Our knowledge is usually incomplete, but this does not absolve us from taking them seriously. Considering the difficulties involved, it is not surprising that so little empirical research has been done in this area, although it is by no means an impossible task. Neither should the problem be viewed as "pulling another skeleton out of the closet" because, it is hoped, the results of such an undertaking will show that in many cases the effects of errors "in real life" tend not to be very dramatic and need not undermine confidence in our empirical findings.

Expectancy effects

Expectancy effects can affect the quality of data in different ways. Two major aspects of such effects will be discussed here; namely, expectancy effects influencing the operationalization of variables and expectancy effects influencing ratings.

Expectancy effects in the operationalization of constructs. It has been pointed out many times that expectancy effects may lead to a bias in that results tend to be produced that are consistent with the prevailing beliefs or theories within the area. Greenwald, Pratkanis, Lieppe, and Baumgardner (1986) call this "confirmation bias." This phenomenon operates on many levels, including the level of data quality.

Let us assume that a researcher, when analyzing a data set, has used a complicated coding or quantification procedure, which is only one of many possible ones. It is then natural that he or she might be hesitant about the appropriateness of the measurement procedures if the results of the analyses exhibited strange properties (usually meaning that the results were contrary to expectations). The danger then becomes using these contrary results as the sole justification for changing a coding or quantification procedure. Such a process would lead to an expectancy bias. The risk is increased by the availability of powerful computer programs that make such changes easy to implement. The otherwise well-founded requirement for saving basic raw data in longitudinal studies can also facilitate this bias in that the necessary data remain available for performing alternative codings, and so forth.

It is doubtful that the researcher's awareness of this expectancy effect constitutes a sufficient safeguard against it. In a longitudinal research program it is presumably a wise procedure to require a written plan for the coding and operationalization of the variables made before any computations are performed and to insist upon some sort of more formal decision before a changed coding or operationalization is accepted.

Expectancy effects in ratings. It is well known that ratings, although a very powerful tool for data collection, can also lead to bias (e.g., errors of halo, severity, and leniency; see Kerlinger, 1973). It has also been emphasized repeatedly that raters should not be given information concerning (a) to which of clinical or control groups each ratee belongs and (b) the hypothesis being tested. The background to this rule is the assumption that raters can be influenced by such information in the direction of confirming the hypothesis in cases when they are in doubt.

A rather dramatic example from the second author's research demonstrates this expectancy effect. Two psychologists rated, independent of each other, drawings from the Bender psychomotor test given to 30 subjects in an experimental group and 30 matched subjects in a control group. It was then believed that all indications of group belongingness had been removed from the test protocols. The results showed that for 27 out of 30 matched pairs the differences were in the expected direction and that the interrater correlation was also high. Thus, the hypothesis was confirmed at a high level of significance. The raters asserted that they had not known to which of the groups each individual belonged. However, a scrutiny of the test protocols revealed that, by mistake, a red mark had been left on the test protocols for the experimental group, whereas a blue mark remained on the test protocols for the control group. In order to rule out the importance of this information for the ratings, a new rating was performed by a third psychologist after removing the colored marks. This yielded results in which only 18 out of 30 matched pairs showed differences in the expected direction. The result was not significant, and thus the hypothesis was not confirmed.

Though the rule just discussed is often reiterated, it is too often neglected in empirical research. The above example demonstrates how important it is that the rule be maintained.

Interviewer effects in standardized interviews

Of course, there are means other than expectancy effects through which bias or error can be introduced into ratings or interviews. In fact, it might well appear in a situation in which one might believe that the scope for interviewer effects on the results would be small, namely, the standardized interview with standardized response alternatives. The effects of the interviewer on the response variation in this situation have been studied within the survey research area where it has been shown that interviewer effects can introduce serious errors of measurement (Kish, 1962).

Interviewer effects refer to the different ways in which the interviewer as a person can affect the responses obtained; for instance, via social desirability effects or via different interviewers' having different ways of expressing the questions. Among other things, it has been shown that in many survey studies the mean squared error of an estimated mean is considerably underestimated because interviewer variance is not incorporated in the ordinary variance formula. The critical factor here is the number of interviews per interviewer. The higher this number is, the higher the response variance due to individual differences among interviewers will be. In a constructed example, Bergman and Wärneryd (1982) showed that, with 40 interviews per interviewer, it is not unreasonable to expect the real standard deviation of the mean to be about one and a half times higher than that given by the ordinary formula, which assumes that no systematic interviewer effects exist. Thus, having one interview per interviewer in this case would imply that only half the sample size would give the same standard error of measurement.

Naturally, the size and nature of the interviewer effects depend on the kind of question asked and on the interviewers' expertise. Generally speaking, the effects are less pronounced for simple factual questions and more pronounced for complicated questions where the instructions for the interviewers are unclear or for questions where social desirability factors may operate (Collins, 1980). However, even for factual questions interviewer variance can be troublesome if the interviewers cannot be properly trained. This is exemplified by Statistics Canada's changing from interviews to self-enumeration in the census of 1971, a decision that led to a substantial decrease in the correlated error variance (Krotki & Hill, 1978). In our opinion, this is an important area for applied statistical and psychometric research, one that has been rather neglected outside the survey area.

In certain situations, it may be a good idea to avoid interviewer effects by supplementing or replacing interviews with a questionnaire; for instance, replacing the interview survey with a mail survey (with interview follow-up to reduce the drop out) or using a handout within an interview for certain sensitive or social desirability-loaded questions. It should thus be recognized that the interview, although it is a powerful, versatile tool for data collection, should not be the first choice in all situations. Sometimes a questionnaire is not just a cheap substitute but a better alternative.

Retrospective data

In a developmental setting an important issue concerning errors of measurement is the question of whether retrospective data of sufficient quality can be obtained in a certain area, thus making the collection of time-consuming and expensive prospective longitudinal data unnecessary. Undoubtedly, this is the case in certain situations, but in many situations retrospective data will contain sizable errors of which we have very incomplete knowledge (Moss & Goldstein, 1979). If retrospective data are used, it is important that the questions be carefully constructed, for instance, by using some method of aided recall (Cannell, Marquis, & Laurent, 1977) and that a validation procedure be incorporated into the design. The burden of proof is on the user of this kind of instant data to show that the data are of sufficient quality. (An example of such a discussion is given by Mayer & Huinink in chapter 12 when discussing the life event data they collected using a retrospective method.) A general discussion of retrospective data, undesirable behavior, and the longitudinal perspective is given by Janson in chapter 6.

General comments

As emphasized by several other authors in this book, the most important issue concerning errors of measurement is, of course, to minimize them by careful design of the study and also by skillful execution of the data collection. Subsequently, it is important to model the errors and to analyze their effects in an appropriate way. One should, however, not forget the less theoretically exciting part of this work, which is a down-to-earth analysis of the actual measurement situation and what happened there. (This is exemplified by Farrington et al. in chapter 7 in their analysis of the data collection.) For this purpose it is important to have access to raw data in its most basic form, as is exemplified in Bergman's (1988) analysis of errors in self-reported factors measuring intrinsic adjustment. It is also essential that an extensive and accurate documentation exists. This need for basic raw data in longitudinal studies and for careful documentation has been emphasized by several authors in this volume.

Time aspects of longitudinal data

The fact that the time dimension is included in a prospective, longitudinal study gives it its unique value for studying development. As emphasized before, only this kind of study can provide the necessary data for effective analyses of many aspects of individual development. Although the time perspective is an asset, it also implies some problems for longitudinal research. Two such problems, commonly discussed, will be briefly touched upon.

Cohort effects

Cohort effects have been the focus of much attention within different disciplines, and in this context the reader is referred to Baltes (1968) and to chapter 12 in this volume. One restriction of longitudinal studies performed on only one age cohort representing a certain generation is that the results in some respects may not be generalizable to other cohorts raised and living under other social and physical environmental conditions. For example, a change in the labor market and in its demand for theoretical education and professional training from one generation to another may have profound effects on youngsters' interest in higher education and in vocational training and on their choice of educational and vocational careers. Consequently, for the elucidation of some aspects of individual development it is necessary to control for cohort effects by including several cohorts in the study. The appropriate difference in age between the cohorts then depends upon the character of the problem under study.

Two other aspects of the issue about differences among cohorts are important to have in mind.

First, differences among cohorts not only reflect measurement errors; they also contain important information that is an essential outcome of a longitudinal study. For example, information about the nature of the effects of changing labor markets on the youngsters' willingness to go into vocational training or into higher theoretical education will contribute to a better understanding of the factors involved in the process underlying individuals' educational and vocational careers. Excellent studies, using the information on differences among generations to elucidate essential issues, have, for instance, been presented by Elder and his coworkers (see, e.g., Elder & Rockwell, 1979).

Second, though differences among cohorts exist for many aspects of individual development, there are important aspects that are not influenced by such differences. For example, it is difficult to see how cohort effects could influence the lawfulness of the interactions in which cognitions, neurotransmitters, and behaviors in individuals are involved. The necessity of making allowance for cohort effects in a longitudinal design is thus dependent on the problem under study. In some cases even just cross-sectional information from a new cohort about relevant variables and the relationships between them can considerably increase the knowledge about the possibilities and limitations of generalizing the results from the longitudinal study to the new generation.

Fading relevancy of longitudinal data

Sometimes the following has been argued. Because a long-term longitudinal study takes a long time to carry out, there is a risk that the theoretical framework that served as the basis for the design of the study, for the choice of variables, and for the construction of indexes, and so forth, has become obsolete by the time the data collection is complete and the results can be published. This problem of possible fading relevance is discussed by Janson in chapter 6. It is one aspect of the danger in pursuing too narrow-minded a theoretical approach in developmental research, an approach in which the value of the results of testing specific hypotheses is too strongly time dependent and is tied to specific procedures. Especially when performing longitudinal research, one must be theoretically broad-minded or even in many cases eclectic. Data should be collected with the purpose of their being useful within different theoretical perspectives, and for this purpose it is important to retain data in their most basic form so that they can be adapted to other coding procedures, and so forth. This issue has been discussed by several other authors in this volume.

In this connection, the importance of careful observation and description per se should be stressed (Magnusson, 1988). A solid work of this kind is the only sound basis for theory and hypothesis generation. In our opinion, too often this very important preliminary step has been skipped and the researcher has started theorizing directly. This might, for instance, lead to wasting research efforts on the construction of formal theories that careful observation could have ruled out from the beginning as being not consistent with the phenomena. The above position does not mean that we advocate a mere atheoretical stocking of facts. Naturally, observation and description should be guided, but not blinkered, by reference to existing knowledge and theories and a careful analysis of the phenomena under observation. As already emphasized, the outcome of such observations and description forms the best basis for sound theorizing (Cronbach, 1975). Theories are transitory, but good longitudinal data are not; it should be recognized that a longitudinal research program, with

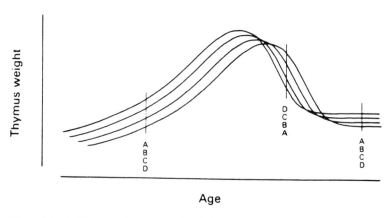

Figure 1.5. Fictitious growth curves for four individuals A–D with respect to thymus weight. From Magnusson (1988).

its investments in time, funding, and members' long-term commitment, is too valuable to risk for a theoretical one-shot.

Perhaps the possible risk of fading relevancy of longitudinal data is something of a blessing in disguise if the researcher is aware of the risk and takes the relevant countermeasures. This can lead to research of more general value. Such research will also be less contaminated by the confirmation bias that is considered by some to be a major problem in the accumulation of knowledge in research (Greenwald et al., 1986).

Chronological and biological age as markers of development

The central marker of development in biological and psychological research on developmental phenomena is chronological age (cf. Magnusson, in press). It has been used as a dependent variable (e.g., the age at which a certain behavior typically occurs) but in most cases serves as the main independent variable or as a control variable (e.g., height is studied as a function of chronological age). The main stages of development are almost exclusively discussed with reference to chronological age, and this is true for research on phenomena at all age stages, from infancy to aging. This approach however, is not without serious problems.

The limitation of using chronological age as the marker of individual development has its basis in the existence of strong individual differences in biological growth rate (Magnusson, 1985). Let us look at a developmental curve for a somatic individual variable that can be studied objectively, namely, the weight of the thymus. This curve is characteristic for the lymphoid system, including lymph nodes and intestinal masses (Tanner, 1978). The typical growth curve for the weight of the thymus gland is shown in Figure 1.5 for four hypothetical individuals, A–D, who differ with respect to biological age, as indicated by the chronological age at which the growth curve reaches its peak. (The weight of the thymus reaches a peak at around 12 years of age and then declines rather rapidly to about half that weight at the age of about 20.)

For various chronological ages, Figure 1.5 shows the rank orders of the individuals with respect to the weight of the thymus. It is seen, for instance, that although the rank order of individuals with respect to thymus weight varies dramatically across ages, there is perfect stability and consistency once biological age is taken into account. What is demonstrated in Figure 1.5 regarding individual differences is also indicated for other psychological as well as biological variables (see, e.g., Bateson, 1978; Ljung, 1965; Loevinger, 1966).

This fact of individual differences in maturational tempo has far-reaching methodological consequences (see Magnusson, 1985; Wohlwill, 1970). What will be discussed here, where we are concerned with the quality of data, are the consequences of neglecting the existence of individual differences in growth rate when using chronological age as the marker of development, especially in cross-sectional studies.

In all cross-sectional matrices of data for aspects of individual functioning that are related systematically to biological maturation, a portion of the variance will be determined by individual differences with respect to biological growth rate. This is also true for data sets in which all subjects are of the same chronological age. Thus, for example, coefficients reflecting relationships among adjustment variables during puberty will be partly determined by individual differences in biological maturity. Such, of course, will be the case even if data for biological maturation are not included in the matrix of data.

Schaie's (1965) model for development maintains that "a response is a function of the age of the organism, the cohort to which the organism belongs, and the time at which measurement occurs" (p. 93). (As Baltes, 1968, noted, Schaie's model implies that two dimensions are free to vary and that data can be explained by a two-dimensional plane in the three-dimensional space.) By age, Schaie here obviously means chronological age. What has been demonstrated above indicates that adding biological age will increase the variance that can be explained in a matrix of developmental data, and using biological age as a complement to chronological age as a marker of development will help us better understand developmental processes per se.

What has been said here about the importance of using biological age as a marker for development is not only applicable to research on early stages of individual development. It is also applicable to research across the life span, for example, to the study of aging. The use of chronological age as the main marker of development in traditional research on aging is a major limitation in that type of research, because individual differences in biological age may be even greater in older age than in infancy, childhood, and/or adolescence. Using biological age as a central marker of development in research on aging, for example, by standardizing data with reference to the endpoint of life or to the total length of life, would certainly contribute to more effective empirical research and to a fuller comprehension of the psychological and biological processes involved.

Conclusions

Good longitudinal data are a precious commodity, uniquely suited for the purpose of analyzing and understanding individual development. It is therefore of great importance that one has the following in mind when planning a longitudinal study:

1. Achieving high data quality is of paramount importance, with particular attention paid to the collection of a broad set of relevant information and to the conservation of basic information. Given the costs and investments in longitudinal studies, it should be possible to use longitudinal data for purposes other than those that could be envisioned in terms of theories that were current at the time the longitudinal project was planned. This has already been discussed and is mentioned in several chapters in this volume.

2. The adequate use of longitudinal data often demands the use of sophisticated and complex methods of analysis that correspond to the substantial problem under study. This will be the topic of a forthcoming volume in the same series as the present one. Of course, the choice of analytic method should be related not only to the theoretical problem under study but also to the kind of data collected. In this book, data and design issues are discussed by Fox and Fogelman in chapter 13, with regard to data collection strategy in a large English longitudinal study, and by Mayer and Huinink in chapter 12, with regard to studying life events.

3. Longitudinal projects are often interdisciplinary, and the results can therefore be of interest within many research areas. It is thus a communication problem that researchers searching for information about individual development often have no overview of the longitudinal research field outside their own discipline. The dissemination of such results therefore demands particular attention; hence the allocation of resources within the European Science Foundation for this purpose.

4. Another important aspect of dissemination is the possibility of sharing data with other researchers outside the longitudinal project, as discussed by Colby and Phelps in chapter 14. They point out that data sharing can increase the usefulness of longitudinal data, but issues are then raised about how to preserve data quality (in the sense of the secondary analysis researcher's using and interpreting the data in a correct way) and how to ensure that the rights of the participants are protected.

5. Legal and ethical issues are involved in performing longitudinal research, because it usually demands the long-term storage of information about persons. While some participants might (erroneously) experience such a data base as a potential threat to their privacy, this concern must be balanced against the duty of the researcher to perform good research based on solid data. This issue will be further discussed in a coming volume focusing on legal and ethical issues in longitudinal research.

Considering the stony road of conducting long-term longitudinal research, one is sometimes surprised that any researcher chooses to follow that path. Long-range commitment and persistence are needed to carry it through. For instance, it can be quite difficult to secure continuous funding, because the granting agencies have a tendency to calculate the estimated total cost for a longitudinal project during its entire life and compare this cost with the cost of a short-lived project based on cross-sectional data. They might deem the longitudinal project expensive, not noticing that (a) the cost per year is often not high, (b) an invaluable data base is created for future research, and (c) the total production of a well-planned longitudinal research program can often be counted in hundreds of publications. However, there is an increasing awareness that well-planned longitudinal research is the lifeblood of studying individual development. Consequently, we believe that data quality-oriented research should be given a high priority to improve the overall quality and efficiency of longitudinal research.

Notes

1 Because C_x and C_y are constants added to obtain x and y, it is clear that the size of the constant systematic error does not influence r_{xy}.
2 This can be seen if it is noted that, for standardized variables, we have

$$r_{xy} = S_{T_x}S_{T_y}R_{T_xT_y} + S_{T_x}S_{V_y}R_{T_xV_y} + S_{T_y}S_{V_x}R_{V_xT_y} + S_{V_x}S_{V_y}R_{V_xV_y} + \text{e-terms (assumed to be approximately zero).}$$

References

Bailar, B. A., & Dalenius, T. (1969). Estimating the response variance components of the census' survey model. *Sankhya,* Series B, 1–20.

Baltes, P. B. (1968). Longitudinal and cross-sectional sequences in the study of age and generation effects. *Human Development, 11,* 145–171.

Bateson, P. P. G. (1978). How does behavior develop? In P. P. G. Bateson & P. H. Klopfer (Eds.), *Perspectives in ethology* (Vol. 3: *Social behavior*). New York: Plenum Press.

Bergman, L. R. (1972). Inferential aspects of longitudinal data in studying developmental problems. *Human Development, 15,* 287–293.

Bergman, L. R. (1988). Modeling reality: Some comments. In M. Rutter (Ed.), *Risk and protective factors in psychosocial development.* Cambridge: Cambridge University Press.

Bergman, L. R., & El-Khouri, B. (1986). *On the preparatory analysis of multivariate data before (longitudinal) cluster analysis: Some theoretical considerations and a data program.* Reports from the Department of Psychology, The University of Stockholm, No. 651.

Bergman, L. R., Hanve, R., & Rapp, J. (1978). Why do some people refuse to participate in interview surveys? *Statistisk Tidskrift, 5,* 341–356.

Bergman, L. R., & Wärneryd, B. (1982). *Om datainsamling i surveyundersökningar. Vilken metod är bäst och vad får vi egentligen veta?* (About data collection in survey investigations. What method is the best and what information do we really get?). Stockholm: Liber Distribution.

Björkman, N.-M. (1979). *Social önskvärdhet som felkälla i frågeundersökningar.* (Social desirability as a source of error in survey investigations). Doctoral dissertation, Sociology Department, The University of Stockholm.

Cairns, R. B., & Green, J. A. (1979). How to assess personality and social patterns: Observations or ratings. In R. B. Cairns (Ed.), *The analysis of social interactions: Methods, issues and illustrations.* Hillsdale, NJ: Lawrence Erlbaum.

Cairns, R. B., Cairns, B. D., & Neckerman, H. J. (1987). *Early school dropout: Configurations, determinants, and aftermath.* Report from the Social Development Laboratory, Carolina Longitudinal Study, Department of Psychology, University of North Carolina at Chapel Hill, Vol. 1, No. 11.

Cannell, C. F., Marquis, K. H., & Laurent, A. (1977). *A summary of studies of interviewing methodology: Vital and health statistics.* Series 2, No. 26, Public Health Service Publication No. 1000.

Collins, M. (1980). Interviewer variability: A review of the problem. *Journal of the Market Research Society, 22,* 77–95.

Coombs, C. H. (1964). *A theory of data.* New York: Wiley.

Cox, A., Rutter, M., Yule, B., & Quinton, D. (1977). Bias resulting from missing information: Some epidemiological findings. *British Journal of Preventive Social Medicine, 31,* 131–136.

Cronbach, L. J. (1975). Beyond the two disciplines of scientific psychology. *American Psychologist, 30,* 116–127.

Cronbach, L. J., Gleser, G. C., Nanda, H., & Rajaratnam, N. (1972). *The dependability of behavioral measurements: Theory of generalizability for scores and profiles.* New York: Wiley.

Dalenius, T. (1962). Automatic estimation of missing values in censuses and sample surveys. *Statistisk Tidskrift, 11,* 395–400.

Edwards, A. L. (1957). Social desirability and personality test construction. In B. M. Bass & I. A. Berg (Eds.), *Objective approaches to personality assessment.* Princeton, NJ: D. van Nostrand.

Elder, Jr., G. H., & Rockwell, R. C. (1979). Economic depression and postwar opportunity in men's lives: A study of life patterns and health. In R. Simmons (Ed.), *Research in community and mental health* (Vol. 1, pp. 249–303). JAI Press.

Fergusson, D. M., & Horwood, L. J. (1988). The uses and limitations of structural equation models of longitudinal data. In M. Rutter (Ed.), *Studies of psychosocial risk.* Cambridge: Cambridge University Press.

Gleason, T. C., & Staelin, R. (1975). A proposal for handling missing data. *Psychometrika, 40,* 229–252.

Goldstein, H. (1979). *The design and analysis of longitudinal studies.* London: Academic Press.

Greenwald, A. G., Pratkanis, A. R., Lieppe, M.R., & Baumgardner, M. H. (1986). Under what conditions does theory obstruct research progress? *Psychological Review, 93*(2), 216–229.

Jöreskog, K.G. (1979). Statistical estimation of structural models in longitudinal developmental investigations. In J. R. Nesselroade & P. B. Baltes (Eds.), *Longitudinal research in the study of behavior and development.* New York: Academic Press.

Kerlinger, F. (1973). *Foundations of behavior research.* New York: Holt, Rinehart & Winston.

Kish, L. (1962). Studies of interviewer variance for attitudinal variables. *Journal of the American Statistical Association, 57,* 92–115.

Krotki, K. P., & Hill, C. J. (1978). A comparison of correlated response variance estimates obtained in the 1961, 1971, and 1976 censuses. *Survey Methodology, 4*(1), 87–99.

Ljung, B.-O. (1965). *The adolescent spurt in mental growth.* Stockholm: Almqvist & Wiksell.

Loevinger, J. (1966). *Models and measures of developmental variation* (Vol. 34, No. 2, pp. 585–590). New York: Academy of Sciences.

Magnusson, D. (1967). *Test theory.* Reading, MA: Addison-Wesley.

Magnusson, D. (1976). The person and the situation in an interactional model of behavior. *Scandinavian Journal of Psychology, 17,* 253–271.

Magnusson, D. (1985). Implications of an interactional paradigm for research on human development. *International Journal of Behavioral Development, 8*(2), 115–137.

Magnusson, D. (1988). Individual development from an interactional perspective: A longitudinal study. In D. Magnusson (Ed.), *Paths through life* (Vol. 1). Hillsdale, NJ: Lawrence Erlbaum.

Magnusson, D. (in press). Personality development from an interactional perspective. In L. A. Pervin (Ed.), *Handbook of personality, theory, and research.* New York: Guilford Publications.

Marx, M. (1951). *Theories in contemporary psychology.* New York: Macmillan.

Mednick, S. A., Harwary, M., & Finello, K. M. (1984). *Handbook of longitudinal research.* New York: Praeger.

Moss, L., & Goldstein, H. (1979). *The recall method in social surveys.* London: University of London, Institute of Education.

Nunnally, J. C. (1978). *Psychometric theory.* New York: McGraw-Hill.

Nystedt, L., & Magnusson D., (1973). Cue relevance and feedback in a clinical prediction task. *Organizational Behavior and Human Performance, 9,* 100–109.

Rutter, M. (1981). Longitudinal studies: A psychiatric perspective. In S. A. Mednick & A. E. Baert (Eds.), *Prospective longitudinal research: An empirical basis for the primary prevention of psychosocial disorders.* Oxford: Oxford University Press.

Saris, V. E. (Ed., 1988). *Variation in response functions: A source of measurement error in attitude research.* Amsterdam: Sociometric Research Foundation.

Scarr, S. (1981). Comments on psychology: Behavior genetics and social policy from an anti-reductionist. In R. A. Kasschan & C. N. Cofer (Eds.), *Psychology's second century: Enduring issues.* New York: Praeger.

Schaie, K. W. (1965). A general model for the study of development problems. *Psychological Bulletin, 64,* 92–107.

Spearman, C. (1907). Demonstration of formulae for measurement of correlation. *American Journal of Psychology, 18,* 161–169.

SPSSX (1986). *Users' guide.* New York: McGraw-Hill.

Tanner, J. M. (1978). *Foetus into man: Physical growth from conception to maturity.* London: Open Books.

Wohlwill, J. (1970). The age variable in psychological research. *Psychological Review, 77,* 49–64.

Wohlwill, J. (1980). Cognitive development in childhood. In O. Brim & J. Kagan (Eds.), *Constancy and change in human development.* Cambridge, MA: Harvard University Press.

2   Improving the quality of psychiatric data: Classification, cause, and course

MICHAEL RUTTER AND ANDREW PICKLES

Conceptual approach to measurement

During the 1950s and 1960s most psychiatric researchers had a rather relaxed approach to measurement issues. Standardized inverviews were the exception, diagnostic criteria tended to be impressionistic and implicit, and there was little acceptance of any need for systematic, let alone operationalized, rules for classification. All of that has changed. Highly structured standardized interviews are the order of the day, research diagnostic criteria have become mandatory, and the classification is the focus of a great deal of attention. It is compulsory to submit measures to reliability studies with chance agreement taken into account. Kappa levels rule the choice of instruments. This virtual revolution in attitudes to psychiatric measurement has led many people to conclude that structured standardized instruments of good reliability, giving rise to research diagnostic criteria applied to operationalized classification systems, are sufficient to ensure high quality data, and that these approaches provide a solution to measurement problems. In this paper we aim to show that this is far from the case. We welcome the improvement in measurement instruments, but we question some of the assumptions that underlie their development, and, more particularly, we argue that much more is required. Specifically, we suggest that issues of measurement necessarily require attention to research design, demand that theories and concepts be made explicit, have inevitable implications for choice of data sources and time points, and unavoidably involve decisions on styles of data handling and statistical analysis. In our discussion of these matters we focus on the use of longitudinal data to tackle questions of classification, cause, and course of psychiatric disorders.

To attempt to combine the measurement implications of such a range of considerations, from theory to data analysis technique, is no small task. Bringing them together can be made simpler by using concepts that unify our thinking of abstract qualities in their context of theoretical interrelationships, and of operational measures in their context of empirical interrelationships. One concept that is fundamental is that of a latent variable – meaning a quantified characteristic or quality (having continuous or discrete values) that cannot be directly observed or measured. The use of latent variables is now commonplace within data analysis; for example, in structural equation, item response, and latent class models. However, the distinction

32

between the actual and the observable that is at the core of the concept of latent variable is also fundamental to most psychiatric concepts.

Thus, in genetics the genotype (that which is inherited) is an abstraction and cannot itself be directly observed. Indeed, so too is the phenotype (the expression in the individual of the genotype); for although it is dependent upon the genotype, it may also require other factors, such as the occurrence of certain environmental conditions to achieve physical manifestation in observables. The same observables may also arise as the result of other quite different processes. Note that this will remain the case even when molecular genetics has succeeded in locating the gene. We will know much more about the ways in which the genetic predisposition is manifest, but in the individual case we will not be able directly to measure whether this particular episode of, say, depression is a result of the known gene anomaly or whether it has resulted from other risk factors.

Note too that research diagnostic criteria do not provide a solution. We may agree, for example, that autism is defined by the presence of a particular type of language deviance, abnormal social relationships, and stereotyped repetitive behavior, but this is a convention. As Popper (1959, 1972) pointed out years ago, definitions should be read from right to left and not the reverse. In other words, we have agreed that we shall use the term *autism* to refer to this particular constellation of behaviors, but this does not define autism (Rutter, 1978). Autism is, in reality, an hypothesis – a theoretical notion that there is some meaningful condition that we think tends to be manifest by these particular symptoms. But it remains a latent variable the validity of which has to be tested. Genetic evidence that has become available in recent years, in fact, strongly suggests that the behavioral expression of the genotype extends more widely than the conventional diagnostic criteria (Folstein & Rutter, 1987), with the implication that methods of diagnostic measurement need to be rethought (Rutter, Le Couteur, Lord, Macdonald, Rios, & Folstein, 1988).

The same considerations not only apply to other diagnoses, but are equally applicable to psychosocial and cognitive concepts. Thus, for example, the concept of "insecure attachment" has been crucial in the study of the early development of social relationships (Bretherton & Waters, 1985). A particular experimental paradigm, "the strange situation," was devised to assess the quality of a child's attachment to particular individuals (Ainsworth, Blehar, Waters, & Warr, 1978). It has proved a gratifyingly robust measure (although one that is not free from problems; Lamb, Thompson, Gardner, Charnov, & Estes, 1984), but no one supposes that a child's particular behavioral response to separation and reunion *is* insecurity. Rather, it reflects an unmeasured latent variable or theoretical concept. The same applies to the whole range of other concepts that pervade risk research in psychiatry, such as marital discord, social support, learned helplessness, and self-esteem.

Some people may prefer to use the term *hypothetical construct* to refer to the underlying variable in a psychological or psychiatric model, retaining *latent variable* for its statistical equivalent. We prefer to use the same term for both in order to emphasize that the latter is simply a numerical expression of the former. Statistical latent variables do not derive automatically from empirical analyses until the model defining the psychological construct has been specified. The same data set will give rise to several quite different latent variables according to differences in the hypothetical construct that is specified.

A common response to these arguments on the need to deal with latent variables is that, although that may be so, we have no alternative but to rely on measures of observables. Moreover, the very fact that they are imperfect reflections of the latent variable means that the observed associations must constitute *under*estimates of the true association. This assumption leads to the use of correlations corrected for unreliability, which necessarily produce much stronger associations (see, e.g., Olweus, 1979). However, it is crucial to recognize that what is being taken into account is the less than perfect agreement between two measures of observables, and *not* the relationship between those measures and the relevant latent variable. That might not matter if the only source of unreliability (with respect to measurement of the latent variable) stemmed from random error, but that is far from the case. Systematic errors or biases are extremely common just because the observables usually reflect *multiple* latent variables, and not only the one that is the focus of interest. Thus, for example, the concept of insecure attachment refers to the quality of a dyadic relationship, but children's response to the strange situation will also reflect their temperamental qualities, their general emotional state, their feelings at the time as influenced by earlier happenings on that day, and situational responses to the experimental situation (deriving from aspects separate from the dyadic relationship). Thus, the question is – insofar as the security measure predicts to, say, later peer relationships – whether this is a consequence of the latent variable of the dyadic relationship or the latent variable of temperament or some other latent variable. It is obvious that this is no semantic quibble or mere academic distinction but, rather, something that is absolutely crucial to the type of inferences that we draw from all our empirical data.

If we cannot avoid a focus on latent variables, we cannot avoid the need for theory to define them. Statistics are of little help in the absence of theory. Factor analysis can bring out the latent variable that accounts for the largest proportion of the variance shared by the combination of some set of observables, but that is a statistical, not a conceptual, abstraction. Perhaps the pertinent concept should instead refer to the features that provide a differentiation from some other set of features and not just those that are common to the first set. The derivation of that latent variable would require a different statistical approach. Statistics are indispensable, but they are the servant and not the master. The guiding principle must come from the concept to be used or tested, and this requires that the researcher be quite explicit both on what notion or theory is being employed and on how that notion may be conceptually operationalized. The emphasis here is on the conceptual basis. Behavioral scientists have tended to assume that operationalization means specification that there should be a score of x from a list of specified symptoms, but that is not what is meant. In the first place, such specification rarely includes precise rules on how such symptoms are to be assessed (Cantwell, 1987). But, of more importance, this operationalization concerns only the observables and not the latent variables that they are intended to measure.

Let us return to the example of autism. The usual research diagnostic criteria (RDC) approach would specify how many of which particular language, social, and behavioral abnormalities must be present for the condition to be coded as present. A more sophisticated application of RDC might go on to specify that certain instruments must be used to assess those symptoms and that unreliability be reduced by demanding that the abnormalities be found on two applications of those instruments by two independent clinicians blind to each other's findings. That sounds like a really tough-minded, highly rigorous approach, but it would miss the point if the latent variable conceptualized was that of a genetically determined condition in which the phenotype included a range of language and social deficits that did not fulfill DSM-III or ICD-10 diagnostic criteria for autism. The point that emerges from this consideration is not just the need for theory but also the need to use research design to test the theory so that the criteria can be improved in the light of these tests. In other words, the real concern is not for the reliability of our measures but rather for their validity – with the recognition that the term *validity* means nothing until the concept against which validity is judged is made explicit. In the field of diagnosis, the essential is that the validating criteria must concern features external to the behavioral characteristics that define the disorder (Rutter, 1978) – such as response to some specified treatment, familial correlates, course, or outcome. It is immediately apparent that this consideration brings together the three elements in the title of this paper: classification, cause, and course. It is also evident that few of our current diagnostic concepts are more than working hypotheses at the moment (Rutter, Tuma, & Lann, 1988).

A necessary consequence of this fact is the recognition that any commitment in a longitudinal study to the classification that happens to be currently in vogue will, with the benefit of hindsight, often be seen to be premature. Unless it is possible to use earlier data to reconstruct diagnostic distinctions that become appreciated only some years after the initial data collection, much of the value of a longitudinal study can be lost. Source data sets organized on the basis of considerable disaggregation of behaviors, rather than diagnoses or behavioral composites, may seem cumbersome, but they will offer greater long-term security. A particular need in that connection is the avoidance of hierarchical approaches to diagnosis that presuppose some unestablished relationship between different types of symptomatology (Leckman, Weissman, Merikangas, Pauls, & Prusoff, 1983). That has been a substantial limitation in many of the existing classification systems, which has required diagnostic unpicking as new data show that the initial assumptions were mistaken.

The latent variable concept is, of course, not the only one that is necessary in improving the quality of psychiatric data. In the study of causal hypotheses and of longitudinal course, there are equivalent needs to define the causal and course concepts if they are to be tested adequately. There is the basic need to search for "experiments of nature" if causes are to be differentiated from noncausal correlates

(Rutter, 1980; 1988b; 1989), but that is not sufficient. We need to go on to ask *how* risk variables operate, whether the effects are direct or indirect, and whether the consequences are contingent on the co-occurrence of other variables that serve as vulnerability catalysts. This often involves the determination of whether risk factors operate in similar ways in different populations and whether there are interactions of various sorts (Rutter, 1983; in press). If we are to capture within our data the often complex nature of the course of a disorder and of the causal mechanisms that such course reflects, we must have concepts that define both. Statistical process models have a language for describing at least some aspects of course. In so doing, they provide formal concepts such as "sufficiency" and "identifiability" that allow us to specify the minimum data required to distinguish among alternative models and explanations. In promoting this use of statistical models for defining data requirements, we must make an immediate qualification – indeed, the same qualification as for the selection of a classification system. A premature commitment to a particular conceptualization of the process can also leave one with inadequate data as ideas develop during a study. Both current classification systems and statistical process models represent an accumulation of knowledge and experience that must be drawn upon in the design of studies, but which it would be foolish to believe necessarily to be true. Rather, the requirement is that the data should allow systematic testing of the systems and models so that the process of data analysis leads to a progressive refining of the concepts and hence of the ways that the data are used to assess such concepts.

We have deliberately labored these points because they are fundamental to our discussion of the various steps that may be taken to improve the quality of psychiatric data. Let us now turn to a more detailed consideration of the specifics involved in order to put both psychiatric and statistical flesh on the conceptual skeleton.

Methods of handling measurement error

There are three rather different approaches to measurement error. First, there are the attempts to improve the reliability of individual instruments through increased structure and a focus on unambiguous observables. Although there is merit in this approach for some variables, we reject it as a general solution. The requirement of rigid structure in questionnaire or interview format necessarily places reliance on respondents' having the knowledge necessary to make the required distinction, as well as the appropriate range of experience, to make judgments on the severity of particular behaviors. That seems in principle a dangerous assumption, and in practice it has sometimes proved unwarranted (Breslau, 1987). Investigator-based interviews and observations may more likely be able to tap behaviors that require subtle distinctions (Rutter et al., 1988). However, of more importance, single measures are in a weak position to deal with systematic biases. Accordingly, we will not consider this approach further.

Second, data sources may be pooled in order to reduce the bias or the effect of latent variables other than those of interest for the hypothesis to be tested. This approach has proved of substantial value, and we give several examples of its application. However, it cannot provide an assessment of measurement error. That is provided by the application of structural modeling to derive measurement of the latent variable (Fergusson & Horwood, 1988), the third approach, and one that we discuss with examples of its use.

Pooling data sources

The approach to measurement error through the pooling of data sources stems from the recognition of the fact that any single measure is likely to reflect a complex mixture of that which we wish to assess (i.e., the latent variable), specific biases due to other influences that we wish to exclude from the measure (i.e., other latent variables), and random error due to the imperfect nature of any assessment. Repeat measurements or statistical corrections for known measured unreliability deal with random error, although corrections based on data from other standard populations require the assumption that the two are equivalent, which often is not the case (hence the not infrequent embarrassing finding that corrected correlations exceed 1). However, they fail entirely to deal with systematic error or bias. The solution here is to use multiple measures that differ in their likely sources of systematic bias, perhaps combined with the avoidance of sources most prone to biases that will seriously jeopardize the intended measurement.

Persistent versus transient disorders. For example, in a prospective study of the effects of parental mental disorder as a risk factor for psychiatric disturbances in the offspring, Rutter and Quinton (1984a) avoided measurement based on parental reports. Although these reports were likely to be the most detailed, they were also most subject to the biases in perception or reporting that could stem from the parent's mental state. Instead, teacher questionnaire scores were used, but, in order better to tap persistent disturbance, this was defined in terms of a score that was deviant on at least 3 out of the potential 5 occasions of measurement. This composite measurement of persistent behavior deviance substantially sharpened the contrast between the cases and the control group, suggesting that the pooling of data sources across time (and across situations, because the teachers completing the scales usually varied over the years) had been effective in reducing the effect of transient disturbances due to other factors. However, as with most composite measures, a price had to be paid. As in any longitudinal study, some children missed data at some time points over the four years of the study. Should 3 out of 4 measures be treated as equivalent to 3 out of 5? Also, there is an inevitable arbitrariness in cutoff points, so that a score of "8" is classed as nondeviant but one of "9" as deviant.

Pervasive versus situational disorders. Another example is provided by Schachar, Rutter, and Smith's (1981) use of the Isle of Wight study data to compare "pervasive" and "situational" hyperactivity. The stimulus for the study lay both in the theoretical concept that the hyperkinetic syndrome required hyperactivity that was pervasive across situations and in Sandberg, Rutter, and Taylor's (1978) empirical finding, from a clinic sample, that the correlates of pervasive hyperactivity differed from those of hyperactivity as measured on just a single parent or teacher questionnaire. Schachar et al. (1981) defined hyperactivity as that which exceeded a particular cutoff on both the parental and teacher questionnaires. The result indicated once again that the correlates of pervasive hyperactivity differed from those of situational hyperactivity, showing the utility of the composite approach. Of course, this could have been simply a function of the two measures providing a more valid reflection of "serious" hyperactivity, rather than a distinction between pervasive and situational hyperactivity as such. If repeat measures on the two scales had been available, this could have been tested more directly, but, as they were not available, comparison was made between pervasive and situational measures of a different behavior (unsociability), where there was not the marked difference found for hyperactivity. The finding suggested that the pervasive–situational distinction might have a meaning for hyperactivity that did not necessarily apply to other behaviors. However, there were the same problems of arbitrariness and missing data noted in the parental mental disorder study.

Combination categories. Sometimes the concept of the latent variable involves the combination of two rather different measures on the assumption that the meaning of the two together differs from that of each considered in isolation. That circumstance is a comonplace in medicine, with the recognition of patterns of symptomatology being central to diagnosis. However, the possibility has been rather ignored in psychology, where analyses have tended to be undertaken separately variable by variable. The need to combine is evident, for example, in the concept of personality disorder as conceptualized in terms of a pervasive, persistent disorder of social functioning that is shown across a range of social contexts (Rutter, 1987a). The concept, or latent variable, requires the assessment of a person's functioning across a range of situations involving different forms of social interactions, such as work, love relationships, and negotiations outside the family (as with doctors, shopkeepers, and neighbors). Such an instrument has been developed and tested (Hill, Harrington, Fudge, Rutter, & Pickles, 1989). It is possible from assessments (giving rise to scores) on six broad areas of functioning to derive a composite measure of personality disturbance that serves reasonably well. However, the straightforward summative combination is complicated by the expectable finding that the sensitivity and specificity of the six areas differ in complex ways and that the relationships between the areas differ somewhat across both groups and sexes. The finding emphasizes the importance of systematic biases. In a real sense, that is a strength of the instrument in terms of the need to differentiate malfunction in specific relationships from a generalized malfunction across social contexts and relationships. Nevertheless, the question is how the data should best be combined and utilized in order to do this.

Severity of disturbance. A further issue arises with the frequent need in risk research to differentiate between some less common "severe" psychiatric manifestation of interest and some much more common phenomenon that is phenomenologically similar. For example, that has been a major problem in studying depression in either childhood or adult life. Thus, Weissman et al. (1987) sought to compare psychiatric disorders in the offspring of depressed parents with those in the offspring of community controls. In spite of the fact that the age range extended from 6 to 23 years (so that most offspring will have had only a short time at risk for depression) a quarter of controls (and 37.6% of the offspring of depressed parents) met the DSM-III criteria for depression. Moreover, 64.8% of controls (vs. 72.8% of cases) received some psychiatric diagnosis. Necessarily, it is worrying if the majority of a normal population are classified as "abnormal," and some means of picking out more severe disorders would seem desirable. Psychiatric contact is often a useful index in that connection, but it would be hazardous here in view of the likely bias towards early referral stemming from the fact that the parents were already under psychiatric care. Weissman et al. (1987) sought to deal with the problem by employing a somewhat stricter set of diagnostic criteria, but the rate of depression in controls remained very high. A variety of other indices could have been added in order to provide some composite estimate based on, say, duration and severity of social impairment, frequency of recurrence, presence of more severe symptoms, and occurrence of hypomania. However, these features are rather unreliable with lifetime assessments (Bromet, Dunn, Connell, Dew, & Schulberg, 1986).

Co-morbidity. A related, but somewhat different, problem is posed by co-morbidity. This may arise in two ways. First, when an RDC approach is employed (as with DSM-III) it is usual for people to have multiple diagnoses for any one episode of disorder. Thus, clinical samples of children with depression frequently also meet the criteria for conduct disorder, separation anxiety, anorexia nervosa, or educational retardation (Rutter, in press). With the World Health Organization (1987) ICD-10, that occurs less often because of the tendency to diagnose on the basis of the preponderant symptom pattern; however, the price paid is uncertainty on how to decide on the preponderant pattern (Rutter, 1988a). In addition, with lifetime appraisals co-morbidity may arise, because individuals with one pattern at one episode may show a different pattern at other episodes. Thus, in the Weissman et al. (1987) study of 6- to 23-year-olds the mean number of diagnoses in the *controls* was 1.7, and in the *cases* it was 2.4. Similarly, in Keller et al.'s (1986) study of the offspring of depressed parents, a third of the children had at least three diagnoses. One key issue here is whether these multiple diagnoses reflect variable expression of the same basic disorder or rather a risk process that leads to an increased vulnerability to several quite different disorders. What, for example, does the Weissman et al. (1987) finding of a relative risk of 2.3 for substance abuse compared with 1.6 for major depression in the offspring of depressed parents mean? Does this imply two separate risk processes, or are both substance abuse and major depression reflections of some integrating underlying disorder (if so, what)? The co-morbidity of anxiety and depression (Weissman, 1987) presents a particular problem here for genetic analyses; and, as Carey (1987) points out, it is necessary to use methods of measurement that allow anxiety and depression to be pooled *or* kept separate, and that statistical modeling must test for both homogeneity and heterogeneity.

What is the phenotype? A particularly severe problem in psychiatric genetics is the uncertainty of what symptom pattern constitutes the phenotype for various disorders thought to have a genetic basis (Rutter, Bolton, Harrington, Le Couteur, Macdonald, & Simonoff, in press a; Rutter, Macdonald, Le Couteur, Harrington, Bolton & Bailey, in press b). We have referred already to this issue in relation to autism, but it applies similarly to schizophrenia and so-called schizotypal personality disorders (Kendler, Materson, Ungaro, & Davis, 1984), and to obsessional disorders and Tourette's syndrome (Pauls, Towbin, Leckman, Zahner, & Cohen, 1986), to give but two examples. The conventional solution has been to rely on structured methods of assessment applying agreed diagnostic conventions. However, although this is likely to increase interrater reliability, it may do so at the price of invalidity with respect to the relevant latent variable (i.e., the "true" phenotype). The need here is not for either "purer" or more composite measures (or for improved statistics) but rather for research designs that will use genetic relationships to test alternative concepts of the phenotype (Rutter et al., in press a & b). Thus, in the case of autism the approaches include study of the features of nonautistic co-twins with some sort of disability in discordant monozygotic pairs; and the study of the cognitive and/or social deficits that aggregate in the families of autistic subjects to a much greater extent than in the families of controls and which coaggregate with each other (i.e., cognitive with social, etc.) on both a family and individual basis. In that connection it is relevant to note that significance may lie in the *conjunction* of several disparate features that do not have the same meaning when they occur in isolation. It is important to analyze on a "person" as well as a 'variable" basis (Magnusson & Bergman, 1988). Thus, Hanson, Gottesman, and Heston (1976) found that poor motor skills *and* large cognitive test-score variance *and* schizoid behavior at both 4 and 7 years occurred only in the offspring of schizophrenics (17% vs. 0%), although each of these items on its own was present in substantial proportions of controls.

The same issue of a single latent variable being manifest in apparently heterogeneous clinical pictures is a common concern in longitudinal studies. Thus, recent evidence suggests that conduct disturbance in childhood leads not only to antisocial personality disorders in adult life but also to a broader range of psychiatric and social malfunctions (Rutter & Quinton, 1984b; Quinton, Rutter, & Gulliver, in press; Robins, 1986). Furthermore, the pattern in adult life seems to differ between the sexes. Whereas it is important to recognize the reality of this heterotypic continuity and to use measures and research designs that can detect it, it is also crucial to appreciate the problems in understanding it. It could be that the heterogeneous manifestations are all reflections of the same basic psychopathological process, but equally it is possible that the heterogeneity arises from a multiplicity of overlapping risk variables or from a multiplicity of direct and indirect longitudinal causal processes. Even if the former is the case, there is the further need to determine how to identify when these varied clinical manifestations reflect the same latent variable and when they do not.

We posed this issue initially in terms of the definition of phenotypes; but, of course, as the conduct disturbance—personality disorder example made clear, in reality the problem extends much more widely. For example, there has been a concern to delineate the particular patterns of disturbance specifically associated with both physical hazards (the fetal alcohol syndrome provides a good example here; Porter, O'Conner, & Whelan, 1984) and psychosocial risk factors (the particular pattern of social relationships that may follow an institutional upbringing is a case in point; Hodges & Tizard, 1989 a & b). Of course, it may be that the risks lead to a general, nonspecific vulnerability to all manners of psychiatric/psychological problems, but it is essential to test for specificities if they are to be detected. If this is to occur, three needs must be met. First, the data gathering must be both theory led (in looking for patterns thought to be possibly specific) and sufficiently sensitive and open to pick up the unexpected. The latter requirement means the use of investigator-based measures by which clinically experienced researchers can note the unusual in a standardized way. Second, it is necessary to use research designs in which two different risk populations are compared (and not just a comparison with a normal control group). Only in this way will it be possible to separate specific from general risk processes. The history of psychiatric risk research shows that a failure to follow this principle has often led to mistaken inferences (Rutter & Garmezy, 1983). The third need is for replication with further built-in tests for the hypothesized specificity. This is essential not only because of the impossibility of controlling for all competing risk mechanisms in any one study but also because, inevitably, the search for the unexpected capitalizes on chance; and replication and cross-validation is the only satisfactory means of ruling out chance associations (statistics provides a measure of chance expectations only for that one population or sample and, in any case, there are problems applying probabilities when multiple comparisons are being undertaken).

It is obvious from the various examples given that there can be no single answer to the questions of how to improve the quality of psychiatric measures. There are unavoidable implications for research design, for the choice of measuring instruments, and for the data handling. However, what is required throughout are multiple data sources, sensitive and wide-ranging measures, an ability to disaggregate and recombine measures in different ways and, above all, the possibility to test competing explanatory models.

Latent variable analyses

We have pointed to the several ways in which data sources may be combined in order to get nearer to the latent variable being considered and to reduce sources of both systematic bias and random error. The use of composite variables has the great advantage of simplicity in handling and in data presentation, and in some circumstances this approach may suffice. However, it has three major disadvantages. First, almost inevitably there is a certain abitrariness in how variables are combined and in how cutoffs are chosen. Second, it provides no satisfactory means of dealing with missing data (a major issue in long-term longitudinal studies with many time points and many data sources). Third, it does not allow any estimate of the error in measurement that remains.

The problem that this last limitation generates cannot be overemphasized, because there are relatively few general rules to indicate what the expected effect of measurement error should be. What is clear is that measurment error is rarely simply absorbed into the ordinary error terms of our statistical analyses but more usually generates potentially misleading results. For this reason measurement error has to be addressed within each study directly. The general recommendation is therefore usually made that multiple measures of disorder and risk factors should be obtained. These multiple measures are then used to construct latent disorder and risk factor variables by means of structural equation modeling, and the relationship between these latent variables is then examined. The key point is that several unreliable measures used to construct a latent variable can provide estimates of the risk factor free of bias, something that no externally calculated composite of these variables could ever do. Where an instrument/schedule includes a considerable number of redundant items (each item response rather than the total being recorded in the data set) this redundancy can be exploited by appropriately dividing the items to form multiple measures of the same latent variable. More usually, however, it will be necessary to seek additional measures that involve repetition or the use of different methods or situations. Each of these may introduce new systematic effects that differentiate them from the original measure; accordingly, the estimation of additional parameters will be needed to account for them. Whether or not there are enough data to estimate all these parameters, that is, whether the model is "identifiable," depends critically upon the design of the study and the details of the data collected. The determination of the identifiability of complex models can be a tedious algebraic exercise. The process can, however, provide a formal indication of which sorts of additional data are required and where in the model they are needed.

This need for multiple measures can be relieved somewhat by appreciating that we do not necessarily need them for the whole sample. Clayton (1985) provides a very persuasive, though hypothetical, case-control example in which the risk factor is measured with error. He found that even having repeat measures only for some of the control group was sufficient to remove the downward bias in the estimate of the effect of the risk factor, although the addition of repeat measurements for some cases helped to restrict the upper bound of the estimate. This would suggest that a sensible strategy might be to select a quite small subsample for intensive measurement, and these relatively few individuals could be appropriately cosseted and rewarded to achieve their full compliance.

It will be appreciated that this strategy is heavily reliant on the relationships between measures being the same in the subsample as in the total population. For the reasons already given, it is a commonplace to find major differences between cases and controls in the persistence over time of disturbance (Rutter & Quinton, 1984a) or in the extent of pervasiveness across situations (Brown, Chadwick, Shaffer, Rutter, & Traub, 1981). Different patterns of continuity/discontinuity across age periods may also characterize high risk groups (Maughan & Pickles, in press). Accordingly, it is always necessary to test for heterogeneity before extrapolating from one group to another.

It may be argued that the derivation of error-free estimates simply provides statistical elegance but does not alter the basic conclusions that may be obtained by much less complicated analyses. However, that is to misunderstand the nature of what is being done. The *analysis* of measurement error (as against just the inflation of correlations through correction for unreliability) may alter the *pattern* of associations found once the latent variable has been separated from sources of systematic bias. An example is provided by Fergusson and Horwood (1987) in their use of structural equation modeling to derive a latent variable of a conduct disturbance trait, which was distinguished from situational effects and measurement error (an important need in view of the consistently low correlation between parent and teacher questionnaire measures). The findings showed that the correlations between the latent trait and male sex, social disadvantage, and family breakdown were all about twice as high as those with the observed variable. In contrast, the correlations between latent trait and both maternal depression and family life events were reduced (because of the major differences in the correlations between these variables and teacher and parent measures of conduct disturbance).

As is always the case, a price must be paid for this precision. In the case of structural equation modeling, the main price lies in the fact that the findings are necessarily dependent on the nature of the highly restricting assumptions that have to be made in undertaking the modeling (Biddle & Marlin, 1987; Martin, 1987; Mulaik, 1987). This is particularly marked when dealing with the small samples that are the consequence of the need for intensive data collection that is characteristic of much longitudinal research (Tanaka, 1987). The flip side of this constraint, however, provides the strength of this approach; namely, the need for the investigator to be explicit about the latent variable to be studied and about the assumptions to be made, together with opportunity to test competing models to account for the pattern of associations in the particular data set.

The study of cause and course

The investigation of risk and protective factors for psychiatric disorder necessarily involves the testing of causal hypotheses. Statistical associations provide no guide to policy or practice unless inferences about causal mechanism or processes can be made. Every student is aware of the hazards inherent in making causal inferences from correlational data, but there is no escaping the need to make, and test, such inferences. Numerous design considerations are involved in this enterprise, but here we concentrate on the issues that apply to the improvement of the measures needed to study causal hypotheses. Cause and course are brought together for this purpose because, except when dealing with risk factors that have already had their effects before birth, cause implies that change within an individual from one state (normality) to another (disorder), and that means the study of longitudinal course. This forces a focus on the measurement of onset and offset of disorder.

Onset and offset of disorder

If we need to assess the transition from normality to abnormality the implication is that, without making difficult assumptions about equilibria or distributions of propensities in the population in any longitudinal study, subjects who are continuously well or continuously disordered may be uninformative for testing the causal hypothesis. That is a serious matter, because such children typically make up the great majority of risk samples when dealing with a chronic risk variable. For example, in Rutter and Quinton's (1984a) four-year prospective study of the children of newly referred psychiatrically ill parents, a third of the offspring already showed disorder at the time of first research contact, and more than a third never showed disorder at any time during the four years of study. That was a consequence of the fact that, although the sample was defined in terms of referral for a new psychiatric disorder, it turned out that most parents had in fact had a disorder for many years. This means that the children had already been exposed to the hypothesized risk factor for a long time and, not surprisingly, many had succumbed. Still some had not, and it would be possible to focus on this minority group to examine the causal hypothesis. This strategy was used to considerable effect by Richman, Stevenson, and Graham (1982) in their five-year follow-up of 3-year-olds. Out of their total sample of 91 control children without disorder at the age of 3, 20 had developed disorder by age 8. The finding that the risk of developing disorder was increased threefold in those exposed to family discord measured at age 3 provided powerful support for the hypothesis that discord played a part in the causation of child psychiatric disorder.

That strategy paid off in a sample where the children were infants during the period of risk that applied before the first data point, but the approach is not trouble free. Necessarily, it relies on the assumption that the children without disorder at the start of the study are representative of those in the general population who might be viewed as at risk. A moment's consideration indicates that this assumption is extremely problematic in the common circumstance that there has been a long period of risk exposure before the study began. Why had the children not succumbed already? Let us take the analogy of children's exposure to some chronic, highly infectious parental disease such as tuberculosis. The probability is that the children who are uninfected after some years exposure are atypical because they had already acquired immunity before their parents became ill. Analysis of the onset of tuberculosis in this subgroup during a follow-up study would give a highly misleading impression of the importance of exposure to parental tuberculosis as a risk factor for the same infection in the children. That provides a very considerable limitation to any focus on subgroups of children showing the normality–disorder transition during the period of data collection. Such a focus probably creates more problems than it solves when dealing with chronic risk variables that are likely to have created their main risk at an age period earlier than the age of most of the children in the sample to be studied. Nevertheless, the longitudinal study of onset of disorder remains the most powerful research strategy if the age period when risk factors first operate is chosen.

What about the strategy of focusing on the offset of disorder – that is, the examination of the factors associated with remission or recovery on the grounds that a reduction in the risk factors associated with onset should lead to offset once the disorder is established? The problem with this approach is that the variables associated with continuation of a disorder are not necessarily the same as those associated with its origins. Thus, the Richman et al. (1982) study that showed that marital discord was a significant risk factor for onset of disorder in those initially free of disorder found no significant association between a reduction in discord and remission in disorder. This could be a consequence of the reduction in discord being too slight to make much impact, of the discord not constituting the relevant risk mechanism (a reduction in maternal criticism did show a significant effect on remission), or of different variables (such as child temperament) playing a greater role in the perpetuation or remission of disorder. The study of offset is a worthwhile strategy, but it does not necessarily provide findings relevant to onset.

If we return to the onset research strategy, we face two rather different needs: first, the use of samples in which it is possible to begin study either before or at a very early stage in the operation of a risk variable (Pickles, 1987); and, second, the accurate measurement of onset. The first need may be met by focusing on acute hazards that are readily identified, such as head injury (Rutter, Chadwick, & Shaffer, 1983) or bereavement (van Eerdewegh, Bieri, Parilla, & Clayton, 1982). Alternatively, it may be met by longitudinal studies from birth to infancy in which the development of disorders may be studied prospectively in relation to already identified risk variables, or through longitudinal studies of large samples with the opportunity to focus on the subgroups without the risk factor initially but in which the risk develops during the course of study.

The measurement of onset of psychiatric disorder has received surprisingly little attention up to now, and it deserves greater research investment. Relatively few disorders have a sharp transition from normality to disorder and, hence, it is not self-evident which time point should be used to label the beginning of disorder. For example, children with an affective disorder have often had a prolonged period of chronic dysthymia before a major depressive episode develops (Kovacs et al., 1984). Also, the major episode often involves a gradual buildup of symptoms that ultimately lead to substantial social impairment. Should the onset be regarded as the first time the low-grade dysthymia features were present, the first appearance of major depressive symptoms, the time when the constellation of symptoms first meet RDC, or the time when there was first substantial social impairment? Of course, the exact timing may not matter if chronic risk factors are being studied or if onset is treated dimensionally as an increase in symptoms or social impairment, but it is crucial if the hypothesis is that some acute risk factor has provoked onset of disorder (as is typical of life events research; Brown & Harris, 1978). The implication is that the measures of disorder should include standardized evaluations of the timing of the different concepts of onset.

Onset and offset of risk factor

Differentiation of risk indicators from risk mechanisms. Generally comparable issues arise in relation to the study of risk factors. The crucial point in this connection is the need to differentiate between risk *indicators* and the risk *mechanisms.* It is essential in risk research to have measures that come as close as possible to the hypothesized risk mechanisms. It is inevitably hazardous to have to derive the latent variable from correlations with indirect risk indicators when the latent variable can only be inferred from what is left over after removing the effects of unwanted correlations with other variables. For example, the early research on low birth weight (LBW) as a risk factor for cognitive impairment through its supposed connection with brain damage was extremely difficult to interpret, because there was no way of knowing which LBW babies had and which had not in fact suffered brain damage. That situation has been transformed by the availability of modern brain imaging techniques, such as ultrasound, which can visualize periventricular hemorrhage and parenchymal echodensities (Stewart et al., 1987).

The same need applies with psychosocial risk variables. For example, at one time marriage was thought to lead to a reduction in criminal behavior, causing delinquent individuals to "settle down" into a more prosocial style of life. However, it now seems that the prosocial effect comes from marrying a nondeviant woman; marriage to a deviant spouse has the reverse effect (West, 1982). Similarly, family breakup or parental loss in early or middle childhood was once regarded as a potent risk factor for psychiatric disorder arising both at the time and later. It may well be that the acute experience of loss creates a degree of risk in its own right, but empirical findings have shown that the main risk derives from the chronic family discord that precedes and follows the breakup (Rutter, 1971) or from the inadequate parental care that may follow parental loss (Brown, Harris, & Bifulco, 1986). Similarly, research has clearly shown that short-term admissions of children into foster homes or institutional care is associated with a substantially increased risk of child psychiatric disorder (Wolkind & Rutter, 1973). However, longitudinal data have been instrumental in showing that the risk was already much increased *before* the admissions took place (St. Claire & Osborn, 1987), suggesting that the main risk stemmed from factors (probably chronic family adversities) associated with the admission, rather than from the admission itself. The same has been reported for acute life stressors in adolescents (Aro, 1987), suggesting that it may be associated chronic adversity that constitutes the risk. The same inference might be drawn from the repeated finding that acute life stressors remain increased after as well as before the onset of disorder (Brown & Harris, 1978; Billings & Moos, 1984), as well as from the finding that although the number of life events is raised in children with psychiatric disorder, there is little temporal association between their occurrence and the onset of child psychiatric disorder (Goodyer, Kolvin, & Gatzanis, 1987).

Sequential and indirect risk processes. The study of divorce (Hetherington, Cox, & Cox, 1982, 1985) brings out the further points that the longer-term sequelae may depend on a sequence of further risk factors that stem from the first (i.e., a series of negative life experiences) and that the effects may vary by sex (parental remarriage seemed to reduce the risk in boys but increase it for girls) and by correlates (the effects of remarriage depended on the quality of the stepparent-child relationship that is established). Other longitudinal studies also bring out the finding that the long-term consequences of exposure to risk variables are often a consequence of a chain of connecting circumstances that require analysis link by link if the risk process is to be understood (Quinton, Rutter, & Liddle, 1984; Quinton & Rutter, 1988). Moreover, it may be necessary to examine counterbalancing protective mechanisms as well as risk processes (Rutter, in press). In that connection, it is important to analyze the mechanisms underlying change or discontinuity as well as those associated with perpetuation of risk. Frequently, this will necessitate a specific focus on subgroups where this has occurred, and always it will require attention to turning points when a risk trajectory alters onto a more adaptive path. The main essential here is a concept or model of how risk and protective mechanisms might operate so that this may be put to the test. Obviously, this also demands appropriate measurement of the hypothesized intervening variables. As with psychiatric measures, there is the need to focus on the postulated latent variable rather than on the measured observable.

Overlap between risk factors. It is a common problem that the hypothesized latent risk variable overlaps greatly with some other risk variable that might constitute the true risk factor. Longitudinal data help in sorting out time relationships, and statistics can be of assistance in determining the extent to which the risk associated with factor A still holds after taking into account the effect of factor B. However, statistical manipulations are of limited use when there is major overlap between the competing risk variables because of the inadequate number of subjects for whom one risk is present without the other and because of the need for various assumptions about the relationships between variables. It is in that circumstance that the next step needs to be the choice of some other population that does not have the same overlap between competing risk factors. Thus, for example, the early investigations of raised lead levels as a risk factor for cognitive impairment (through its hypothesized effect in causing brain damage) were severely hampered by the fact that children with higher lead levels (in blood or teeth) tended to come from socially disadvantaged families (Rutter, 1980; Rutter & Russell-Jones, 1983). The studies of populations where this is not the case have been helpful in demonstrating that a small lead effect on cognitive functioning still applied, suggesting that there may indeed be a true direct toxic effect of lead (see, e.g., Fulton et al., 1987).

Sample size. It is commonplace in psychiatric and psychological risk research to expect a small risk effect. This is inevitable in situations where multifactorial causation is the rule. Critics frequently point to the small proportion of the population variance accounted for by factors such as lead exposure or the experience of negative life events, but that is to ignore the reality of what is known. If there are other powerful risk factors, if there are important modifying variables, or if the risk factor in question applies only to a small segment of the total population, it is inevitable that the percentage of variance accounted for by the risk factor will be small. Moreover, it follows from these considerations that statistics on the proportion of variance accounted for provide a very poor guide to the strength of a risk effect at an individual level (Rutter, 1987b).

Nevertheless, if small effects are to be detected, it is essential to have sample sizes with the power to detect them. Extraordinarily few published studies offer any justification for the sample size achieved, making no attempt at calculations of power even where this would have been straightforward (see Meinert & Tonascia, 1986). It is well known that smaller samples will result in higher rates of false negatives (the failure to find a significant effect for a real risk). However, by maintaining a constant significance level (say .05) from large to small samples, we are maintaining the same level of false positives (the finding of an irrelevant risk factor as significant) at one in 20. Thus, as Pocock (1983) pointed out, because we are inevitably testing a mixture of real and irrelevant risk factors, the number of false positives, as a proportion of all significant effects found, can increase substantially on reducing sample size. When the propensity to have published only positive findings is included, the so-called publication bias, the problem is exacerbated. As a consequence, Pocock seriously put forward the view that, in the context of clinical trials, no small studies should be published because more than half of them are likely to be false positives! The unpleasant, but inevitable, conclusion is that sample size must be taken rather more seriously than it is and that the task of replication, dull though it may be, is crucial. We do not doubt that we shall join the others who have made these same points in being ignored.

Modeling of course and causal processes

The data necessary to characterize course inevitably depend upon the complexity of the process thought to be operating; in other words, the model. The timing of onset begins the characterization of course, but many more data are usually required to

ers are familiar with these various formalizations, and this reflects as much a limited knowledge of statistics as an unwillingness to commit themselves to thinking about precise mechanisms. At the same time the class of statistical models that are readily computed represents only a fraction of the causal mechanisms that researchers might contemplate. Extending and matching the range of models that both statisticians and applied researchers use will help in study design as well as in analysis.

References

Ainsworth, M. D. S., Blehar, M. C., Waters, C., & Warr, S. (1978). *Patterns of attachment: A psychological study of the Strange Situation*. Hillsdale, NJ: Lawrence Erlbaum.

Allgulander, C., & Fisher, L. D. (1986). Survival analysis (or time to an event analysis) and the Cox regression model: Methods for longitudinal psychiatric research. *Acta Psychiatrica Scandinavica, 74,* 529–535.

Aro, H. (1987). Life stress and psychosomatic symptoms among 14–16 year old Finnish adolescents. *Psychological Medicine, 17,* 191–201.

Biddle, B. J., & Marlin, M. M. (1987). Causality, confirmation, credulity and structural equation modelling. *Child Development, 58,* 4–17.

Billings, A. G., & Moos, R. H. (1984). Chronic and non-chronic unipolar depression: The differential role of environmental stressors and resources. *Journal of Nervous and Mental Disease, 172,* 65–75.

Breslau, N. (1987). Inquiring about the bizarre: False positives in diagnostic interview schedule for children (DISC). Ascertainment of obsessions, compulsions and psychotic symptoms. *Journal of the American Academy of Child and Adolescent Psychiatry, 26,* 639–644.

Bretherton, I., & Waters, E. (Eds.) (1985). Growing points of attachment theory and research. *Monographs of the Society for Research in Child Development, 50* (1–2, Serial No. 209).

Bromet, C. J., Dunn, L. O., Connell, M. M., Dew, M. A., & Schulberg, H. C. (1986). Long-term reliability of diagnosing life-time major depression in a community sample. *Archives of General Psychiatry, 43,* 435–440.

Brown, G., & Harris, T. (1978). *Social origins of depression*. London: Tavistock.

Brown, G., Chadwick, O., Shaffer, D., Rutter, M. & Traub, M. (1981). A prospective study of children with head injuries. III. Psychiatric sequelae. *Psychological Medicine, 11,* 63–78.

Brown, G. W., Harris, T. O., & Bifulco, A. (1986). The long term effects of early loss of parent. In M. Rutter, C. E. Izard, & P. B. Read (Eds.), *Depression in young people: Clinical and developmental perspectives* (pp. 251–296). New York: Guilford Press.

Cadoret, R. J., Troughton, E., Moreno, L., & Whittles, A. (in press). Early life psychosocial events and adult affective symptoms. In L. N. Robins & M. Rutter (Eds.), *Straight and devious pathways from childhood to adulthood*. Cambridge: Cambridge University Press.

Cantwell, D. P. (1987). Clinical child psychopathology: Diagnostic assessment, diagnostic process and diagnostic classification: DSM-III studies. In M. Rutter, A. Tuma, & I. Lann (Eds.), *Assessment and classification in child and adolescent psychopathology*. New York: Guilford Press.

Carey, G. (1987). Big genes, little genes, affective disorder and anxiety: A commentary. *Archives of General Psychiatry, 44,* 486–491.

Chesher, A., & Lancaster, T. (1983). The estimation of models of labour market behavior. *Review of Economic Studies, 50,* 609–624.

Clayton, D. (1985). Using test-retest reliability data to improve estimates of relative risk: An application of latent class analysis. *Statistics in Medicine, 4,* 445–455.

Cox, D. R. (1972). Regression models and life tables. *Journal of the Royal Statistical Society, Series B*, Vol. 34, 187–220.

Fergusson, D. M., & Horwood, L. J. (1987). The trait and method components of ratings of conduct disorder: Part I, Maternal and teacher evaluations of conduct disorder in children; Part II, Factors related to the trait composition of conduct disorder scores. *Journal of Child Psychology and Psychiatry, 28,* 249–272.

Fergusson, D. M., & Horwood, L. J. (1988). Structural equation modelling of measurement processes in longitudinal data. In M. Rutter (Ed.) *Studies of psychosocial risk: The power of longitudinal data* (pp. 325–353). Cambridge: Cambridge University Press.

Folstein, S., & Rutter, M. (1987). Family aggregation and genetic implications. In E. Schopler & G. Mesibov (Eds.), *Neurobiological issues in autism* (pp. 83–105). New York: Plenum Press.

Fulton, M., Raab, G., Thomson, G., Laxon, D., Hunter, R., & Hepburn, W. (1987). Influence of blood lead on the ability and attainment of children in Edinburgh. *Lancet, i,* 1221–1226.

Goodyer, I. M., Kolvin, I., & Gatzanis, S. (1987). The impact of recent undesirable events on psychiatric disorders of childhood and adolescence. *British Journal of Psychiatry, 151,* 179–184.

Griliches, Z. (1979). Sibling models and data in economies: Beginnings of a survey. *Journal of Political Economy, 87,* S37–S64.

Hanson, D. R., Gottesman, I. I., & Heston, L. L. (1976). Some possible childhood indicators of adult schizophrenia inferred from children of schizophrenics. *British Journal of Psychiatry, 129,* 142–154.

Hetherington, E. M., Cox, M., & Cox, R. (1982). Effects of divorce on parents and children. In M. E. Lamb (Ed.), *Nontraditional families* (pp. 223–288). Hillsdale, NJ: Lawrence Erlbaum.

Hetherington, E. M., Cox, M., & Cox, R. (1985). Long-term effects of divorce and remarriage on the adjustment of children. *Journal of the American Academy of Child Psychiatry, 24,* 518–530.

Hill, J., Harrington, R., Fudge, H., Rutter, M., & Pickles, A. (1989). Adult personality functioning assessment (APFA): An investigator-based standardised interview. *British Journal of Psychiatry, 155,* 24–35.

Hodges, J., & Tizard, B. (1989a). IQ and behavioural adjustment of ex-institutional adolescents. *Journal of Child Psychology and Psychiatry, 30,* 53–75.

Hodges, J., & Tizard, B. (1989b). Social and family relationships of ex-institutional adolescents. *Journal of Child Psychology and Psychiatry, 30,* 77–97.

Hoem, J. M. (1985). Weighting, misclassification, and other issues in the analysis of survey samples of life histories. In J. J. Heckman & B. Singer (Eds.), *Longitudinal analysis of labour market data* (pp. 249–293). Cambridge: Cambridge University Press.

Keller, M. B., Beardslee, W. R., Dorer, D. J., Lavori, P. W., Samuelson, H., & Klerman, G. R. (1986). Impact of severity and chronicity of parental affective illness on adaptive functioning and psychopathology in children. *Archives of General Psychiatry, 43,* 930–937.

Kendler, K. S., Materson, C. C., Ungaro, R., & Davis, K. L. (1984). A family history study of schizophrenia-related disorders. *American Journal of Psychiatry, 41,* 424–427.

Kovacs, M., Feinberg, J. L., Crouse-Novak, M. A., Paulaukas, S. L., Pollack, M., & Finkelstein, R. (1984). Depressive disorders in childhood. II. A longitudinal prospective study of risk of a subsequent major depression. *Archives of General Psychiatry, 41,* 643–649.

Lamb, M. E., Thompson, R. A., Gardner, W. P., Charnov, E. L., & Estes, D. (1984). Security of infantile attachment as assessed in the "Strange Situation": Its study and biological interpretation. *Behavioral and Brain Sciences, 7,* 127–147.

Lancaster, A., & Nickell, S. J., (1980). The analysis of re-employment probabilities for the unemployed. *Journal of the Royal Statistical Society, 143A,* 141–165.

Lavori, P. W., Keller, M. B., & Klerman, G. L., (1984). Relapse in affective disorder: A reanalysis of the literature using life tables methods. *Journal of Psychiatric Research, 18,* 13–25.

Leckman, J. F., Weissman, M. M., Merikangas, K. R., Pauls, D. L., & Prusoff, B. A. (1983). Panic disorder and major depression. *Archives of General Psychiatry, 40,* 1055–1060.

Magnusson, D., & Bergman, L. R. (1988). Longitudinal studies: Individual and variable based approaches to research on early risk factors. In M. Rutter (Ed.), *Studies of psychosocial risk: The power of longitudinal data* (pp. 45–61). Cambridge: Cambridge University Press.

Manski, C., & McFadden, D. (1981). Alternative estimates and sample designs for discrete choice analysis. In C. Manski & D. McFadden (Eds.), *Structural analysis of discrete data: With econometric applications* (pp. 2–50). Cambridge, MA: Massachusetts Institute of Technology Press.

Martin, J. A. (1987). Structural equation modelling: A guide for the perplexed. *Child Development, 58,* 33–37.

Maughan, B., & Pickles, A. (in press). Adopted and illegitimate children grown up. In L. Robins & M. Rutter (Eds.), *Straight and devious pathways from childhood to adulthood.* Cambridge: Cambridge University Press.

Meinert, C. L., & Tonascia, S. (1986). *Clinical trials: Design, conduct and analysis.* New York: Oxford University Press.

Mulaik, S. A. (1987). Towards a conception of causality applicable to experimentation and causal modelling. *Child Development, 58,* 18–32.

Olweus, D. (1979). Stability of aggressive reaction patterns in males: A review. *Psychological Bulletin, 86,* 852–875.

Pauls, D., Towbin, K. E., Leckman, J. F., Zahner, G. E. P., & Cohen, D. J. (1986). Gilles de la Tourette's syndrome and obsessive-compulsive disorder: Evidence supporting a genetic relationship. *Archives of General Psychiatry, 43,* 1180–1182.

Pickles, A. R., (1987). The problem of initial conditions in longitudinal data analysis. In R. Crouchley (Ed.), *Longitudinal data analysis* (pp. 129–149). Aldershot: Avebury.

Pocock, S. J., (1983). *Clinical trials: A practical approach.* Chichester: Wiley.

Popper, K. (1959). *The logic of scientific discovery* (2nd ed.). London: Hutchinson.

Popper, K. (1972). *Conjectures and regulations: The growth of scientific knowledge* (4th ed.). London: Routledge & Kegan Paul.

Porter, R., O'Conner, M., & Whelan, J. (Eds.) (1984). *Mechanisms of alcohol damage in utero.* Ciba Symposium No. 105. London: Pitman.

Quinton, D., & Rutter, M. (1988). *Parenting breakdown: The making and breaking of intergenerational links.* Aldershot: Gower Publishing.

Quinton, D., Rutter, M., & Liddle, C. (1984). Institutional rearing, parenting difficulties and marital support. *Psychological Medicine, 14,* 107–124.

Quinton, D., Rutter, M., & Gulliver, L. (in press). The social functioning in early adulthood of the children of psychiatric patients. In L. N. Robins & M. Rutter (Eds.), *Straight and devious pathways from childhood to adulthood.* New York and Cambridge: Cambridge University Press.

Richman, N., Stevenson, J., & Graham, P. (1982). *Preschool to school: A behavioural study.* London: Academic Press.

Ridder, G., (1984). The distribution of single-spell duration data. In G. R. Neumann & L. Westergaard-Nielson (Eds.), *Studies in labour market dynamics* (pp. 45–73). Berlin: Springer-Verlag.

Robins, L. N. (1986). The consequences of conduct disorder in girls. In D. Olweus, J. Block, & M. Radke-Yarrow, (Eds.), *Development of antisocial and prosocial behavior: Research, theories and issues* (pp. 385–414). New York: Academic Press.

Robins, L. N., Davis, D. H., & Wish, E. (1977). Detecting predictors of rare events: Demographic, family and personal deviance as predictors of stages in the progression towards narcotic addiction. In J. C. Strauss, H. N. Babigian, & M. Roff (Eds.), *The origins and cause of psychopathology: Methods of longitudinal research* (pp. 379–406). New York: Plenum Press.

Rutter, M. (1971). Parent-child separation: Psychological effects on the children. *Journal of Child Psychology and Psychiatry, 12,* 233–260.

Rutter, M. (1978). Diagnostic validity in child psychiatry. *Advances in Biological Psychiatry, 2,* 2–22.

Rutter, M. (1980). Raised lead levels and impaired cognitive/behavioural functioning: A review of the evidence. *Developmental Medicine and Child Neurology, 22,* Supplement No. 42.

Rutter, M. (1981). Epidemiological/longitudinal strategies and causal research in child psychiatry. *Journal of the American Academy of Child Psychiatry, 20,* 513–544.

Rutter, M. (1983). Statistical and personal interactions: Facets and perspectives. In D. Magnusson & V. Allen (Eds.), *Human development: An interactional perspective* (pp. 295–319). New York: Academic Press.

Rutter, M. (1987a). Temperament, personality and personality disorder. *British Journal of Psychiatry, 150,* 443–458.

Rutter, M. (1987b). Continuities and discontinuities from infancy. In J. Osofsky (Ed.), *Handbook of infant development* (2nd ed.) (pp. 1256–1296). New York: Wiley.

Rutter, M. (1988a). DSM-III: A Research Postscript. In M. Rutter, A. Tuma, & I. Lann (Eds.), *Assessment and classification in child and adolescent psychopathology* (pp. 453–464). New York: Guilford Press.

Rutter, M. (1988b). Epidemiological approaches to developmental psychopathology. *Archives of General Psychiatry, 45,* 486–500.

Rutter, M. (1989). Age as an ambiguous variable in developmental research: Some epidemiological considerations from developmental psychopathology. *International Journal of Behavioural Development, 12,* 1–34.

Rutter, M. (in press). Psychosocial resilience and protective mechanisms. In J. Rolf, A. Masten, D. Cicchetti, K. Nuechterlein, & D. Weintraub (Eds.), *Risk and protective factors in the development of psychopathology.* New York: Cambridge University Press.

Rutter, M., & Garmezy, N. (1983). Developmental psychopathology. In E. M. Hetherington (Ed.), *Socialization, personality and social development* (Vol. 4 of *Handbook of child psychology,* 4th ed.), pp. 775–911. New York: Wiley.

Rutter, M., & Russell-Jones, R. (1983). *Lead versus health: Sources and effects of low level lead exposure.* Chichester: Wiley.

Rutter, M., & Quinton, D. (1984a). Parental psychiatric disorder: Effects on children. *Psychological Medicine, 14,* 853–880.

Rutter, M., & Quinton, D. (1984b). Long-term follow-up of women institutionalized in childhood: Factors promoting good functioning in adult life. *British Journal of Developmental Psychology, 2,* 191–204.

Rutter, M., Chadwick, O., & Shaffer, D. (1983). Head injury. In M. Rutter (Ed.), *Developmental neuropsychiatry* (pp. 83–111). New York: Guilford Press.

Rutter, M., Tuma, A., & Lann, L. (Eds.) (1988). *Assessment and diagnosis in child psychopathology.* New York: Guilford Press.

Rutter, M., Bolton, P., Harrington, R., Le Couteur, A., Macdonald, H., and Simonoff, E. (in press a) Genetic factors in child psychiatric disorders: I. A review of research strategies. *Journal of Child Psychology and Psychiatry.*

Rutter, M., LeCouteur, A., Lord, C., Macdonald, H., Rios, P., & Folstein, S. (1988). Diagnosis and subclassification of autism: Concepts and instrument development. In

F. Schopler & G. Mesibov (Eds.), *Diagnosis and assessment in autism* (pp. 239–259). New York: Plenum Press.

Rutter, M., Macdonald, H., Le Couteur, A., Harrington, R., Bolton, P. and Bailey, A. (in press b) Genetic factors in child psychiatric disorders: II. Empirical findings. *Journal of Child Psychology and Psychiatry.*

St. Claire, L., & Osborn, A. F. (1987). The ability and behaviour of children who have been "in-care" or separated from their parents. *Early Child Development and Care, 28*(3), whole issue.

Sandberg, S. T., Rutter, M., & Taylor, E. (1978). Hyperkinetic disorder in psychiatric clinic attenders. *Developmental Medicine and Child Neurology, 20,* 279–299.

Schachar, R., Rutter, M., & Smith, A., (1981). The characteristics of situationally and pervasive hyperactive children: Implications for syndrome definition. *Journal of Child Psychology and Psychiatry, 22,* 375–392.

Stewart, A. L., Reynolds, E. O. R., Hope, P. L., Hamilton, P. A., Baudin, J., Costello, A. M. de L., Bradford, B. C., & Wyatt, J. S. (1987). Probability of neurodevelopmental disorders estimated from ultrasound appearance of brains of very preterm infants. *Developmental Medicine and Child Neurology, 29,* 3–11.

Tanaka, J. S., (1987). "How big is big enough?" Sample size and goodness of fit in structural equation models with latent variables. *Child Development, 58,* 134–146.

van Eerdewegh, M. M., Bieri, M. D., Parilla, R. H., & Clayton, P. (1982). The bereaved child. *British Journal of Psychiatry, 140,* 23–29.

Weissman, M. M. (1987). *Evidence for co-morbidity for anxiety and depression: Family and genetic studies of children.* Paper presented at a conference on symptom co-morbidity in anxiety and depressive disorders. Sterling Forest Conference Center, Tuxedo, NY, September 28, 1987.

Weissman, M. M., Gammon, G. D., John, K., Merikangas, K. R., Warner, V., Prusoff, B. A., & Sholomskas, D. (1987). Children of depressed parents: Increased psychopathology and early onset of major depression. *Archives of General Psychiatry, 44,* 847–853.

West, D. J. (1982). *Delinquency: Its roots, careers and prospects.* London: Heinemann (Cambridge, MA: Harvard University Press).

White, H. (1982). Maximum likelihood estimation of misspecified models. *Econometrica, 50,* 1–25.

Wolkind, S., & Rutter, M., (1973). Children who have been in care. *Journal of Child Psychology and Psychiatry, 14,* 97–105.

World Health Organization (1987). *ICD-10 1986 draft of Chapter V, Categories F00 and F99: Mental, behavioural and developmental disorders.* Geneva: W.H.O.

3 Data in epidemiological longitudinal research

GUNNAR EKLUND

Introduction

Textbooks define epidemiology as "the study of the distribution and determinants of health-related states and events in populations, and the application of this study to control of health problems" (Last, 1983). Today, the most important topic of epidemiology concerns etiology of diseases with long latency time (induction time). Thus, between exposure and diagnoses, 10–25 years may have elapsed. In modern epidemiological research rare diseases dominate; for example, the risk of contracting leukemia during the whole life span is less than 1%. Given that long latency time is common, that the majority of diseases seem to have multiple causes, and that rare diseases dominate epidemiology today, the choice of study design is a crucial question for epidemiological research.

In the field of cancer epidemiology, it is possible to survey the ordinary design and data sources used. A publication of ongoing projects (Muir & Wagner, 1986) has shown that case-control studies based on interview data are the most common, followed by historic cohort data with, for instance, register data, followed by prospective cohort data studies (including random control trials) and correlation studies on an aggregated level, for instance, comparisons between statistics from regions or time periods.

From the Nordic point of view, retrospective, historical cohort studies are of special interest because the access to many computerized demographic registries, with a unique person number as the key for linkage, has provided the opportunity to carry out a great variety of epidemiological studies. These registries are of special value because they often cover the whole population and because they have been stored since 1960. With respect to cancer epidemiological research, the access to the National Swedish Cancer Registry since 1958 (National Board of Health and Welfare, 1984) is of great importance, especially because the reporting is compulsory. The same is true with respect to registration of the causes of death. For these reasons it can be claimed that cancer epidemiology constitutes a Nordic research niche.

The register sources from the early 1960s are not free of problems. From the Swedish census of 1960 (FoB 60) it is possible to identify data concerning occupation, industry, and place of residence for every Swedish inhabitant in 1960. In some respects the data are of limited value because they refer to a certain time period (e.g., occupation during a certain week in October 1960). Further, the occupation data are sometimes wrongly reported or miscoded (Brivkalne, 1964).

As the latency time (induction time) is of great importance in cancer studies as well as in many studies of other chronic diseases, it is preferable to have access to data over a long period, not only from a single occasion. Thus, it is suggested that the cancer incidence between 1961 and 1979 could be matched to occupation data during the period 1950–1970. The data from FoB 60 could at most be regarded as a suitable "proxy" for the occupational status during the surrounding 20 years.

Nevertheless, a special registry called the cancer-environmental registry (CER), including approximately 600,000 cancer cases (e.g., malignancies), has been constructed with the purpose of identifying occupational cancer risks (Wiklund, Einhorn, Wennström, & Rapaport, 1981). The cancer sites, occupation, age, sex, industry, and place of residence in 1960 are recorded, along with the year and cause of death for those persons who are deceased. The same information is given for the population at risk, that is, the population in Sweden according to FoB 60. A great number of analyses have been carried out using the CER. These analyses have identified many excessive risks for some tumor sites and for some occupations, as well as identifying underrisks for other occupations and sites (Malker & Weiner, 1984). In a similar way, it has been stated that some geographical regions show considerable over- or underrisks (Eklund & Carstensen, 1986).

The aims

The main aim of this chapter is to illustrate the defects in the quality of data in historic prospective studies, especially if they have measured the main predictor on only a single occasion. Another aim concerns the consequences of defects in data quality with respect to the choice of study design and data-gathering strategies. The presentation starts with a survey exemplifying the problem.

Examples of data quality problems

Occupation

As mentioned above, CER has been obtained by a combination of data from FoB 60 and the cancer register from 1961 to 1979. The occupation data in FoB 60 were self-reported and referred to a certain week in October 1960. The occupational classification in FoB 60 is a revised version of the standards from the International Labour Office, 1958. The list contains 291 specific occupations (3-digit codes) that are grouped into 60 general occupations (2-digit codes). By combining occupation and tumor site, 10,000 risk ratios are obtained. A great number of these are found to be statistically significant over- or underrisks.

Can we really trust the occupation data to be adequate? A control study made in connection with the 1960 census revealed that classification errors comprised nearly 20% of the total number of occupations classified at the most detailed level and 13% of the total at the general occupational level (Brivkalne, 1964). The main problem is whether or not the occupation data according to FoB 60 is a good "proxy" for the whole period 1950–1970. As occupational changes are common, it is reasonable that data from a single occasion are not representative for the whole period (Olsson & Brandt, 1982). The extent to which the occupation data of 1960 are correlated with those of 1950 is unknown because the classification was altered between these census opportunities. On the other hand, detailed tables exist regarding industry changes between 1950 and 1960. For occupations, however, we do have information between FoB 70 and FoB 75 (Statistiska centralbyrån, 1979). Among other data illuminating changes of occupational situation, a set of tables based on large interview investigations, including the cohorts 1895–1955, deserves to be considered (Östlin, Lindberg, & Thorslund, 1985). With the assistance of these tables, one can decide whether or not the number of people in a certain occupation has changed substantially. For some individual occupation groups, among them bakers and confectioners, a manual comparison between FoB 60 and a sample from 1950 was made concerning occupation changes from 1950 to 1960 (Wicksell, Carstensen, Eklund, & Gustafsson, 1988). However, it is difficult to estimate the time period over which persons who declare themselves as bakers in FoB 60 have, on the average, been active as bakers during the period 1950–1970.

Individual occupation data that consider the whole period 1950–1970 are, otherwise, very limited. In spite of the fact that occupation and industrial data have been collected at the census opportunities in 1950, 1960, 1965, 1970, and 1975, only a few tabulations illuminating occupation changes and including the group "leaving working life" have been published. These age-classified tables illuminate what happened between 1950 and 1960. In another publication (Statistiska centralbyrån, 1979), the economically active population in 1960, 1965, 1970, and 1975 is divided into 74 occupation groups for which occupation changes between 1970 and 1975 are accounted.

Having the occupation data from FoB 60 as a basis, as in the CER and in the cause of death registry, the question concerning stability arises. For an occupation with considerable reduction between 1960 and 1970, the proportion of the group leaving work must be considerable. For example, in the area of argicultural work, the number of active workers was 362,000 according FoB 60, and 224,000 according to FoB 70, thus demonstrating a considerable (38%) reduction.

For forest workers the 37% reduction is of the same magnitude. For textile work and sewing, the reduction is 33%, for mining and quarrying 21%, for shoemaking and leather work 53%, and for bakers and confectioners 35%. For the other occupational groups the reduction is less than 20%, and for most of them the numbers are increasing between 1960 and 1970. From this it is evident that many of the agricultural workers, according to FoB 60, have been active only a few years during the

Table 3.1. *Population in 1960 in some occupations/industries. Correction with respect to occupational morbidity 1950–1960 and 1960–1970.*

Occupation/Industry	A 1960 active population	B Both 1950 and 1960	Kvot B/A	Correction $\dfrac{1 + B/A}{2}$	Correction 1960–1970
Agricultural workers	277,863	248,901	0.896	0.95	0.66
Forest workers	64,867	34,698	0.535	0.77	
Fishermen	8,576	7,127	0.831	0.92	
Waiters	9,755	5,708	0.585	0.79	0.50
Mining and quarrying workers	48,801	26,757	0.548	0.77	0.43
Beverage and tobacco workers	7,430	3,683	0.496	0.75	
Sawyers, planers, etc.	68,612	40,014	0.583	0.79	
Medical workers, nurses, nurses' assistants	12,774	17,667	0.723	0.86	
Printing and publishing workers	28,781	19,942	0.693	0.85	0.68
Shoemakers and leather workers	6,371	3,987	0.626	0.81	
Rubber workers	8,577	4,409	0.514	0.76	
Chemical, pulp, and plastic workers	19,177	7,731	0.403	0.70	0.52
Secretaries, typists, etc.					0.67
Bakers and confectioners			0.90[a]		0.60

[a]The source is Wicksell et al., 1988

period 1961–1970. Agricultural workers, according to FoB 60, have been at most active in the same occupation 81% of the 10 years during the period 1961–1970. This is, however, an overestimation, because some of them may have changed to another occupation and been replaced by others. For the period 1974–1979 Wiklund states (Wiklund & Holm, 1986) that for all sites the relative risk for agricultural male workers is 0.84 in relation to the whole country, after standardization with respect to age. The estimate is based on CER data. The period 1961–1970 seems to be reasonable with regard to the cancer induction period for cancer observed from 1974 to 1979. A correction of 0.84 can be obtained as $1 - 0.16/0.81 = 0.80$, where 0.16 is the underrisk and 0.81 (81% above) is a rough correction factor due to leaving agricultural work. It is evident that the underrisk is underestimated and that the correction is not negligible.

With the help of available data (Central Bureau of Statistics, 1965) it can be determined how many workers in a certain occupation have been active in the occupation both in 1950 and in 1960. For some selected occupations information has been extracted and is given in Table 3.1. The table is limited to persons born between 1896 and 1935. The share of workers who were in agricultural work at both measurement times was 90% (ratio *B/A*). For fisherman the corresponding figure is 83%, for forest workers and various industrial workers, miners, waiters, and so forth, between 40% and 60%. Thus, the agricultural workers show high stability, but it must be remembered that the estimate is based on agricultural workers in 1960 and that the majority were already in the same occupation in 1950. If the basis had been 1950 instead of 1960, a considerable reduction should have been noted.

In a special column in Table 3.1 a rough estimate of the correction factor for the period 1950–1960 is given. This factor is chosen so that it is proportional to the share of the time period 1950–1960 during which the 1960 adult population in a certain occupation belonged to the same occupation group as in 1960. In this estimation, it has been assumed that changes in occupation took place in the middle of the period for those who were not already in the same occupation in 1950. The same result is obtained if it is assumed that the starting date among the agricultural workers active in 1960, but not in 1950, were evenly distributed over the 10 years between. This approximation implies that changes to other occupations and deaths during the period are negligible and indicated that the correction factor is somewhat too high. For agricultural workers the correction of observed over- and underrisks seems to be without importance; but for other groups of occupations, the application of the correction factor implies multiplications of over- and underrisks by 1.33; that is, an observed overrisk of 30% is raised to 40%.

Starting from 1975 one can in a similar way make a comparison with 1970. The proportion of persons in the occupation during the whole period is found to be 87% for agricultural workers, 63% for forest workers, 52% for workers involved in the manufacture of pulp, chemical, rubber, and plastic products, 66% for waiters, and 75% for workers in printing and publishing. The main impression is that the annual mobility between occupations has slightly increased. The difference in occupational mobility between the periods 1950–1960 and 1970–1975 is, however, so small that a reconstruction for 1960 and 1970 is regarded as possible.

This calculation is carried out, assuming that the transition 1970–1975 can be applied and that the number of workers in various occupations is known in 1960, 1965, and 1970. The guessed mobility between 1960 and 1965 is based on estimates of the share leaving working life from 1970 to 1975, changing occupation from 1970 to 1975, remaining in occupation in 1975, and newly reentering from 1970 to 1975. Applying this information, it is possible to give a rough estimate of the persons active in a certain occupation in 1960 who were in the same occupation during the sixties. This share is given in the last column of Table 3.1. The shares are between 43% and 68% of the whole period and can be used as a rough correction. It is then evident that the earlier suggested correction factor for agricultural workers is sharpened from 81% to 66%. As a consequence, the observed relative risk 0.84 is corrected to $1 - 0.16/0.66 = 0.76$. For the period 1964–1969 the observed relative risk for agricultural workers is 0.80 after correction – now with respect to correction figures for the period 1950–1960; the risk value becomes $1 - 0.20/0.95 = 0.79$. Thus, the original trend from 0.80 to 0.84 is substituted with a decreasing trend from 0.79 to 0.76. If correction is extended to the whole period 1950–1970, the mean value of the correction number for the two periods can be recommended; for example, this mean is 0.805 for agricultural workers.

The choice of the correction number depends on the induction time. Various induction times are suggested for cancer initiators and for cancer promoters. For the initiators, the induction time is often chosen as 5–20 years before diagnosis, with a top level between 10 and 15 years. Thus, the chosen induction time is from 1950 to 1970 if cancers observed during the period 1961–1979 are studied. For some tumor types, as, for instance, with leukemia, and for promoters, shorter induction times are recommended but difficult to specify.

It has here been assumed that the effffect on cancer is proportional to the number of years in the occupation. This corresponds to the idea that a simple linear relationship exists between the number of years in the occupation and the cancer risk. If the length of the induction time is decreased or if the interval between induction and diagnosed cancer is decreased, the change is of importance for the magnitude of the correction.

Cancer risks and other mortality and morbidity rates change with age. Therefore, it should be reasonable to give greater weight to persons aged 55–65 years than to persons aged 25–35 years, if the intention is to study cancer risks during the following 10 or 20 years. Generally speaking, the younger age group has, for the majority of the tumor sites, not yet reached the age groups characterized by high cancer rates. In Table 3.1 it has not been possible to take age distribution into account. However, for the majority of the occupations – agricultural work possibly excepted – the age distribution is so similar that it seems to be of little importance whether age is taken into consideration in the estimate of the correction ratios or not. The over- and underrisks are often not specified for age groups or birth cohorts, but as a rule are given only as age-standardized relative risks.

The confounding problem has, for the most part, not been considered in this report. However, the high mobility among occupations may be followed by confounding bias, especially if the change has been dominated by mobility from one occupation to another and this other occupation is characterized by high or low cancer risk. Another confounding effect of importance can be suspected if the correction is strong (or the dilution is widespread), and this type of bias is especially common if the real overrisk is small. The above section can be summarized in the following consequences caused by effects in data quality:

1. Over- and underrisks could be considerably sharpened if corrections were carried out.

2. Occupational cancer trends can be biased if no correction is carried out.

3. Conclusions (absence of over- or underrisks) are not to be recommended when corrections are not undertaken.

4. The need of adequate correction estimates is great.

5. The need for improved estimates of changes between occupations from 1960 to 1970 is urgent and can be obtained by linkage between FoB 60 and FoB 70. By this linkage it is possible to divide the population according to the number of years in the same occupation. Those with 10 years or more can be separated from those with some, but probably fewer, number of years. In this way it is possible to add an

analysis of "dose-response" with respect to years in an occupation and to carry out corrections especially for birth cohorts and age groups.

Cholesterol in serum and succeeding cancer

In a health screening during the years 1963–1965, 92,839 persons under the age of 75 participated (Socialstyrelsen, 1971). The screening was carried out by a mobile unit using standardized serum sampling and included, among other parameters, serum cholesterol measurements (Zak, Dickenman, White, Burnett, & Cherney, 1954), which were analyzed by using an automatic serum analyzer device (Jungner & Jungner, 1968).

The cohort was matched with the Swedish Cause of Death Register and with the Swedish Cancer Register (National Board of Health and Welfare, 1984) in the end of 1979 to obtain data on succeeding cancer and on the cause of death of deceased subjects. The record linkage was made possible by the unique identification number used in Sweden whereby each person is assigned an identification number consisting of 10 digits (i.e., year, month and day of birth, supplemented with digits indicating region of birth, sex, and one control digit). The numbers are not affected by possible changes in names.

As the result of an analysis, a statistically significant positive relationship was observed between the incidence of colorectal cancer and baseline serum cholesterol level among men during a 17-year follow-up period (Törnberg, Holm, Carstensen, & Eklund, 1987; Törnberg, Holm, Carstensen, & Eklund, 1986). This study as well as other studies (Stemmermann, Nomura, Hellbrun, Pollack, & Kagan, 1981; Williams et al., 1981) were based on a single blood sample, and the relevance of a single serum cholesterol value in a study of cancer risks may be questioned.

Thus, it may be indicated that the relevant period due to cancer induction corresponds, for example, to 1955–1965 and that the measurement of the predictor at a single occasion is not representative for the serum cholesterol average for this period. However, if the values are stable, a single value can be regarded as acceptable.

The stability of serum cholesterol could be studied in another Swedish population in which repeated cholesterol samples were taken at intervals of six weeks and two years (Socialstyrelsen, 1979). This repeated sampling enabled an analysis of both the short-term and long-term variations of the measured serum cholesterol values.

The correlation coefficient between the cholesterol values in 1969 and in 1971 in this cohort was 0.66. The correlation coefficients for the cholesterol samples taken at a six-weeks interval were 0.71 in 1969 and 0.78 in 1971; that is, the mean value of the correlation coefficients for those two occasions was 0.74 (Törnberg, Jakobsson, & Eklund, 1988). In order to classify how to estimate the stability, a path analysis model (Blalock, 1961) is given in Figure 3.1.

The correlation between the "true" cholesterol value and the observed value at any time is designated by r_0 and is expected to be less than 1.0, mainly because of random errors in the chemical analysis.

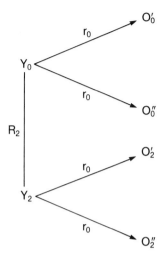

Figure 3.1. Path analysis scheme. Y refers to true and O to observed values. O' and O'' refer to the first and second observations within a short interval. r_0 and R_2 are correlations, and the subscripts refer to time (years). Time_0 was the initial examination and Time_2 the repeated examination two years later.

The correlation between the true cholesterol value at the time of the initial examination and the true value at a later point of time $(=t)$ is designated R_t. If it is assumed that R_t diminishes with time in accordance with a simple stationary autoregressive model (Kendall, 1948), then

$$R_t = R_1{}^t$$

An estimate of the correlation r_0, could be obtained by the use of the path analysis scheme shown in Figure 3.1. According to path analysis the correlation between O'_0 and O''_0 as well as between O'_2 and O''_2 corresponded to $r_0{}^2$. This value can be estimated approximately as the correlation between two observed values on the short term, that is, as 0.74.

The correlation between determinations separated by two years is obtained in Figure 3.1 by following paths between O'_0 and O'_2. Using the path analysis scheme this correlation is $r_0{}^2 R_2$ and is estimated to be 0.66.

Since $r_0{}^2$ was known to be approximately 0.74 and $r_0{}^2 R_2$ to be approximately 0.66, substitution can be used to obtain a value for R_2 ($R_2 = 0.66/0.74 = 0.89$). The ratio $0.66/0.74 = 0.89$ is an estimate of the correlation between the true cholesterol values, at two-year intervals, free of measurement errors and intraindividual variations in dietary habits. It is also possible to estimate R_1 (time $= 1$ year) from the equation as $\sqrt{0.89} = 0.94$, since $R_2 = R_1{}^2$.

The values for R_t are high in any case when $t < 6$ years, because $R_6 = R_1{}^6 = 0.709$. From this it follows that the cholesterol values were stable, at least in the sense that it is highly probable that individuals with high cholesterol values in the middle of a twelve-year period had high values over the whole period.

On the basis of these preconditions the correlation is obtained between "the true value at the single occasion" and "the average value over a period of $\pm k$ years" as $R_{k/6}$.

An approximate correction of the overrisks is obtained by dividing the overrisk by the square of the correlation between the observed single determinations and the period averages. The R-values correspond to the correlation between the true single determination and the period average, and represent a measurement that replaces single determinations with period ones.

To summarize, the results indicate a high long-term stability of cholesterol. However, in general, the lack of stability might result in a considerable bias. If the correlation between single determination and period averages can be estimated, a correction of the bias is possible.

Further examples of data quality problems due to substitution of single measurements for period data

A survey of predictors based on single measurement is given in Table 3.2. The predictors are chosen mainly because they are of interest in cancer epidemiology, but they are also relevant as factors for other morbidity or mortality. Most of the predictors are recorded for the whole population in a census. Other predictors are obtained in a sample by questionnaire or measurements. For some important factors, such as birth year and sex, the single determination can be generalized over a long period. Other factors are by definition at least partially known; "never married in 1960" and "level of education" in 1960 are predictor values giving information concerning the past. For therapeutic ionizing radiation the single observation is often adequate.

Table 3.2 is specified whether individual data exist or can be obtained before and after the basic time point or access is limited to group level (aggregated level).

It is evident from the table that the predictors in register and retrospective cohort data often are characterized as single measurements and that a correction often seems to be possible.

How to measure data quality

In the above examples, bias due to a special type of data quality has been described, and a correction factor has been suggested. The main aim with the correction factor is to consider errors due to substitution of single measurements for period ones. If the mean value over the period was the relevant measurement, the correction factor is appropriate because it is simply related to the bias. With respect to occupation, it may be difficult to separate the errors because of deviation between observed and true single measurements.

In Figure 3.2 the relationship between occupation and succeeding cancer is given

Table 3.2. *Examples of data quality problems due to substitution of single measurements for period data.*

Predictor	Individual single measurements, year	Data 10 years before		Data 10 years after	
		Individual data known?	Group data known?	Individual data possible to obtain?	Group data known?
County, living (Central Bureau 1965)	1960	Known 1947[a]	–	Yes	–
Marital status (Central Bureau 1965)	1960	Partially[b]	Yes	Yes	Yes
Education (Central Bureau 1965)	1960	Partially[c] 1960		Partially[c] 1960	Yes, high stability
Occupation (Statistika centralbyrån, 1979)	1960	No	Yes, partially[d]	Yes	Partially[d]
Cumulated fertility (Johansson & Finnås, 1983)	1970	For women born 1925	–	For women born 1925	–
Smoking habits (Wicksell et al., 1988)	1963	Yes[e]	–	No	No
Serum cholesterol (Törnberg et al., 1987)	1962–65	No	Yes, estimated	No	Yes, estimated
Dietary habits	1968	No	No	No	No
Ionizing radiation (therapy or diagnosis)		Not relevant	–	Not relevant	
Radon in dwellings (Lanctot, 1985)	1987	No	No		
Alternating magnetic fields (Wertheimer & Leeper, 1979)		Rough[f] estimates	No		

[a]County known 1947, part of person number.
[b]Never married 1960 – never married 1950.
[c]Education level can change in only one direction.
[d]Group data, not for all occupations.
[e]Retrospective information, obtained by questionnaire.
[f]Dose during limited period. Living near power lines correlated to magnetic fields.

in the form of a path analysis scheme in order to illustrate the generation of bias. The correlations between variables are given close to the corresponding arrows.

Figure 3.2 shows how the correlation between observed occupation and cancer can be explained. The path scheme indicates that the correlation is obtained as a product between the correlations corresponding to each arrow. Because only the observed

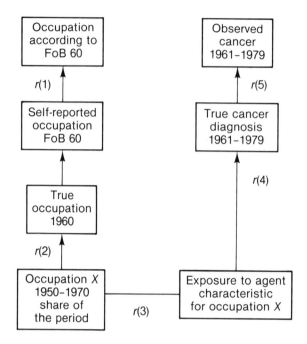

Figure 3.2. The correlation between observed occupation and observed cancer diagnosis: A path analysis model.

occupation and the observed cancers are known, the correlation between these variables, R, can, according to the model, be written as:

$$R = r(1) \times r(2) \times r(3) \times r(4) \times r(5)$$

The correlation corresponding to the most relevant arrow is $r(4)$. Thus, it is evident that the dilution is considerable. Now, it is reasonable to presume that $r(5)$ and $r(1)$ are almost equal to 1. The correlation $r(2)$ is roughly estimated, for example, by the aid of the correction factor in Table 3.1. Hereby, $r(1) \times r(2)$ equals the correction factor because of the lack of data for the period 1950–1979, while the correlation $r(3)$ is unknown and is assumed to change considerably from occupation to occupation. The weak correlations, $r(2)$ and especially $r(3)$, give a considerable contribution to the dilution effect.

Conclusions

The bias due to the use of single-occasion data as substitute for period data can be approached in three different ways:

1. A correction is carried out by estimation on an aggregated – not individual –

level of the predictor stability over the relevant period. This stability can be expressed as a correlation coefficient, as in the cholesterol-cancer example, or as the average agreement between the single-occasion data and the period data, as illustrated in the occupation-cancer example. In this type of approach the source concerned with individual predictor and cancer data must be supplemented with other sources, often obtained from a subpopulation of the original one or from an external population.

2. The single-occasion value is supplemented with another single-occasion value or by period data. This is possible in some longitudinal cohort/register studies; for example, through linkage of individual census data from two opportunities, 1960 and 1970. However, supplementing historic sources is rare. Supplementary data can, however, also be obtained from a randomly selected subcohort from the part of the target population (Persson, Bergkvist, & Adami, 1987), which had positive predictor values at the single occasion. Only for this subcohort and for the new detected cancer cases is more detailed information gathered concerning the predictor over a long period.

3. An ordinary case-control study is carried out instead of a longitudinal cohort/register study. By a questionnaire or by measurements, data for the predictor is obtained. Contrary to the cohort/register study, the case-control study, based on a questionnaire, is sometimes not free from recall bias and from information and observation bias due to an absence of blinding.

There are, however, other reasons to recommend the case-control design; namely, that data can be gathered for plenty of factors, especially factors recently identified as of possible importance.

Until now, the confounding bias has been regarded as the main drawback in longitudinal cohort/register studies. The bias due to single-occasion data has been almost ignored. However, it appears to be common in this type of study, and the above approaches 1 and 2 can sometimes be used to eliminate or reduce the bias. It is also possible to estimate the bias through a cast-control study, because in such a study the (stability) correlation or agreement between period and point values can be estimated. In this way the historic longitudinal studies have a raison d'être in the end.

References

Blalock, H. M. (1961). *Causal inferences in non-experimental research.* Chapel Hill, NC: University of North Carolina Press.

Brivkalne, M. (1964). *The control study made in connection with the 1960 census of population.* Statistical Report B, No. 16. Stockholm: The National Central Bureau of Statistics.

Central Bureau of Statistics. (1965). Census of the population in 1960. XI. *Sample surveys: Families, income, internal migration and change of industry.* Stockholm.

Eklund, G., & Carstensen, J. (1986). Cancer incidence in Sweden 1959–1980: A geographic evaluation. In *Cancer incidence in Sweden 1983.* Stockholm: National Board of Health and Welfare.

International Labour Office. (1958). *International standard classification of occupations.* Geneva: International Labour Office.

Johansson, L. & Finnäs, F. (1983). *Fertility of Swedish women born 1927–1960.* Stockholm: Statistiska Centralbyrån.

Jungner, G., & Jungner, I. (1968). Chemical health screening. In C. L. E. H. Sharp & H. Keen (Eds.), *Presymptomatic detection and early diagnosis: A critical appraisal* (pp. 67–108). London: Pitman.

Kendall, M. G. (1948). *The advanced theory of statistics* (Vol. 2). London: Charles Griffin & Co. Ltd.

Lanctot, E. M. (1985). *Radon in the domestic environment and its relationship to cancer.* Stony Brook: State University of New York.

Last, J. M. (1983). *A dictionary of epidemiology.* Oxford: Oxford University Press.

Malker, H. & Weiner, J. (1984). The Cancer-Environment Registry 1961–1973: Examples of the use of register epidemiology in studies of the work environment. Arbete och hälsa, No. 9. Solna: National Board of Occupational Safety and Health. (Summary in English).

Muir, C. S., & Wagner, G. (1986). *Directory of on-going research in cancer epidemiology.* IARC Scientific Publ. No. 69, Lyon.

National Board of Health and Welfare. (1984). The Cancer Registry: Cancer incidence in Sweden 1961, 1962, 1963, . . . , 1984. Stockholm.

Östlin, P., Lindberg, G., & Thorslund, M. (1985). Yrke och ohälsa: En studie av sambandet mellan yrkeserfarenhet och hälsa. (Occupation and ill health. A study on the association between occupational experience and disease.) Report No. 4. Department of Social Medicine, University of Uppsala. (In Swedish with English summary).

Östlin, P., Lindberg, G., & Thorslund, M. (1985). Yrke och ohälsa: En studie av samband et mellan yrkeserfarenhet och sjukdom. (Occupation and ill-health: A study on the association between occupational experience and disease). Department of Social Medicine, University of Uppsala.

Olsson, H., & Brandt, L. (1982). Hur säkra är resultat erhållna via cancer-miljöregistret? *Läkartidningen, 79*(30–31), 2290.

Persson, I., Bergkvist, L., & Adami, H.-O. (1987). Reliability of women's histories of climacteric oestrogen treatment assessed by prescription forms. *International Journal of Epidemiology, 16*(1).

Socialstyrelsen redovisar 23. (1971). The Värmland Survey. Stockholm: Allmänna Förlaget.

Socialstyrelsen redovisar 11. (1979). Försöksverksamhet med upprepade allmänna hälsoundersökningar i Gävle 1971–72. Projekt X-71. Uppföljning av projekt X-69. Stockholm: Liber Distribution. (In Swedish).

Statistiska centralbyrån. (1979). Miljöstatistisk årsbok 1978. Arbetsmiljön. (Yearbook of environmental statistics 1978. Working environment). Stockholm: Statistiska centralbyrån. (In Swedish with English summary).

Stemmermann, G. N., Nomura, A. M. Hellbrun, L. K., Pollack, E. S., & Kagan, A. (1981). Serum cholesterol and colon cancer incidence in Hawaiian Japanese men. *Journal of the National Cancer Institute, 67,* 1179–1182.

Törnberg, S. A., Holm, L.-E., Carstensen, J. M., & Eklund, G. A. (1986). Risks of cancer of the colon and rectum in relation to serum cholesterol and beta-lipoprotein. *The New England Journal of Medicine, 315,* 1629–1633.

Törnberg, S. A., Holm, L.-E. Carstensen, J. M., & Eklund, G. A. (1987). Serum cholesterol and the risk of colorectal cancer. Letter to the editor. *The New England Journal of Medicine, 317,* 114.

Törnberg, S. A., Jakobsson, K. F. S., & Eklund, G. A. (1988). Stability and validity of a single serum cholesterol measurement in a prospective cohort study. Including a statistical appendix by G. Eklund. *International Journal of Epidemiology, 17,* 797–803.

Wertheimer, N., & Leeper, E., (1979). Electrical wiring configurations and childhood cancer. *American Journal of Epidemiology, 109,* 273–284.

Wicksell, L., Carstensen, J. M., Eklund, G., & Gustafsson, J.-Å. (1988). Lung cancer incidence among Swedish bakers and pastrycooks: Geographical variation. *Scandinavian Journal of Social Medicine, 16,* 183–186.

Wiklund, K., Einhorn, J., Wennström, G., & Rapaport, E. (1981). A Swedish cancer-environment register available for research. *Scandinavian Journal of Work, Environment and Health, 7,* 64–67.

Wiklund, K., & Holm, L.-E. (1986). Trends in cancer risk in 1961–1979 among Swedish agricultural workers. *Journal of National Cancer Institute* (JNCI), *56:* 505–508.

Williams, R. R., Sorlie, P. D., Feinleib, M., McNamara, P. M., Kannel, W. B., & Dawber, T. R. (1981). Cancer incidence by levels of cholesterol. *Journal of the American Medical Association, 245,* 247–252.

Zak, B., Dickenman, R. C., White, E. G., Burnett, H., & Cherney, P. J. (1954). Rapid estimation of free and total cholesterol. *American Journal of Clinical Pathology, 24,* 1307–1315.

4 Data in pediatric longitudinal research

ROLF ZETTERSTRÖM

Introduction

Human growth and development under normal and pathological conditions forms the basis of pediatrics. The various aspects of this field are numerous. Growth can be studied from the anthropometric view in which are included various parameters such as length during infancy and height during childhood, sitting height, body weight, head circumference, and skinfold thickness. For the understanding of the biology of growth it is also of importance to know about the growth of various tissues and organs such as brain, heart, liver, kidneys, thymus, and various endocrine organs. Human growth and development is influenced by genetic instruction and environmental factors. The basis of preventive health care in children is to promote optimal somatic and psychological development by beneficial factors and by preventing children from being subjected to adverse environmental factors such as infectious diseases, nutritional deficiences, deprivation, and psychosocial stress.

Anthropometric parameters can easily be measured continuously in prospective longitudinal studies. Information about changes in weight of different organs during growth can be obtained only by cross-sectional studies of material coming from autopsies, whereas volume changes of, for instance, the heart can be determined by X-ray examinations. Discussions of measurements concerning growth must consider whether the values have been obtained in longitudinal or cross-sectional studies.

The situation becomes more complicated in studies with the aim of elucidating the effect of beneficial or adverse factors on genetically predetermined somatic growth or physiological and psychological development. The effect of environmental factors operating in early life may not be possible to identify until adult age; and if it can be investigated only prospectively and longitudinally, a considerable part of the active lifetime of the scientist will pass before the results can be evaluated.

When studying child health and development in relation to the psychosocial and socioeconomic situation, as in, for example, the family, the following factors are of great importance:

1. The cohort being studied must be representative for the problem that will be studied.

2. The information about factors that are of importance for the hypothetical model

must be as accurate as possible. During long-term prospective longitudinal studies these factors may change considerably. Because the information about important psychosocial stress factors in the family, such as criminality, alcohol addiction, and psychiatric disease, which can be obtained by interviews, are extremely unreliable, other methods must be used to get accurate data when the study is started and during the follow-up.

3. Attrition must be kept as low as possible both at the start of the study and during the follow-up. Attrition is selective in most studies, particularly in those that attempt to investigate the effect of psychosocial factors in multiproblem families. When attrition is high there is a risk that the most interesting group is lost.

4. The methods for assessment must be accurate for the aim of the study. Because the methodology for the assessment of somatic, psychological, and social development is changing with scientific progress, the reliability of the methods being chosen must be well established.

5. Because of secular trends, reference values for anthropometric data, such as height, as well as physiological and psychological data may change during the concept of a long-term study.

Aspects of longitudinal studies in pediatric research will be exemplified by short summaries of some projects.

Growth and maturation

Growth and development is an extremely broad subject that can be looked upon in various ways. It is the result of various biological processes and can be discussed in terms of size, maturity, and time. The process starts at conception and ends when the adult state has been attained.

When we speak about adult state, we generally mean that the individual has reached adult stature and is sexually mature. Adult height is attained when the metaphyses in the skeletal bones are closed, a process that occurs because of stimulation by estrogen in women and testosterone in males. The peak excretion of these sexual hormones occurs when the state of sexual maturity is being reached. Even if maturity has then come accordingly to an end, this does not mean that the individual has reached a steady state from the physiological point of view. The function of various organs may change continuously even if the growth in height has stopped, although the rate of change may be different.

The most commonly used method of studying maturity prospectively and longitudinally is to follow skeletal maturation, eruption of deciduous and permanent teeth, and somatic pubertal development.

In addition to these parameters of maturation, there are numerous physiological and psychological parameters that change during human growth and development. Some of them can easily be measured without causing too much discomfort for the child and can thus be followed prospectively, but others can only be measured in connection with diagnostic procedures that are clinically motivated. In connection with chronic medication, developmental changes in the kinetics of drugs can be longitudinally studied.

Age and longitudinal studies

Chronological age

Chronological age, meaning age from birth, is not always accurate when studying growth and development, particularly in infants. Anthropometric data and physiological development may vary to a great extent in newborn infants. To mention extremes, a newborn preterm infant can be born with a very low birth weight after a gestation of only 25 weeks, or a newborn can be postmature with a gestational age of up to 45 weeks. The range of the birth weights can be from 500 g (in very low birth weight preterm babies) up to about 6 kg. The mean weight of Swedish infants born at term is 3,700 g for boys and 3,500 g for girls and is higher than in most other countries. Under certain conditions – for example, if the mother has toxemia during pregnancy – the weight of the newborn infant may be much lower than expected according to gestational age. In such instances we use the term *small for gestational age* in contrast to when the infant has a weight appropriate for gestational age. Under some conditions, as in offspring of diabetic mothers, birth weight may exceed the expected one. In such instances we speak about *large for gestational age* infants. Since the rate of growth and development is highest during fetal life, consideration must be given to the gestational age of each individual infant. In preterm infants it may be necessary to use *conceptional age* (or postmenstrual) instead of chronological age during infancy and early childhood when considering growth and development.

For every individual, predetermined growth pattern is set by genetic factors operating from conception. This pattern may be modified by various environmental factors that may be operating prenatally as well as postnatally. Birth is an episode in a continuous biologic process that has started with conception. The fact that the changes are dramatic during birth and the immediate adaptation to extrauterine life, and that environmental factors such as obstetric complications are of great influence during this period does not influence this basic concept.

Longitudinal studies of anthropometric, physiological, and psychological parameters during human growth and development have been started at various ages, depending upon the project or the availability of material. In some studies, the first year or years of life have been considered to be rather uninteresting, and the studies may have been started after the age of one year. Other studies may have begun when the children are in kindergarten or primary school. When the topic has been pubertal growth, the study may have begun when the subjects are 9 to 10 years old.

During the last decades it has become quite obvious that the most dramatic changes, not only of growth but also of physiological and psychological parameters, occur during infancy and that longitudinal studies should be started as soon as possible after birth to obtain accurate information. This fact became obvious in developmental physiology about two decades ago and in developmental psychology about 10 years ago. In fact, in recent years enormous progress has been made in developmental psychology during infancy. Our concepts about the ontogeny of the brain have changed completely due to the progress in transdisciplinary research involving neurobiology and psychology. Our previous rather static concept regarding the organization and funciton of the central nervous system has changed because of new knowledge about the plasticity of the brain during early life.

The recent discoveries within the fields of early infant neurology and behavior point to the importance of starting longitudinal studies of growth and development as early as feasible. Subjects entering longitudinal studies should be recruited as soon as possible, in some instances even during early gestation.

Because the survival rate of infants born after only two trimesters has improved markedly during the last decade, it has become possible to make observations from which we can deduce aspects on growth and development during the last trimester of fetal life. Previous anthropometric data during fetal growth were based on measurements on aborted fetuses or relatively mature preterm babies. Because of the rapid development of ultrasound technique it has now become possible to make longitudinal anthropometric measurements during fetal life. Accurate information can be obtained, not only of the bitemporal diameter of the head and crown–rump length, but also of the size and shape of various organs.

Because of the recent tremendous improvement of our abilities to obtain correct information about growth and development during fetal life, the collection of much longitudinal data can be started already before birth.

Aspects of growth and development under normal conditions

Physical growth

Data on physical growth based on longitudinal studies have been obtained only recently. Earlier growth charts are mainly based on cross-sectional studies in which the material may have been selected. For instance, in a Swedish study by Broman, Dalhberg, and Lichtenstein (1942) in the 1930s a group of kindergarten children represented preschool children, 7–10-year-old children comprised a primary school group, and teenagers were represented by children from a high school.

In 1955 a longitudinal growth study including anthropometry and development was started in Stockholm by Karlberg and co-workers (Karlberg et al., 1968; Klackenberg, 1971; Karlberg, Taranger, Engström, Lichtenstein, & Svennberg-Redegren, 1976; Karlberg, Engström, & Karlberg 1981). This study was coordinated with similar studies in Brussels, London, Paris, and Zürich by the International Children's Center in Paris. Antenatally, 183 children were recruited by asking the participation of every fourth pregnant woman at the antenatal clinic in the community in which the study was conducted. Another 29 children constituted a pilot group and were selected antenatally or neonatally. All the 212 children (122 males and 90 females) were born between 1955 and March 1958. The representativeness of the sample was thoroughly discussed. At the time of birth, the sample was considered to be representative for an urban Swedish society with 17% of the families belonging to the upper class, 37% to the middle class, and 46% to the lowest social class. Analyses of various perinatal factors showed good agreement with a nationwide investigation of all live-born newborn infants performed in 1956. The follow-up to an age of 16 years was 85% (179 children). Out of the 33 children leaving the study, three-fourths of them did so because of lack of interest. Subsequent analyses demonstrated that some children were excluded for medical reasons, for example, those having an aberrant growth pattern.

To elucidate the real growth pattern it is, of course, important that the examinations are performed at appropriate ages and intervals. In this study the children were examined at 1 month, 3 months, 6 months, 9 months, 12 months, 18 months, 2 years, and subsequently once a year. Since velocity of growth is highest during infancy, the infants were examined at short intervals during this period. The examination comprised not only somatic but also psychological and social investigations. In order to get accurate information regarding the growth spurt in puberty, standing and sitting height and body weight were measured every third month from the age of 10 years up to the end of puberty.

In order to get accurate data, the body measurements were made according to a standardized program recommended by the International Children's Center in Paris. The measurements included body weight, length, and crown–rump length during infancy, standing and sitting height with a stretching upward, circumferences of head, chest, upper arm, and calf, the size of the anterior fontanel, and the layer of subcutaneous tissue assessed by measuring a skinfold over biceps and triceps, subscapulary and suprailiacally. Most of the measurements were made in the morning between 8 and 10 a.m. and by only two examiners.

After analyzing the data, charts for Swedish boys and girls have been prepared on a logarithmic scale. Mathematically, the charts have been based on conceptional age, which means that a full-term infant has a gestational age of 38 weeks at birth. Since velocity of growth will decrease gradually after birth, a logarithmic age concept will give a biological description of growth.

Although the material in the study of Karlberg and co-workers is limited, the results have been of great clinical importance because of the accuracy by which the measurements have been performed and because of the representativeness of the material. By use of the data, accurate figures for increment, that is, growth velocity or growth in centimeters per year, can be given. They are also of great importance for the identification of infants and children who have been subjected to abuse or neglect, because such conditions very often are associated with "failure to thrive."

The growth charts can also be used as reference data in longitudinal studies of selected groups of infants and children; for example, those belonging to special ethnic groups, to special socioeconomic or psychosocial family groups, or in children with particular diseases or handicaps.

From the results of studies of the normal growth pattern Karlberg, Engström, Karlberg, and Fryer (1987) have elucidated the regulation of three different phases of growth. The first, which starts after conception and lasts up to an age of 12–18 months, is stimulated by insulin; the second, which lasts to puberty, is mainly stimulated by human growth hormone; and the last, that is, the growth spurt in puberty, is regulated by the sex hormones.

Longitudinal studies of maturation and other physiological parameters

The possibilities of performing such longitudinal studies depend upon whether or not they are ethically acceptable and also upon the cooperation of the family. If each individual child can be studied only once because of ethical reasons, only cross-sectional studies can be performed.

Numerous studies on different physiological parameters during the growth of healthy children have been performed during the last 50 years. Some examples will be mentioned.

Skeletal maturity has been measured by means of X-ray investigations of different bones. The numbers of bone centers have been assessed by X-ray examination of one or several parts of the skeleton, for example, the wrist. Another method of following skeletal maturity has been to follow the structure of certain joints such as the knee joint. During recent years methods have also been developed to make it possible to follow the density of mineralization in the shaft of a long bone. Because of the concern we now have about the risk of exposing children to unnecessary doses of X-ray, such longitudinal studies can no longer be performed.

For the differentiation between normal and abnormal hematological findings, information about changes of various hematological parameters such as hemoglobin concentration, packed erythrocyte volume, and red and white cell counts during infancy and childhood must be known. If blood samples are taken at relatively long intervals, a longitudinal study may be acceptable. On the other hand, if repeated samples must be taken with short intervals, which is the case during the first month after birth when the hemoglobin concentration declines rapidly, cross-sectional or a combination of cross-sectional and longitudinal studies may be necessary. Longitudinal studies performed by a technique that is noninvasive and not associated with obvious discomfort are, of course, more easily performed than other studies. Blood pressure is easy to perform without negative consequences. Thus, it is surprising that we have not had any accurate longitudinal studies of this very important physiological parameter until very recently.

Developmental neurology and psychology in longitudinal studies

As already mentioned, rapid progress has been made in recent years in the field of developmental psychology during infancy.

Our understanding of the development of speech has improved considerably during recent years. Until a few years ago, linguists interested in speech in early childhood ignored prespeech vocalization. In fact, less than 10 years ago authorities in the field of the development of speech refused to see any connection between so-called babbling and early speech. The gradual continuous development that different physiological parameters undergo and that can proceed at different rates has only recently been generally recognized in developmental psychology. The lack of differentiated longitudinal studies from early infancy has made it difficult to understand that the ability to perform, like the ability to walk, appears rather suddenly, although the neurobiological background for such a performance develops continuously.

A full-term newborn infant can only cry, but there are different kinds of crying in newborn infants. We can differentiate between at least four different types of crying, such as the birth cry, hunger cry, cry of pain, and the fourth type, which may be called the pleasure cry (Lind, Vuorenkoski, Forsberg, Partanen, & Wasz-Höckert, 1970; Michelsson, 1986). Prespeech vocalization has been studied by Holmgren, Lindblom, Aurelius, Jalling, and Zetterström (1986). At a postconceptional age of 44 weeks, when infants start with glottal articulation, the sounds they produce are usually named cooing. From about 50 weeks' postconceptional age, infants start with supraglottal articulation. The frequency of glottal articulation declines gradually from this time. At a postconceptional age of 70 weeks, that is, 5½ months after birth in term infants, about half of the utterances are glottal and the rest supraglottal. The typical babbling is produced by means of supraglottal articulation. At an age of 8 months the infant starts to change syllables in the babbling. In the ordinary babbling, that is, canonic babbling, the same syllables are repeated with a frequency of three per second. The first words are formed when babbling of the type ma-ma-ma-ma starts to mean the word *Mama*, which is when the infant has obtained a cognitive memory. From longitudinal studies of the development of prespeech vocalization it becomes quite obvious that this is a continuous process from cooing to babbling.

The milestones in prespeech vocalization are associated with the involvement of successively higher structures in the brain (Ploog, 1979). Crying is controlled by ponto-mesencephalic structures, cooing and syllabic babbling by the cingulate area, and imitation of speech by neocortical areas.

To the parents it is quite obvious that their baby communicates by the way of cooing. According to them, infants start to answer by cooing at a postconceptional age of 45½ weeks. The parents can also describe how cooing changes with age and when the infants start to play with the voice. On the other hand, parents are rather uncertain about the time when canonic babbling starts.

The best information about the development of prespeech vocalization, and thus also of speech, may be obtained by longitudinal studies from the time of birth by means of repeated interviews of the parents and by phonetic and acoustic analyses of recorded sounds. The response of the infant to speech or other ways of communication that may be motoric and/or vocal also has to be considered. For longitudinal studies of this type, advanced cooperation with the parents is necessary.

Longitudinal studies in pathological conditions

Such studies may be performed without any difficulties by physicians who are in charge of the patients. The investigations are then part of the clinical follow-up. Longitudinal studies with the primary aim of benefiting the patients may also give results of physiological, pharmacological, or psychological implications.

Longitudinal studies of children with risk of developing somatic disease or mental and psychosocial illness

The main goal of curative and preventive pediatric care is to prevent somatic and mental illness as well as social maladjustment due to health problems. In child health centers, infants and children are regularly checked, and the mothers are informed about how to prevent various diseases. Infectious diseases are prevented by immunization programs. Information is also given about the prevention of accidents and behavioral disorders.

To improve the efficiency of child health centers, much work has been done to develop methods that will make it possible to identify children who are at risk for becoming psychosocially maladjusted or for having accidents or being subjected to child abuse and neglect. The reliability of different predictors in identifying risk families has been studied at many centers by means of long-term longitudinal studies, many of which have begun in the maternity hospital. Although much progress has been made in this field, sensitivity and specificity are still rather low for the methods that have been developed for the identification of infants who are at risk of being subjected to child abuse and neglect.

From retrospective studies it is well documented that children of alcoholic parents live under severe conditions and that they run a great risk of being subjected to child abuse, neglect, and sexual molestation. In a nationwide Swedish study from the period 1970–1971 (National Board of Health and Welfare, 1975), in which all cases of child abuse and neglect reported to the social welfare authorities were included, it was found that out of a total number of 1,206 cases the father was an alcoholic in 53% and the mother in 34% of them. The serious consequences of alcohol abuse among the parents have been confirmed in a more recent study from North America by Korcok (1981). About 60% of the children of alcoholic parents had been subjected to severe physical maltreatment, and about 30% of the girls had been the victims of incest.

Nylander (1960) performed a study in 1960 of Stockholm children in the 4–12-

year age group where the father, but not the mother, was an alcoholic. The survey showed that both boys and girls in these families very often had various nervous symptoms. The children also had difficulty in getting through school. According to the teachers, 75% of the boys in the prepuberty age group could be regarded as problem children. They were unable to follow the curriculum, although they were of normal intelligence. The children studied by Nylander were followed to adult age (to 26–32 years of age) by Rydelius (1981), who noted that many of them had, when they reached adulthood, both medical and social handicaps with different reaction patterns for boys and girls. Statistically confirmed differences were found between proband boys and the control boys with regard to social adjustment in later years. The behavior of the proband boys was found to be characterized by aggressiveness and in adult age by serious adjustment problems with high rates of criminality and alcohol abuse. In contrast, the proband girls did not differ from the controls with regard to social adjustment. The only difference between proband girls and their controls was more frequent visits to gynecologists. In retrospective and semi-prospective studies it has thus been well established that parents with addictions in their history may have children who deviate with regard to their mental development and behavior, and that these children to a high frequency are subjected to abuse and neglect. A similar effect on psychological development and behavior may occur in families with parental mental disease (Rutter & Quinton, 1984) or criminality (Johansson, 1981).

With the aim of investigating the relation between mental disease, addictions, and criminality in addition to a high life stress score in the parents and early deviations in the child's health, development, and behavior, a longitudinal prospective study was started in a new Stockholm suburb in 1980 (Nylander & Zetterström, 1983). The primary material included all the pregnant women who during the period between September 1, 1980 and August 31, 1981 made their first visit to the welfare center. Out of a total number of 640 women, 532 (83%) were interviewed. The primary drop out constituted a negative selection from the social viewpoint. Information was collected at the maternity health center from consecutive structured interviews on the basis of a questionnaire. A general assessment of the psychosocial situation of the family was also made. Based on the results of the interviews, a life stress score was calculated, as is shown in Figure 4.1 In addition to the information obtained at the interviews and from the general assessment of the families, information was collected from hospital records, social welfare records, and police records. The poor relation between various methods of assessing the psychosocial situation of the families by means of soft data is demonstrated in Figure 4.2. Only eight families were classified as high-risk families by all three methods. Only two of these families had been identified as risk families during the course of routine care in the maternity hospitals.

A compilation of all information showed that 11.8% of the fathers and 3.4% of the mothers were known to be alcohol addicts (Table 4.1). However, only a few of the mothers were more generally known to be addicts, and only a few of them were

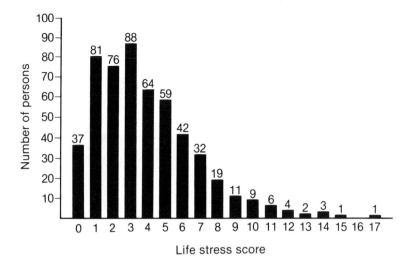

Life stress score

Figure 4.1. Distribution of life stress points among the pregnant women interviewed (Nylander & Zetterström, 1983). The average number of points for the entire material was 3.9. Fifty-six out of 532 women (10.5%) had a life stress score of >7 points, which was considered to indicate psychosocial stress.

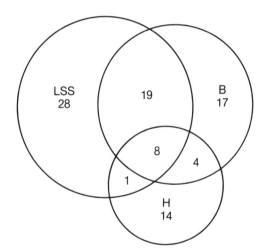

Figure 4.2. Relation between the results of three different soft data methods of predicting psychosocial stress during infancy and childhood (Nylander & Zetterström, 1983). The total material consists of 532 women who were interviewed and followed at the maternity health center.

LSS circle: 56 women with a life stress score of >7 points.

B circle: 48 women considered to have insufficient behavior when examined at the maternity health center.

H circle: 27 families in which the home situation was considered unsatisfactory when visited by a child health center nurse after the mother and child had been discharged from the maternity hospital.

Table 4.1. *Information from various sources concerning addiction to alcohol in the family.*

Source	Cohabiting men ($n = 483$)	Interviewed women ($n = 532$)
Interview	13	6
Hospital records	6	4
Police records	18	2
Social welfare records	31	13
Number of alcohol addicts	57	18

Source: Nylander and Zetterström (1983).

Table 4.2. *Information from various sources concerning criminality in the family.*

Source	Cohabiting men ($n = 483$)	Interviewed women ($n = 532$)
Interview	3	0
Hospital records	0	0
Police records	61	17
Social welfare records	14	6
Number of criminal records	69	21

Source: Nylander and Zetterström (1983).

known with certainty to have been alcoholics during pregnancy. At the interviews, 6 mothers out of 18 admitted that they had problems with alcohol. Only three of the women had been treated in a clinic for alcoholism, and they showed serious changes indicative of chronic alcoholism. Only 13 out 57 alcoholic fathers were identified at the interviews with the mothers. The information regarding criminality, which was obtained at the interview and as is shown in Table 4.2, was as inaccurate as that regarding alcohol addiction. In a prospective study of the offspring of alcohol-addicted mothers (Nylander, Rydelius, Nordberg, Aurelius, & Zetterström, 1988), the consequences for the child were found to differ from those reported from studies of proband samples or when the material is selected due to inaccurate background factors (Zetterström & Nylander, 1985).

Conclusions

In a longitudinal study of a cohort with the aim of identifying predictors of risk situations for the children in the family, it is extremely important to have accurate information about the occurrence of such adverse factors as addiction to alcohol and drugs, criminality, and severe psychiatric disease.

When the results of the interviews in the study of Nylander and Zetterström

(1983) were compared with the data from official records, there were obvious differences indicating that the answers to certain questions were not reliable. Questions about emotionally neutral matters and socially accepted behavior such as physical diseases, working conditions, housing, and financial situation were answered fully and truthfully, whereas those related to "delicate matters," such as gynecological and mental illnesses, social welfare assistance, addictions, and criminality often were not.

The results of our study have shown that various sources about the family situation complement each other. Information concerning diseases was obtained from interviews and from both hospital and social welfare records. Addiction to alcohol and drugs was noted mainly from hospital, police, and social welfare records, whereas the interviews did not give reliable information. Criminality was noted mainly in the police and social welfare records. However, the interviews also yielded useful information as to how members of the individual families felt about disease, addiction, and criminality, and as to the consequences of these problems.

The interview and record examination methods complement each other. Together they give a many-sided and detailed picture of the home situation, although each method in itself includes relatively serious sources of error.

When the longitudinal study was started, 17% of those invited refused to enter. From information obtained in registers it was obvious that the families who did not participate had the highest number of adverse factors.

References

Broman, B., Dahlberg, G., & Lichtenstein, A. (1942). Height and weight during growth. *Acta Paediatrica Scandinavica, 30,* 1.

Holmgren, K., Lindblom, B., Aurelius, G., Jalling, B., & Zetterström, R. (1986). On the phonetics of infant vocalization. In B. Lindblom & R. Zetterström (Eds.), *Precursors of early speech* (Wenner-Gren International Symposium Series, Vol. 44, pp. 51–63). New York: Stockton Press.

Johansson, E. (1981). Recidivistic criminals and their families. *Scandinavian Journal of Social Medicine,* Suppl. 27.

Karlberg, J., Engström, I., Karlberg, P., & Fryer, J. G. (1987). Analysis of linear growth using a mathematical model. I. From birth to three years. *Acta Paediatrica Scandinavica, 76,* 478–488.

Karlberg, P., Engström, I., & Karlberg, J. (1981). A method for evaluation of growth. In M. Ritzén, A. Aperia, K. Hall, A. Larsson, A. Zetterberg, & R. Zetterström (Eds.), *The biology of normal human growth* (pp. 321–325). New York: Raven Press.

Karlberg, P., Klackenberg, G., Engström, I., Klackenberg-Larsson, I., Lichtenstein, H., Stensson, J., & Svennberg, I. (1968). The development of children in a Swedish urban community: A prospective longitudinal study. I–VI. *Acta Paediatrica Scandinavica,* Suppl. *187,* 9–121.

Karlberg, P., Taranger, J., Engström, I., Lichtenstein, H., & Svennberg-Redegren, I. (1976). The somatic development of children in a Swedish urban community: A prospective longitudinal study. *Acta Paediatrica Scandinavica,* Suppl. *258,* 5–147.

Klackenberg, G. (1971). A prospective longitudinal study of children: Data on psychic health and development up to 8 years of age. *Acta Paediatrica Scandinavica,* Suppl. 224.

Korcok, M., (1981). Many children overcome difficulties: Survey shows old stereotypes are off base. *Focus on Alcohol and Drug Issues, 4,* 20–24.

Lind, J., Vuorenkoski, V., Forsberg, G., Partanen, T. J., & Wasz-Höckert, O. (1970). Spectrographic analysis of vocal response to pain stimuli in infants with Down's syndrome. *Developmental Medicine and Child Neurology, 12,* 478–486.

Michelsson, K. (1986). Cry analysis in clinical neonatal diagnosis. In. B. Lindblom & R. Zetterström (Eds.), *Precursors of early speech* (Wenner-Gren International Symposium Series, Vol. 44, (pp. 67–77). New York: Stockton Press.

National Board of Health and Welfare, in collaboration with Allmänna Barnbördshuset. (1975). *Abused children in Sweden: A study of child abuse and neglect in relation to the home situation.* Karlshamn: Nya Lagerblads Printing.

Nylander, I. (1960). Children of alcoholic fathers. *Acta Paediatrica Scandinavica,* Suppl. *121,* 1–134.

Nylander, I., Rydelius, P. A., Nordberg, L., Aurelius, G., & Zetterström, R. (1989). Infant health and development in relation to the family situation: A review of a longitudinal prospective study in a new Stockholm suburb. *Acta Paediatrica Scandinavica, 78,* 1–10.

Nylander, I., & Zetterström, R. (1983). Home environment of children in a new Stockholm suburb: A prospective longitudinal study. *Acta Paediatrica Scandinavica,* Suppl. *310,* 1–40.

Ploog, D. (1979). Phonation, emotion, cognition with reference to the brain mechanisms involved. In *Brain and Mind,* Ciba Foundation Series 69.

Rutter, M., & Quinton, D. (1984). Parental psychiatric disorders: Effects on children. *Psychological Medicine, 14,* 853–880.

Rydelius, P.-A. (1981). Children of alcoholic fathers: Their social adjustment and their health status over 20 years. *Acta Paediatrica Scandinavica,* Suppl. *286,* 1–89.

Zetterström, R., & Nylander, I. (1985). Children in families with alcohol abuse. In U. Rydberg et al. (Eds.), *Alcohol and the developing brain* (pp. 153–159). New York: Raven Press.

5   Alcohol data in longitudinal research

AMBROS UCHTENHAGEN

Introduction

Among the critical issues dealt with in recent scientific literature, there are two questions of outstanding importance for longitudinal studies in the field of alcohol abuse: (1) What are the relevant risk factors for behavioral and health problems traditionally connected with alcohol abuse and what is the evidence concerning these factors? and (2) How valid are alcohol data collected by self-reported estimates? In fact, the results of numerous studies that leave these basic questions unconsidered may be inconclusive. It may be helpful, then, to review how the situation has been dealt with and where we stand at present. In this context, I wish to focus on the nature and quality of alcohol data according to the purpose of the study: on measurement of alcohol consumption, on reliability and validity of self-report measures, on sampling methods, on reexamination timing, and on risk constellations.

Research including data on alcohol consumption is not per se research on alcoholism, because epidemiological and clinical studies dealing with alcoholism must start from a concept of alcoholism that goes beyond the measurement of consumption data. Concepts of alcoholism operate on the level of aggregated data and include hypotheses regarding the consequences of alcohol consumption. The dependence syndrome is defined not only by the quantity and frequency of drinking alcoholic beverages; other data are also needed in order to determine quantity and patterns of alcohol consumption in a given population, as compared with determining prevalence and incidence figures for alcohol dependence in a given population. Especially in longitudinal studies, traditional binary assessment models (alcoholics/nonalcoholics) are inadequate for measuring detailed change over time; therefore, it has been repeatedly suggested that these models be replaced by alternative multivariant approaches (Pattison & Kaufman, 1982; Dean, 1985). Use of multivariant assessment models is more appropriate in order to avoid the pitfalls of a unitary concept of alcoholism; in fact, researchers like Jacobson (1976) and Edwards (1977) have already advocated concepts of several "alcoholisms." It has become obvious not to base alcoholism research on clinical diagnosis but on behavioral data, including consumption data. It is also recommended that studies on alcoholics include an adequate measurement of alcohol consumption in order to determine changes in intake patterns and quantities over time. Therefore, I prefer not to deal with various concepts of alcoholism and alcohol dependence but to restrict the review to problems associated with assessing alcohol consumption.

The nature and quality of alcohol data with respect to the purpose of the study

Longitudinal studies in the alcohol field may aim at various purposes with different impacts on methodological issues. We deal here with the following:

1. Consequences of alcohol consumption (health, psychological, social, societal consequences). In these studies, the measurement of quantity, consumption patterns, and type of beverage is a crucial element as well as the measurement of other types of behavior (nutrition, smoking, exposure to environmental hazards, etc.). Because most consequences become observable after a year-long time lag only, retrospective studies risk being invalidated by the difficulties in measuring alcohol consumption based on subjective recollection; prospective cohort studies with adequate control groups are preferred.

2. Prospective evaluation of preventive activities or therapeutic interventions. Alcohol data are used here as dependent variables, on the basis of a pre/postintervention comparison. The nature of alcohol data and the required accuracy depend upon the goals of intervention (e.g., total abstinence, abstinence from specific beverages, controlled frequency/quantity of intake, etc.).

3. Identification of risk factors and populations at risk. We mention studies on the identification of populations at risk for developing alcohol-related problems (occupations at risk, children of alcoholics, marginal groups with increased propensity for substance abuse, etc.), on the identification of risky consumption patterns and risk constellations, and on the identification of risk phases in the biography of various groups (e.g., switching from controlled drinking to harmful drinking, discontinuity of drinking behavior over time, transition periods in the life cycle, etc.). Again, the required nature and accuracy of alcohol data will vary with the aims of the study in question.

Measuring alcohol consumption

Various approaches have been used, and some debate has taken place on topics such as advantages and disadvantages of assessing quality versus quantity of alcohol intake, on the use of indicators (e.g., quantity/frequency indicators, average volume/ maximum per occasion indicators). It may be helpful to discuss which approach should be used for what research purposes. The following is partly based on the excellent review by Greenfield (1986).

Predicting organic damage

According to Cowan, Massey, and Greenfield (1985), a high volume of alcohol intake rather than a high maximum per occasion is discriminated by the results of 35 blood test variables indicating dysfunction in various organ systems. Lelbach (1974) claims that lifetime volume of alcohol intake is most predictive for an increased risk of liver cirrhosis.

Estimating lifetime volume is a method with comparatively little accuracy and will lead to false negative rather than false positive results. A significant correlation of lifetime volume with organic damage may be admissible for interpretation. Still, a cautionary remark is due, especially with respect to retrospective estimation of intake volume. As Simpura and Poikolainen (1983) have demonstrated, retrospective alcohol consumption estimates are biased by actual consumption patterns that are used as a frame of reference and lead eventually to over- or underestimation of the past. We suspect estimates to be less accurate where intake volume varies over the years. This is rather the rule than the exception in typical transition periods, for example, adolescence and young adulthood.

Evidence from studies of Magnussson and Stattin (1982), Andersson and Magnusson (1988), and Temple and Fillmore (1986) demonstrates little continuity in drinking behavior across time from adolescence to adulthood. Also, factors that correlate with alcohol intake do not remain the same during this transition period. Whereas independent variables such as the impact of negative peers, family social class, family support, and high school success were appropriate to predict successfully alcohol involvement at age 18, these factors showed little utility in predicting alcohol involvement at age 31 (Temple & Fillmore, 1986; Windle, 1988 however questions their data interpretation). Jessor (1986) in his longitudinal study found within a seven-year period from adolescence to young adulthood a considerable turnover in drinker status. About 50% of the males who were problem drinkers as adolescents are no longer problem drinkers as young adults; for females the discontinuity is even greater, and the comparable figure is about 75%. This observed discontinuity over time is neither random nor adventitious, but systematic and predictable to a significant degree. Prediction of problem drinking rests on an assessment of antecedent psychosocial proneness to problem behavior in adolescence.

One of the largest surveys, the national U.S. study "Monitoring the Future," was designed to assess drug use in high school seniors, with follow-up surveys after graduation (O'Malley, Bachman, & Johnston, 1983). According to their findings, there is a definite underreporting for drug use including alcohol use during the last 12 months when compared with use in the last 30 days. This systematic underreporting of annual frequency relative to monthly frequency confirms that self-reported consumption data for the past are biased. However, there is a high stability over time in the data concerning use versus nonuse of substances, especially with respect to alcohol, cigarette, and marijuana (annual and 30-day measures). The authors conclude that prevalence estimates may be much less subject to bias than frequency estimates in this age group.

Less attention has been devoted to other transition periods, particularly to the alcoholism and alcohol-related problems of the elderly (Douglass, 1984). Research, if any, concentrates on actual drinking status, mostly separating daily drinkers, occasional drinkers, and abstainers; economic and situational factors are of greater interest than former drinking history and eventual changes in drinking patterns and frequencies (Douglass, Schuster, & McClelland, 1988). One may reasonably presume, however, that assessing lifetime volume of alcohol intake is becoming increasingly difficult and biased with age, with age-related difficulties for adequate recollection, and with alcoholism-related organic brain damage. As abstinence rates increase with age, this may also contribute to underreporting of past alcohol intake.

These findings make it difficult to use lifetime volume estimates, especially for transition periods, and especially for research purposes, which require a higher accuracy of alcohol data. Still open for further investigation is to what extent time concepts and time orientation as found in alcoholics and social drinkers have an impact on retrospective self-reported consumption data (Hulbert & Lens, 1988).

Predicting behavior problems

Patterns of consumption rather than overall volume may be critical here (e.g., when dealing with driving while intoxicated, vandalism). Two main reasons may be cited. First, intoxication, with concomitant impairment of cognitive functions and emotional control is a relevant factor in itself that lowers the threshold for undesirable behavior, including risk-taking behavior followed by accidents (Mäkelä, 1978). Second, circumstantially determined patterns have to be considered here, such as furtive drinking at night in automobiles by adolescents or excessive weekend drinking after dry periods of intensive work (Rabow & Neuman, 1984; Argeriou, 1978). Qualitative factors of availability are also discussed, with particular emphasis on food stores, which account for a major proportion of purchases (Neuman & Rabow, 1986).

Data from a 1984 U.S. national survey indicate higher levels of behavioral problems in the categories of belligerence, accidents, and trouble with the police in the historically drier regions of the southern and mountain states. This is seen in the context of unresolved tensions in the drier regions between relatively high (per drinker) consumption and relatively conservative drinking attitudes (Hilton, 1988).

In the joint Scandinavian Drinking Survey (Hauge & Irgens-Jensen, 1984), the negative consequences at the national level did not reflect well the per capita average consumption; the frequency of intoxication was a better indicator of problem levels across the countries than was volume. One may ask, of course, to what extent such data reflect cultural differences in connotations of intoxication. Knupfer (1984) pointed out this difficulty and compared several "frequency of intoxication" and "quantity per occasion" indicators in relation to prevalence of drinking problems, using data drawn from nine U.S. population samples. She concluded that the best index for risk of behavioral problems seems to be eight or more drinks once a week or more; the best for inclusiveness seems to be a combined index with a longer time period, once a month or more. This method excludes differential interpretation of intoxication, but at the same time it meets the other difficulty of interindividual differences of tolerance for identical amounts of alcohol intake. Mitigation of behavior through tolerance is another issue to be looked at more closely.

The Scottish Study by Kreitman and Duffy (1982) contributes to the methodological question of how to describe drinking patterns. Examining two populations, company directors/executives and brewery shop-floor workers, Kreitman and Duffy used a one-week retrospective diary method instead of the usual quantity/frequency measures considered to be inadequate and inexact descriptors. Also, they distinguished five groups of consequences (general health, alcohol dependence syndrome, marital and family problems, work environment, and public order), on the hypothesis that volume consumed or drinking style relates to these problem areas in a differential way. Logistic linear analysis predicting probabilities of problems in each domain, based on volume plus each pattern variable in turn, allowed identification of the most relevant drinking style variables: maximum amount consumed on a drinking day and speed of drinking. Once the pattern variable was fitted, volume added nothing significant in many instances.

Problems associated with acute intoxication are potentiated or mitigated by set (expectancies specific to the beverage type) and setting (e.g., situation, solitary vs. collective drinking). Although such factors are relevant for subjective experiences independent of the amount consumed (Sher, 1985), eventual effects of these factors on behavior are more difficult to demonstrate. The relative impact of, for example, drinking experience, susceptibility to peers, tolerance, "cushions" in the social and physical environment on the consequences of alcohol consumption needs to be investigated (Greenfield, 1986).

In addition, the period used for assessing alcohol consumption may be too short (not representative for including drinking episodes with long dry intervals) or too long (for reasons such as inaccurate recollection and inadequacy of characterizing the present status). Serious error is expected where the period assessed is not a multiple of at least the dominant wavelength of the cycle in the periodicity of respondents (Argeriou, 1978). A useful combination of a one-month period plus the previous week's drinking quantities by day is recommended, a compromise used in recent surveys conducted by the Alcohol Research Group at Berkeley (Room, 1985).

The widely used quantity/frequency measures are considered to guarantee good comparability of results, but they present serious drawbacks. The original concept of Straus and Bacon (1953) totaled quantity and frequency in one index only, thus making rare excessive drinking equivalent to frequent moderate drinking. Later types of Q-F measures, which ask for typical amounts or usual quantity, result in biased estimates and risk missing changes in drinking behavior. Asking for actual rather than typical reports is a way out recommended, for example, by Armor and Polich (1982).

Efforts to develop useful typologies have been made by Cahalan and Cisin (1968) and Cahalan, Cisin, and Crossley (1969), who proposed the volume-variability method. Its applicability, however, is limited by severe problems of low cell frequency. Greenfield (1986); Greenfield, Karzmark, Haymond, Wyatt, and Gunns

(1980); and Greenfield and Duncan (1985) have developed a volume maximum index, used in a two-year longitudinal study on 1,000 students initially enrolled in a large university in the northwestern United States. They recommend a sliding threshold with variable cut-points, resulting in subgroups of adequate size for analysis. Construct validity was demonstrated and a partial replication performed (Gwartney-Gibbs, 1985).

In conclusion, Greenfield (1986) considers the distinction of overall volume and episodic amount in order to reveal the respective contribution to consequences as a major research issue for the future. For individuals as well as subpopulations, volume alone cannot be a sufficient descriptor of alcohol consumption for establishing risk factors. Volume should be complemented by quantitative measures of drinking style. Furthermore, continuous variables are better than categorical measures because they can be taken as dependent or independent variables in multivariate modeling.

Reliability and validity of self-report measures

Surveys on alcohol use rely mostly on self-reported consumption data. This is true for surveys on population samples, for household surveys, and for surveys on selected populations. In clinical studies the self-reported data are to a certain extent combined with data from collateral informants, earlier documents, direct observations, and so forth. The reliability and validity of self-report measures are therefore crucial and need to be looked at more closely. This is all the more indicated because consumption according to sales figures and estimated consumption from self-reports show a ratio of 2:1.

Various approaches have been used in this regard. Hubbard, Eckerman, and Rachal (1976) distinguish external (or empirical) validity, which refers to the extent to which the self-report data accord with other indicators of behavior; construct validity, which refers to other measures in theoretically predicted ways; and internal validity, which refers to how internally consistent responses are to the same or similar items as measured within or across time. Hesselbrock, Babor, Hesselbrock, Meyer, and Workman (1983) use concurrent for external validity and add discriminant validity, which refers to discriminating subjects in terms of the target behavior, whereas predictive validity relates to predicting future performance.

Reliability and validity of self-reported consumption estimates have been dealt with quite frequently. A review of the literature was presented by Midanik (1982a). In many validity studies, self-reports are considered to be basically valid. Variation exists depending on what is being validated and how its accuracy is measured. Recent reports on consumption are validated more easily than are drinking patterns measured in drinking practices surveys. Collateral reports by significant others do not necessarily yield better information on consumption. Only a few highly visible problems realistically can be validated.

The closer a measure comes to assessing actual quantities consumed during a given period, the more reliable should be the result and the estimates (Alanko, 1981).

In contrast to a widely held notion that alcoholics deny the extent of their drinking, errors in the direction of overreporting were found in some studies (Midanik, 1982b). Studies using official records and collateral reports suggest that self-reports of concrete drinking problems are not biased and that overreports equal or exceed underreports. Overall outcome classifications based on a combination of consumption and other measures were not substantially affected by errors in consumption reports (Polich, 1982). Another study by O'Farrell, Cutter, Bayog, Dentch, and Fortgang (1984) demonstrated substantial agreement of male alcoholics' reports and their wives' reports on the number of the "wet" days and on the number of days spent hospitalized or jailed for alcohol-related reasons; there was less agreement on the number of light and heavy drinking days. Verinis (1983) found an almost exact agreement between the alcoholic and his relatives in 80% of cases; in the remaining cases, the discrepancy between the alcoholic's and the relatives' reports varied according to area asked about and was greatest concerning drinking pattern, family relationships, and longest dry periods.

Finally, the study published by Hesselbrock et al. (1983) evaluated the validity of information obtained by means of self-report questionnaires in male and female alcoholics. Composite measures of alcohol dependence, withdrawal symptomatology, pathological intoxication, and alcohol psychosis were compared with independent and external criteria, such as drinking estimates made by collateral informants, measures of general alcohol involvement, and drinking behavior six months after treatment. Concurrent, discriminant, construct, and predictive validity were supported by the results, and thereby the assumption that alcoholic self-reports were not accurate has been contradicted.

Why then are self-reports so frequently considered to be unreliable? A plausible explanation is that reliability is directly related to eventual consequences the self-report may have for the informant. Such an impact is to be expected in intervention settings but not in the context of research projects protecting those who participate from practical consequences.

Internal validity, which is closely associated with the term *reliability*, was especially examined using longitudinally collected self-report data from the "Monitoring the Future" project, an ongoing nationwide study of high school seniors (O'Malley et al., 1983). Although the authors noted satisfaction with external and construct validity, they report on a consistent discrepancy between data on actual and past substance use. Reported monthly frequency was in general higher than the expected value (one-twelfth of the reported annual frequency). Discrepancy ratios were calculated for each respondent where possible; for alcohol and marijuana, the average discrepancy ratios were about 3.0 or higher. It was concluded that the major part of the discrepancy was due to a systematic underestimation of past use. Variability of discrepancy ratios among individuals was considerable. The authors, therefore, looked for individual characteristics responsible for this variability. They examined individual characteristics such as sex, race, parental education, urbanicity, geographic region, curriculum, educational aspirations, grades, truancy behavior, hours worked per week, weekly income, religious commitment, political beliefs, and amount of social and dating behavior. Among 1980 high school seniors, these potential correlates could account for less than 2% of the variance in the discrepancy ratios for alcohol. The findings suggest that the discrepancy ratios are not related to stable individual characteristics.

Apart from collateral informants, laboratory methods have been used in order to corroborate self-reported data on actual alcohol intake. Breath tests were applied with satisfactory results (Midanik, 1982b). Urine testing is less reliable unless direct observation of urinating is applied. Changes in blood test values from treatment discharge to follow-up can be used to distinguish recovering alcoholics who remain abstinent from those who resume drinking (Irwin, Baird, Smith, & Schuckit, 1988). Introducing faked laboratory testing (bogus pipeline) in a controlled study did not affect significantly self-reports of adolescents on alcohol use and misuse (Campanelli, Dielman, & Shope, 1987).

Midanik (1988) in her most recent review of validity studies concludes that research on the validity of self-reported alcohol use should emphasize the interactions of the respondent, the interviewer, the information being obtained, and the context of the interview to determine under which conditions valid responses can be maximized.

Problems of sampling

Two main problems may be mentioned here. One is the problem in population surveys where those with heavy alcohol use tend to be underrepresented because they are less available (being institutionalized, without fixed abode, or refusing interview). The other problem is the selectivity of identified samples and cohorts of alcoholics, according to the identification process, which is less geared by the dependence syndrome alone, but rather by concomitant health and/or psychosocial consequences. Both problems have an impact on the conclusiveness of studies when it comes to relating consumption patterns and individual consumption volume/frequency to the eventual sequelae of alcohol use.

Population surveys with a longitudinal design will not be representative for determining risk factors and risk constellations for the heavier forms of alcohol consumption or for its eventual consequences unless detailed information is given on those not available for interview. This part of the spectrum has to be complemented by samples of identified heavy users drawn from other sources. On the other hand, longitudinal studies that used samples drawn from patients in general hospitals, psychiatric hospitals, specialized units or organizations, general practitioners, and so forth, are equally deficient. Such samples are not only biased by referral and admission selectivity, but also by inconsistencies in diagnosing. They are not representative for heavy users without health or psychosocial consequences and are, in this respect, prone to provide misleading results.

A study by Singer and Anglin (1986) in a large urban teaching hospital in Ohio demonstrated that only about 25% of expected problem cases were identified during hospitalization. The identification of alcohol-related problems by general practitioners has been a research issue for several years. Studies demonstrated that questionnaire surveys of patients attending general practitioner surgeries always produce higher prevalence rates than those obtained by asking general practitioners how many patients with alcohol-related problems they have on their lists. This suggests that many general practitioners do not identify the majority of the alcohol-related problems that can be found among their patients (Clement, 1986). This has its impact on referrals to specialized units and organizations, which again results in highly selective samples drawn from these units and organizations. Registers are equally biased according to the type of information used to identify subjects for registration.

The difficulties of clinical diagnosing cannot be overcome by using biological methods. Laboratory tests in a sample of 1,121 young alcohol consumers did not succeed in discriminating low and high consumers and, therefore, are not recommended for screening purposes (Bliding, Bliding, Fex, & Tornqvist (1982). On the other hand, multivariate analysis of blood chemistry in 460 alcoholics revealed little or no relationship to drinking history (Evenson, Frankel, & Freedland, 1988).

As a consequence, all studies and surveys must indicate clearly their sampling method and selectivity in order to indicate as well the limitations of the study results.

Time intervals for follow-up

Apart from what has been mentioned concerning assessment periods, it may be helpful to focus on a few issues pertinent to the timing of reexamination.

Adverse effects of alcohol consumption are mostly not immediate effects; according to the nature of effects, we observe an "effect-lag" until the risk of effect manifestation becomes apparent. The effect-lag not only varies with various types of effects (e.g., liver cirrhosis, delirium tremens, alcohol dependence syndrome), but also with biological factors, consumption patterns, and concomitant factors. The relative importance of these variables for the duration of the effect-lag is another research issue for the future. For the time being, one single reexamination is bound to give an incomplete picture.

Excess morbidity and excess mortality related to alcohol consumption are not equally distributed among all age groups, a maximum being found in the age group 40–49 (Mackenzie, Allen, & Funderburk, 1986). To which extent this is due to a corresponding onset of alcohol consumption and timing for consumption patterns or to associated factors is still open for further research. The same age group shows a maximum of hospitalizations for reasons other than treating alcoholism. Whatever the reasons may be, research on adverse health effects of alcohol intake with a longitudinal design has to consider that a maximum of health consequences will not become visible before the age of 40.

Regarding behavioral effects of alcohol intake, the effect-lag is different from the one observable in health consequences. Whereas behavioral effects related to intoxication are immediate ones, those connected with gradual changes in emotional control, perceived consequences of drinking, labeling processes, and so forth, will take more time. A differential analysis of such sequences needs further efforts and meets major methodological difficulties. An outstanding example of how to deal with these research questions in the framework of problem behavior rather than as problematic alcohol use as an isolated phenomenon is Jessors' longitudinal study on problem behavior in adolescence (Jessor & Jessor, 1977; Jessor & Jessor, 1984; Jessor, 1986).

Just as intervals for follow-up may be too short, they may also be too long. Attrition rates vary with length of intervals for reexamination. Specific tracking methods and motivation strategies have been developed in order to minimize attrition rates (e.g., using regular contacts between follow-up examinations, key persons indicated initially by subjects, feed-back strategies). Such methods and strategies may reduce attrition rates considerably, if enough effort and time is provided for in the initial design of the study. Another method to be used in finding a reasonable compromise between frequency of reexaminations and attrition rate is the method of oversampling those with a higher probability of attrition from the very beginning. Such a procedure is recommended when frequent reexaminations meet a growing resistance from those included in the study, a situation that again may become a major source for attrition. It must be kept in mind, however, that the method of oversampling does not overcome the problem of selectivity (loss of subjects who refuse interview), but it is an answer to the problem of low cell frequency.

Risk constellations

Adverse effects of alcohol consumption are observed in rates that differ from sample to sample. One of the central research questions is how to explain these differences on the basis of identified concomitant risk factors, apart from sampling effects and other procedural impacts and apart from variable attrition rates that also account for differences in mortality and morbidity rates.

An overview on excess mortality and morbidity is presented by Mackenzie et al. (1986). Excess mortality rates vary from 1.0 to 6.5 (ratio of number of deaths observed to that expected). A stepwise regression analysis of data demonstrating age and number of previous general hospitalizations for reasons other than treating alcoholism are the best predictors for excessive mortality.

Other intervening variables dealt with in research are social class (Edwards, Kyle, Nicholls, & Taylor, 1978, found higher excess mortality in upper-class as compared to lower-class alcoholics), type of beverage (Mackenzie et al., 1986), occupation (Slattery, Alderson, & Bryant, 1986), cigarette smoking, personal neglect, adverse environmental conditions, emotional factors, influence of skid row status (Ashley, Olin, leRiche, Komaczewski, Schmidt, & Rankin, 1976; Ashley, 1982). Excess mortality due, for example, to liver cirrhosis, neoplasms, suicide, accidents, and so forth, is not related to a uniform risk constellation; on the contrary, it shows a considerable variability in constellations of contributing factors.

Similar considerations and observations have been made with respect to excess morbidity and also with respect to behavior consequences of alcohol consumption. Still more needs to be done in the field of identifying relevant factors and constellations when it comes to evaluating prophylactically or therapeutically intended changes in alcohol consumption or in spontaneous remission from harmful alcohol consumption. A reduction of consumption is only one element, although an essential one.

If progression from abstinence to acceptable forms of alcohol intake, from acceptable forms to harmful styles of alcohol consumption, from harmful drinking to manifest health and social consequences of drinking is favored by variable risk constellations, longitudinal studies will profit considerably from using an adequate combination of collecting alcohol data with data collection on other variables suspected to intervene with the effects of alcohol intake. Also, it may be useful to consider intervening variables that potentiate eventually the effects of alcohol intake as well as intervening variables that are expected to compensate for such effects. For the time being, I do not know of any single effect of alcohol consumption that would not be related to intervening factors; even the incidence of liver cirrhosis, traditionally used as an indicator for the extent of alcohol consumption, is related to intervening factors such as eating habits, and so forth. Future research on alcohol consumption as a risk factor will profit most from transcending to a concept of complex risk situations and constellations.

Conclusions

Recent research in the field has contributed considerably to our knowledge concerning the two initially formulated research questions and supports a number of recommendations for future studies. Among these, the following comprise a priority for researchers' concerns.

Independent of the context in which the study design is using alcohol data, it is recommended that consumption data be assessed separately from eventually assessing clinical diagnosis because the former are a better measure for change over time. It is recommended that continuous variables rather than categorical measures be used in order to provide dependent or independent variables in multivariate modeling. The nature of alcohol data, the type and accuracy of the measure, should be compatible with the nature of hypotheses that the study aims to test. For instance, health consequences, especially organic damage, are correlated to volume of alcohol intake rather than to frequency of intake or to quantity per occasion, whereas unwelcomed behavior is related to patterns of consumption rather than to overall volume. It is recommended that assessment of volume be complemented by quantitatively measuring drinking style. Special indexes and typologies have been proposed in this respect.

The validity of self-report measures has been tested frequently, with various methods and in various contexts. The results are reported to be satisfactory in many instances. Assessing actual intake is more reliable than the measurement of past consumption, the latter being frequently misjudged in the light of recent experience. This has to be taken into consideration when past consumption, especially lifetime volume, are asked for retrospectively. Because there is little continuity in alcohol consumption in typical transition periods (e.g., from adolescence to adulthood, from adulthood to old age), the assessment of past consumption is especially prone to inaccuracy if the assessment period includes such transition stages. On the other hand, external validity of self-report data is often better than expected. If it is admissible, then, to use self-report data, it is advisable to consider prospective designs rather than retrospective ones where the assessment of past alcohol intake is critical for the purpose of the study.

A general warning is expressed concerning eventual biases from sampling procedures, because population surveys tend to underrepresent problematic and heavy alcohol use, and because samples drawn from therapeutic institutions and registers underrepresent drinkers without manifest consequences and, therefore, without reasons for therapeutic or legal intervention. Deficiencies in diagnosing, which are not overcome by using biological testing, should be taken into consideration.

As far as the timing of assessment is concerned, follow-up intervals may be too short or too long for a variety of reasons. It is recommended that intervals be timed in accordance with the purpose of the study and the specific effect-lag of sequelae that are to be investigated. Regarding the interdependence of interval for follow-up and attrition rate, recommendations concern specific methods (oversampling of those most prone for attrition) and strategies (tracking procedures between follow-up interviews).

Finally, it is recommended that specific risk constellations be considered with regard to testing etiological hypotheses in the domain of alcohol-related health and social consequences. Growing evidence discloses complex interaction patterns where alcohol intake is only one among a number of intervening variables that are not identical in the various problem areas.

References

Alanko, T. (1981). An overview of techniques and problems in the measurement of alcohol consumption. In R. G. Smart et al. (Eds.), *Research advances in alcohol and drug problems* (Vol. 8, pp. 209–226). New York: Plenum Press.

Andersson, T., & Magnusson, D. (1988). Drinking habits and alcohol abuse among young men: A prospective longitudinal study. *Journal of Studies on Alcohol, 49*(3), 245–252.

Argeriou, M. (1978). Daily alcohol consumption patterns in Boston: Some findings and a partial test. *Journal of Studies on Alcohol, 36,* 1578–1583.

Armor, D. J., & Polich, J. (1982). Measurement of alcohol consumption. In E. M. Pattison & E. Kaufman (Eds.) *Encyclopedic handbook of alcoholism* (pp. 72–80). New York: Gardner Press.

Ashley, M. J. (1982). Alcohol, tobacco, and drugs: An audit of mortality and morbidity. In

L. H. R. Drew et al. (Eds.), *Man, drugs and society – Current perspectives* (pp. 350–365). Canberra: Australian Federation on Alcoholism and Drug Dependence.

Ashley, M. J., Olin, J. S., leRiche, W. H., Komaczewski, A., Schmidt, W., & Rankin, J. G. (1976). Skid row alcoholism: A district sociomedical entity. *Archives of Internal Medicine, 136*, 272.

Bliding, G., Bliding, A., Fex, G., & Tornqvist, C. (1982). The appropriateness of laboratory tests in tracing young heavy drinkers. *Drug and Alcohol Dependence, 10*(2–3), 153–158.

Cahalan, D., & Cisin, I. H. (1968). American drinking practices: Summary of findings from a national probability sample. II. Measurement of massed versus spaced drinking. *Journal of Studies on Alcohol, 29*, 642–656.

Cahalan, D., Cisin, I. H., & Crossley, H. M. (1969). American drinking practices: A national study of drinking behavior and attitudes. *RCAS Monograph Number 6*. New Brunswick, NJ: Rutgers Center of Alcohol Studies.

Campanelli, P. C., Dielman, T. E., & Shope, J. T. (1987). Validity of adolescents' self-reports of alcohol use and misuse using a bogus pipeline procedure. *Adolescence, 22*(85), 7–22.

Clement, S. (1986). The identification of alcohol-related problems by general practitioners. *British Journal of Addiction, 81*, 257–264.

Cowan, R., Massey, L., & Greenfield, T. K. (1985). Determination of average, binge, and maximum alcohol intake in healthy young men by discriminant function analysis of a panel of blood tests. *Journal of Studies on Alcohol, 46*, 467–482.

Dean, J. (1985). A multivariant assessment and treatment technique for alcohol problems. *International Journal of the Addictions, 20*(8), 1281–1290.

Douglass, R. L. (1984). Socioepidemiology of aging and alcohol problems. In M. Galanter (Ed.), *Recent developments in alcoholism* (Vol. 2). New York: Plenum Press.

Douglass, R. L., Schuster, E. O., & McClelland, S. C. (1988). Drinking patterns and abstinence among the elderly. *International Journal of the Addictions, 23*(4), 399–415.

Edwards, G. (1977). The alcohol dependence syndrome: Usefulness of an idea. In G. Edwards & M. Grant (Eds.), *Alcoholism: New knowledge and new responses* (pp. 136–156). London: Croom Helm.

Edwards, G., Kyle, E., Nicholls, P., & Taylor, C. (1978). Alcoholism and correlates of mortality: Implications for epidemiology. *Journal of Studies on Alcohol, 39*, 1607–1617.

Evenson, R. C., Frankel, M. F., & Freedland, K. E. (1988). What is measured when we identify alcoholics by means of blood tests? *International Journal of the Addictions, 23*(4), 433–436.

Greenfield, T. K. (1986). Quantity per occasion and consequences of drinking: A reconsideration and recommendation. *International Journal of the Addictions, 21*(9 & 10), 1059–1079.

Greenfield, T.K., & Duncan, G. (1985). *Evaluation of an alcohol abuse prevention program correcting for self selection.* Paper presented at the Annual Convention of the American Psychological Association, Toronto, 1984. ERIC Resources in Education No. ED 253807.

Greenfield, T. K., Karzmark, P. B., Haymond, C. J., Wyatt, C. J., & Gunns, D. A. (1980). *Patterns of student drinking: Characteristics, experiences, motivations and problems in College* (SSR Report No. 2). Washington State University: Pullman, Student Services Research.

Gwartney-Gibbs, P. A. (1985). *Alcohol use at the University of Oregon, 1982: Implications for an alcohol education program.* Unpublished manuscript, University of Oregon, Department of Sociology, quoted from Greenfield, 1986.

Hauge, R., & Irgens-Jensen, O. (1984). *The relationship between alcohol consumption and the negative consequences of drinking in four Scandinavian countries.* Paper presented at the Alcohol Epidemiology Section meetings of the International Council on Alcohol and Addictions, Edinburg, Scotland, June 1984.

Hesselbrock, M., Babor, T. F., Hesselbrock, V., Meyer, R. E., & Workman, K. (1983).

"Never believe an alcoholic"? On the validity of self-report measures of alcohol dependence and related constructs. *International Journal of the Addictions, 18*(5), 593–609.

Hilton, M. E. (1988). Regional diversity in United States drinking practices. *British Journal of Addiction, 83,* 519–532.

Hubbard, R., Eckerman, W., & Rachal, J. V. (1976). Methods of validating self-reports of drug use: A critical review. *Proceedings of the American Statistical Association,* 406–409.

Hulbert, R. J., & Lens, W. (1988). Time perspective, time attitude, and time orientation in alcoholism: a review. *International Journal of the Addictions, 23*(3), 279–298.

Irwin, M., Baird, S., Smith, T. L., & Schuckit, M. (1988). Use of laboratory tests to monitor heavy drinking by alcoholic men discharged from a treatment program. *American Journal of Psychiatry, 145*(5), 595–599.

Jacobson, G. R. (1976). *The alcoholisms: Detection, assessment, and diagnosis.* New York: Human Sciences Press.

Jessor, R. (1986). Adolescent problem drinking: Psychosocial aspects and developmental outcomes. In R. K. Silbereisen, K. Eyferth, & G. Rudinger (Eds.), *Development as action in context* (pp. 241–264). Berlin: Springer-Verlag.

Jessor, R., & Jessor, S. L. (1977). *Problem behavior and psychosocial development: A longitudinal study of youth.* New York: Academic Press.

Jessor, R., & Jessor, S. L. (1984). Adolescence to young adulthood: A twelve-year prospective study of problem behavior and psychosocial development. In S. Mednick & M. Harway (Eds.), *Longitudinal research in the United States.* New York: Praeger.

Knupfer, G. (1984). The risk of drunkenness (or ebrietas resurrecta): A comparison of frequent intoxication indices and of population sub-groups as to problem risks. *British Journal of Addiction, 79,* 185–196.

Kreitman, N., & Duffy, J. (1982). *Beyond consumption: The effect of drinking patterns on the consequences of drinking.* Paper presented at the Alcohol Epidemiology Section meetings of the International Council on Alcohol and Addictions, Helsinki, Finland, July 1982.

Lelbach, W. K. (1974). Organic pathology related to volume and pattern of alcohol use. In R. J. Gibbins et al. (Eds.), *Research advances in alcohol and drug problems* (Vol. 1, pp. 193–198). New York: Wiley.

Mackenzie, A., Allen, R. P., & Funderburk, F. R. (1986). Mortality and illness in male alcoholics: An 8-year follow-up. *International Journal of the Addictions, 21*(8), 865–882.

Magnusson, D., & Stattin, H. (1982). *Biological age, environment, and behavior in interaction: A methodological problem.* Reports of the Department of Psychology, University of Stockholm, No. 587.

Mäkelä, K. (1978). Level of consumption and social consequences of drinking. In Y. Israel et al. (Eds.), *Research advances in alcohol and drug problems* (Vol. 4, pp. 303–348). New York: Plenum Press.

Midanik, L. (1982a). The validity of self-reported alcohol consumption and alcohol problems: A literature review. *British Journal of Addiction, 77*(4), 357–382.

Midanik, L. (1982b). Over-reports of recent alcohol consumption in a clinical population: A validity study. *Drug and Alcohol Dependence, 9*(2), 101–110.

Midanik, L. (1988). Validity of self-reported alcohol use: A literature review and assessment. *British Journal of Addiction, 83,* 1019–1029.

Neuman, C., & Rabow, J. (1986). Drinkers' use of physical availability of alcohol: Buying habits and consumption level. *International Journal of the Addictions, 20*(11 & 12), 1663–1673.

O'Farrell, T. J., Cutter, H. S. G., Bayog, R. D., Dentch, G., & Fortgang, J. (1984). Correspondence between one-year retrospective reports of pretreatment drinking by alcoholics and their wives. *Behavioral Assessment, 6*(3), 263–274.

O'Malley, P. M., Bachman, J. G., & Johnston, L. D. (1983). Reliability and consistency in self-reports of drug use. *International Journal of the Addictions, 18*(6), 805–824.

Pattison, E. M., & Kaufman, E. (1982). The alcoholism syndrome: Definitions and models. In E. M. Pattison, & E. Kaufman (Eds.), *Encyclopedic handbook of alcoholism* (pp. 3–30). New York: Gardner Press.

Polich, J. M. (1982). The validity of self-reports in alcoholism research. *Addictive Behaviors, 7*(2), 123–132.

Rabow, J., & Neuman, C. A. (1984). Saturday night live: Chronicity or alcohol consumption among college students. *Substance and Alcohol Actions/Misuse, 5,* 1–7.

Room, R. (1985). *Measuring alcohol consumption in the U.S.: Methods and rationales.* Paper presented at the Alcohol Epidemiology Section meetings of the International Institute on the Prevention and Treatment of Alcohol Problems, Rome, Italy, June 1985.

Sher, K. J. (1985). Excluding problem drinkers in high-risk studies of alcoholism: Effect of screening criteria on high-risk versus low-risk comparisons. *Journal of Abnormal Psychology, 94*(1), 106–109.

Simpura, J., & Poikolainen, K. (1983). Accuracy of retrospective measurement of individual alcohol consumption in men: A reinterview after 18 years. *Journal of Studies on Alcohol, 44*(5), 911–917.

Singer, M., & Anglin, T. (1986). The identification of adolescent substance abuse by health care professionals. *International Journal of the Addictions, 21*(2), 247–254.

Slattery, M., Alderson, M. R., & Bryant, J. S. (1986). The occupational risks of alcoholism. *International Journal of the Addictions, 21*(8), 929–936.

Straus, R., & Bacon, S. D. (1953). *Drinking in college.* New Haven: Yale University Press.

Temple, M. T., & Fillmore, K. M. (1986). The variability of drinking patterns and problems among young men, age 16–31: A longitudinal study. *International Journal of the Addictions, 20*(11 & 12), 1595–1620.

Verinis, J. S. (1983). Agreement between alcoholics and relatives when reporting follow-up status. *International Journal of the Addictions, 18*(6), 891–894.

Windle, M. (1988). Are those adolescent to early adulthood drinking patterns so discontinuous? A response to Temple and Fillmore. *International Journal of the Addictions, 23*(9), 907–912.

6   Retrospective data, undesirable behavior, and the longitudinal perspective

CARL-GUNNAR JANSON

Introduction

Longitudinal studies[1] are often said to be both expensive and time-consuming. They certainly require considerable patience of both researchers and grant-giving agencies. It is no wonder, then, that less patient people look for faster alternatives if they still want to study long-term processes. Our culture is impatient and Americanized, so in addition to instant coffee and instant lawns we have instant longitudinal studies. In one giant interview wave, all the necessary information on the subjects' life histories is obtained retrospectively. Instead of plodding on gathering data for, say, 20 years, one receives all the data at one stroke. Evidently this is much faster. Whether it is much less expensive is another question.

The instant longitudinal study is a great invention – to the extent that it works. As usual, much depends on the technical quality of the design, fieldwork, and data handling, but much also depends on the field of application. Limits on its applicability are essentially set by its retrospective character and by some people's reluctance to reveal their own socially undesirable behavior.

Retrospective design and retrospective data

The attribute "retrospective" is usually attached to designs (or samples) and data.

Retrospective designs (samples) belong to diachronous studies, studies dealing with more than one point in time. If the sample of units to be studied refers to the end of the investigated period,[2] the design (sample) is *retrospective.*. The sample does not contain units that left the system or area under study before the end of the period; that is, a sample of persons does not retain outmovers or those who died during the period. If the sample refers to a time within the period, the design (sample) is retrospective as to the earlier part of the period and again does not contain units that left before the sample's time of reference. On the other hand, a retrospective unit may include units added to the system from the beginning of the period till the time of the sample (i.e., inmovers and the newborn).

Correspondingly, a design with a sample of the units at the beginning of the period is said to be *prospective,* and a sample referring to some time within the period would be prospective in relation to later parts of the period. The prospective sample will include units leaving the system before the end or, generally, sampled persons who moved out or died before the end of the period but after the time of the sample.

Obviously, the instant longitudinal study is retrospectively designed. This puts some restrictions on its field of application, because processes of leaving the system and related topics cannot be analyzed.

In defining "retrospective data" a series of times or phases will be used as they relate to a given item of information in an empirical study.[3] This will not lead to the definition of a contrary concept of "prospective data" because only descriptive items, in contrast to predictive ones, are considered. Perhaps the latter could be called prospective. The times or phases are as follows (cf. Janson, 1978:27f.):

a. The time the item refers to. It describes an aspect at a certain time. This can be a specific point or a period during which conditions are assumed to remain basically constant or within limits narrow enough to make the item valid as an approximation.

b. The time the item is produced. It is produced when materialized as a notation (sentence, word, check mark, or other sign) on paper or tape, a photo, a recording, and so forth. Thus, an observation is "produced" when its relevant aspects are documented.

c. The time the item is collected in the study. Collecting the data may be the same process that documents, "produces," the item. If so, time b and time c are evidently also the same. However, the item may have been produced outside the research project, which later extracts what is considered useful. Both documenting and collecting, whether carried out as one phase or separately, clearly comprise an element of interpretation. Something is observed (i.e., seen, heard, or otherwise perceived) and is given an elementary description in selected aspects. It is here assumed that the selection of aspects and their description are straightforward and simple enough to be basically uncontroversial. It is a question of knowing the language and recognizing what words, figures, and signs were written or spoken. This does not preclude mistakes, but they would be due to carelessness and inadequate instruction rather than to profound semantics. For this to hold true, the kind of item must be restricted to items the recording of which is routinized, such as items in structured interviews and questionnaires used in large-scale surveys and in certain manual and computerized files. In some respect the meaning of the item may be ambiguous or vague, and as recorded it can remain so. Such ambiguities will, to the extent they are discovered, be considered in the next phase.

d. The time the item is codified and made ready for analysis. At least in part this phase may have been carried out in the previous phase, but now necessary classifications and interpretations will be chosen in order to code the item as measuring something, not necessarily one thing only. Presumably there were at least implicit intentions in collecting the item at time c. Now the coding should be made so as to facilitate one or more of the intended uses of the items, not necessarily those that were originally intended. The coding can be such that the usage of the item remains more or less open.

e. The time the item is analyzed and the results interpreted. Here again there is interpretation, this time predominantly in the wider context of the set of variables and the results.

Some of these phases can be carried out in the same operation and thus can be simultaneous, whereas others can follow in an unbroken sequence and be almost simultaneous. However, the phases can also be widely apart in time. Various minor complications can occur in the sequence listed due to checking, recoding, multiple use of the item, and so forth; but they can easily be taken into account and the scheme correspondingly adjusted. The phases are listed in time order. Each phase on the list presupposes those already listed. A seeming exception might be when an observation made (produced) before the end of a period of assumed constant conditions is taken to refer to the whole period or to a later point during that period. Apart from this and possible similar anomalies, no phase can precede a phase listed higher on the list, although it can be practically simultaneous.

An item on a survey by interview or questionnaire on an aspect of the contemporary situation is produced when asked and answered as noted at a time that coincides with the time of reference. On the other hand, a survey item on past conditions has by definition an earlier time of reference than time of production. In both cases, if the survey is carried out within the study, the item is produced and recorded simultaneously. Otherwise, the recording would come later when the survey is put at the disposition of the study. Coding and analysis can come immediately after recording, but both or the analysis on its own can take place much later.

An item as to whether a person was accepted at a certain college can be documented at the time of the acceptance by a note in the person's file at the college. The item is thus produced at the time of reference but is recorded by the study at that later point in time when the file is extracted by the study. Documents such as memoirs are produced after their time of reference to the extent that they do not just reproduce contemporary documents from these times.

An item is called retrospective if it is produced after its time of reference. The longer after the time of reference it is produced, the more retrospective it is.

In the behavioral sciences, by far the most common retrospective data originate in survey questions relating to past circumstances. It should be noticed that questions about how things "usually are" also contain a retrospective element as the respondent is asked to weigh and summarize things over a certain period.[4]

Problems of recollecting

In an interview or questionnaire study there is always the problem of accessibility, that is, to what extent the respondent has the information in conscious form, conceptualized in the terms used by the interviewer or questionnaire (Cannell & Kahn, 1968:535f.). As already indicated, the concern in this chapter is with the accessibilty of items in large-scale surveys using structured interviews or questionnaires. Accessibility depends on the method and instrument of inquiry in several ways. No doubt careful, competent, and protracted probing can give information not accessible under the restrictions of the large-scale survey. If so, this suggests that "not remembering" on a survey item might be a problem of retrieval rather than one of retention (cf. Crowder, 1976:4–12). Some factors will influence learning but not retrieval, and vice versa (cf. Baddeley, Lewis, Eldridge, & Thomsen, 1985).

Neither are we here considering interviews and questionnaires other than those in research (i.e., therapeutic, evaluative, selective, and other administrative interviews and forms) that can also be sources of documentary information used in research. Unlike these other ways of seeking information, the survey interview and questionnaire have only indirect consequences for the respondent outside the situation of actual questioning. With the exception of the census survey, if that is considered a research survey, participation in surveys is voluntary. It is initiated by the research organization, and the respondent's motive in participating is as a rule not to get personal help or advantages or to clear himself from suspicions.

With few exceptions one can assume that respondents, if agreeing to participate, do not positively want to deceive or misinform the study. Although they may not want to answer everything they are asked about, they are prepared to cooperate at least to some extent. There may be some intrinsic motivation to participate. A bored or lonely informant may get something out of the interaction with the interviewer or even from filling out a questionnaire. The focus on the informant as the most important person in the world may also be rewarding. However, to be interviewed or to fill out a form is not usually that much fun, so a more instrumental motivation is generally needed. Since participation has no direct effects apart from participating itself, an element of altruism or civic spirit must be present. There must usually be apparent a trace of a positive attitude to research or the specific study, as, for example, something generating valuable new knowledge. Among factors preventing a respondent from participating or, if participating, to make the necessary effort to recall, would be lack of time, dislike of the subject, embarrassment of showing ignorance, fear of revealing socially undesirable behavior, and dread of possible consequences and leaks (Cannell & Kahn, 1968:538f.).

In this chapter the focus is on retrospective items, especially on exceptionally long-term retrospective items such as can be found in the life-history surveys of instant longitudinal studies (cf. Moss, 1979: 164; Sudman & Bradburn, 1983:42–45). Surveys, of course, involve many problems of validity and reliability (see, e.g., Cherry & Rodgers, 1979:32, on asking about stature). What is specific to retrospective items is the problem of recollecting mostly autobiographical past events, conditions, characteristics, and feelings.

To some questions there may be no recall because there is nothing to recall. The informant has simply never known about the matter asked about. This in itself has nothing to do with the question's being retrospective, because obviously the informant can be ignorant about contemporary as well as past matters. However, it may be easier to make mistakes about what the respondent knows regarding past events and situations than regarding present questions.

The will to participate and to make the effort to recall and to give the correct answer is a strong determinant of the accessibility of the information, with the proviso, as pointed out above, that the respondent ever knew the answer and, it should be added, that he or she can translate it into the terms provided for answering. Again, untranslatable terms have little to do with the specific problems of retrospective data because they can occur in questions concerning the present as well.

With some retrospective items, answering is more a matter of the respondent's recalling something learned than recollecting something experienced, although the learning has been reinforced by experience. This refers mostly to items concerning the respondent's early life and family; for example, birth dates of the respondent himself (herself), the spouse, and parents, parental education and early work history, what father did during the war, and similar family folklore. The recall may not always be correct as fact, but accessibility is usually high.

However, most retrospective items call for the respondent's own recollection of past circumstances. That we all remember and forget is, of course, part of our conception of human nature and firmly established by experience. Recalling and forgetting have been studied by psychologists ever since Ebbinghaus. Although most theories and empirical studies deal with the retention and retrieval of learned material as empirically analyzed in short-term laboratory experiments (e.g., Murdock, 1973), problems of recollecting autobiographical information and other events have also been studied (e.g., Hunter, 1964, ch. 6; Crowder, 1976; Gruneberg & Morris, 1978; Baddeley, 1979, 1986; Rubin, 1986). There is also a fairly substantial literature on retrospective items in surveys (e.g., Sudman & Bradburn, 1973; Moss & Goldstein, 1979; Jabine, Straf, Tanur, & Tourangean, 1984; Bernard, Killworth, Kronenfeld, & Sailer, 1984; Bradburn, Rips, & Shevell, 1987).

The evidence is overwhelming to the point of triviality that recollecting tends to decrease with the time span involved, but that the pace of this recollection decline differs strongly among types of circumstances to be recollected. The rate of recalled information is often described mathematically as an inverse power or exponential of time (cf., e.g., Sudman & Bradburn, 1973; Wagenaar, 1986; for another approach, see Sikkel, 1985). The decline of recall over time is rarely ascribed to time itself but to processes influencing retention and retrieval over time. Although there seems to be no generally accepted model for these processes, proactive and retroactive interference[5] of other experiences are prominent in proposed models (cf. Crowder, 1976, ch. 8; Morris, 1978, ch. 4).

The respondents may use various strategies to reach an acceptable answer to the autobiographical questions asked. For instance, for the questions regarding how often they engaged in a certain type of activity during a given period, one way would be to attempt to recall each time this happened. Perhaps one could add a few occasions for good measure in order to correct for possibly forgotten events. Another way would be to try to remember all recent occasions and then duly enlarge the number to cover the whole period asked about (cf. Bradburn, Rips, & Shevell, 1987). However, all serious strategies build on attempts to recall.

At least since Bartlett's classic analysis (Bartlett, 1932), remembering has been seen as an active process of selecting, (re)interpreting, and (re)structuring, that is productive as well as reproductive (cf. Morris, 1978:71ff.). The respondent may forget or suppress an experience completely, at least so much so that it does not surface when the survey question is asked. One may also recall that something took place in greater or lesser detail. The aspect asked about may or may not be recalled, and the recall may be more or less clear. With Conway and Bekerian (1987) one may speak of "autobiographical memory organization packets." Retrieval of episodes can be seen as occurring in a hierarchical system of contexts, from lifetime periods such as "school days" down to more specific autobiographical categories. Knowledge about classes of events is organized in "scripts" (Jabine et al., 1984:11f.). Activities are also organized according to verbal labels. When a memory is retrieved, its contexts, scripts, and labels to some extent determine what aspects are recalled and color their associations and interpretation (cf. Shweder & D'Andrade, 1980). The more the picture fades, whether from interference or other processes, the more room for rearranging and reinterpreting. Details are left out (cf. Wagenaar, 1986), especially odd pieces that do not fit into an overall pattern, and the pattern and details are changed to a more rational and coherent picture. Postman's hypotheses for perception are also applicable to memory (Postman, 1951). What is recalled will depend on the actual structure of the event or situation experienced but also on the functional factors related to the person perceiving and memorizing. We have hypotheses – expectations and predispositions – according to which we select aspects to be perceived and memorized, interpreted, and adapted. Obviously, we both experience and recall unexpected and disliked phenomena when structural factors are sufficiently strong. That we sometimes learn from experience means that expectations and predispositions are readjusted. However, the less dominant the structural factors are in perception and the less information retained, the more room there is for functional factors (cf. Carlsson, 1954:59–62). To the extent that retained material is actively processed in this way in recall and is recollected several times, it may change serially to a mixture of earlier recollections and the original episode.

The recall can be facilitated by various devices that provide cues and put the item asked about in context by focusing on retrieval techniques. Some probing and cues are better than others (cf. Reiser, Black, & Abelson, 1985). Aided recall can be taken to the point where the respondent is asked to recognize the item rather than recall it. In readership studies such facilitating measures are well established: reading the names of the newspapers, showing their logotypes, showing front pages, skimming the pages of magazines, and so forth (cf. Schyberger, 1965). To facilitate self-reports on delinquency, a list of offenses and other delinquencies is read or shown to the respondent (cf. Hindelang, Hirschi, & Weis, 1981). To refresh the memory of yesterday's alcohol consumption, each meal and each occasion for a drink are gone through. Obviously, the personal interview offers better possibilities of aiding recall than the telephone interview and, especially, the questionnaire.

In asking a certain survey question, the researcher wants information on some state of affairs, with the information couched in the language of the researcher and with its relevance and interpretation decided by the researcher (i.e., "etic" information, cf. Harris, 1980:32–34). Compared with contemporary items, some retrospective items have two complications. First, as the retrieved picture of the circumstances asked about becomes less distinct, structural factors will be less dominating and will give room for functional factors in the recollection. This will introduce a slice of information selected and evaluated according to the informant's standards and frame of reference (i.e., "emic" information; *Ibid.*). Second, by definition the answers will be shaped according to the informant's opinion at the time of answering about the situation at the time of reference. For some items this may make no or little difference; for others the difference can be important.

In the following discussion the respondents are sometimes said "not to recall," but what can be observed in the surveys is that they do not report or say they do not recall. It is seldom possible to check whether they really do not recall or just do not want to report. The research inquiry has some advantages over other types of questioning, but it puts the respondent under no obligation to answer truthfully at all cost. It just relies on the respondent's preference to do so if treated appropriately.

Telescoping

Some circumstances and aspects make recollection more precarious than otherwise. For example, estimating the time a recalled event occurred often turns out to be difficult. This is especially the case with fairly frequent events, each of which is not particularly salient. Estimates tend to be biased towards recency; that is, if a respondent errs, the event is usually reported as having happened more recently than it actually did. Such "telescoping" often leads to overreporting or false positives about events or actions within a specified time period because possible earlier events are recollected as occurring within that period.[6] For instance, when 433 British government employees retrospectively reported their periods of sick leave during each of five months, 55 monthly reports telescoped sick leaves to later months, whereas 27 reports moved them in the opposite direction. Twenty-eight reports contained sick leaves that were either telescoped from before the whole period or were invented, whereas 64 reports overlooked some episodes of sick leave (or placed them before the period under study). Of 205 employees who had no sick leave in the whole period, according to the staff records, 13 reported such leave (Gray, 1955:354–357). Public events have been found to be remembered as more recent the more that is known about them, that is, the more easily accessible (Brown, Rips, & Shevell, 1985).

When some boys give self-reports that they have been picked up by the police, although they have no police reports in the period in question (e.g., Hirschi, 1969:59), telescoping may be one explanation. Bachman & O'Malley (1981) found drug-use estimates based on last-month recalls inconsistently high compared with estimates based on last-year recalls.

In a Stockholm cohort 274 members between 17 and 30 years of age were identified as injecting drug addicts at least once. When examined they were also asked in what year they had started to inject. Forty-four persons refused to answer or did not remember, 88 were examined only once or gave the same answer when asked more than once, but 132, or 48% gave different years. Early in the period differences were few and small but gradually grew with time. The tendency was to give more recent years when interviewed later in the period (Torstensson, 1987:147).

Sudman and Bradburn (1973) went through about 500 studies in which retrospective data on various, mostly economic and, with the exception of voting, socially neutral subjects were validated in a total of about 4,000 codable entries. There is much irregular variation in their results, but overreporting in the nearest period and underreporting in the more remote periods seem to be the rule. One table shows slight overreporting by young respondents and considerable long-term underreporting by older respondents. It was concluded that the use of records in answering reduced telescoping but also the rate of recall to some extent. Using records would thus be "most appropriate for major events where omissions are unimportant and telescoping is the major source of error" (*Ibid.:* 815), whereas aided-recall techniques increased recollection but did not reduce telescoping. They would thus be "most helpful for less important events and for longer recall periods when telescoping effects have become small" (*Ibid.;* cf. Bradburn, 1983:309).

Robbins (1963) compared retrospective data with contemporary data on child development and child-rearing practices taken from a longitudinal study.[7] She found significant differences in the stated age at which several developments and practices took place. The retrospective dates tended to be more in accordance with the child-rearing recommendations by Dr. Spock and to some extent also to be more recent.

Whether the time direction in which questioning is carried out (e.g., starting with the early years and moving toward contemporary items, as in life-history interviewing, or doing it in the reverse direction) has any effect on telescoping is, to my knowledge, not known. However, some experimental results referred to by Bradburn, Rips, and Shevell (1987) suggest that sometimes moving backward from the most recent item may produce somewhat better recall, but that some respondents themselves prefer forward recall, whereas others prefer backward recall.

Questions of the type "Have you ever . . . ?" as well as other retrospective yes-or-no questions can give both false positives (yes-answers that should have been no) and false negatives (no-answers that should have been yes). The risk of errors on yes-or-no questions will, of course, depend on what the question is about and on how the question is put. On the whole, false positives tend to be more prominent in questions about socially valued and ego-enhancing actions, whereas false negatives will mostly appear in questions about socially undesirable behavior. Other questions will lead to a relative balance of positive and negative errors due to telescoping and omissions. However, for "Have you ever . . . ?" questions there can be no telescoping, so one can expect the false negatives to dominate. This was also what Norlén (1977) found when estimating the risk for false negatives and positives on 32 questions in two waves of a large Swedish survey. All except one estimated probability[8] of false positives were below 0.05, whereas the estimated probability of false negatives ranged between 0.05 and 0.89, with 23 of them on or above 0.20 and the median 0.39.

Further problems of recollection

As already mentioned, among factors that make for good recall are saliency and subjective importance, including ego-enhancing aspects. To the important things in life belong firsts of many meaningful events in the life course: change of marital status, change of household, moving, first job, first trip abroad, and so forth. The latest episode will be fairly easily recalled as long as it is the latest. There are also other kinds of such long-accessible items.

For persons with few job changes in their occupational career, the chain of jobs should be rather easy to recall. The average length of a job for a man in the United States has been estimated to be about two years and for a man in Germany to be about six years (Carroll & Mayer, 1986:325). If so, there are not too many jobs in a 20-year period for most men to remember and place in the right order. With what precision dates and other aspects can be recalled is another question (cf. Cannell & Kahn, 1968:541f. for reference to a study from 1961 by Weiss et al. who found inaccuracies increasing with time in work histories).

Comparing unemployment survey data concerning the previous week with such retrospective data concerning the previous year, Morgenstern and Barrett (1974) found considerable underreporting among females and young respondents. For young females the underreporting reached 50%, whereas males in the age category 25–44 and females in the 45+ category had some overreporting. No difference in reporting was found between races. Miller (1976), on the other hand, found little net difference in work status in 1965 and as reported retrospectively in the 1970 census, but quotes a comparison on the individual level of work status in 1963 as reported in 1963 and as reported retrospectively in 1968. It was found that the response rate in 1968 was much lower among 1963 nonworkers than among 1963 workers. About 13% retrospectively reported work status different from that of 1963 (26% for persons below age 30 in 1968).

Cannell and Kahn (1968:548) found that underreporting of hospital episodes varied according to length of stay, time since discharge from hospital, and degree of threateningly diagnosed illness. There was no underreporting found for stays of at least five days on threatening diagnoses and hospital discharge at most 20 weeks before the interview, but 56 and 33% underreporting for stays of less than five days and at least five days, respectively, on threatening diagnoses and hospital discharge more than 40 weeks before the interview. Underreporting was especially high among low-income people (Moss, 1979:161). Cannell and Kahn (1968:542) also mention a study from 1958 by Peters, who found that hospitalized patients had difficulty in reporting their preoperative anxieties only a few days after their surgery. Stunkard, Foster, Glassman, and Rosato (1985), on the other hand, found some patients greatly exaggerating retrospectively their first unpleasant postoperation symptoms.

Considering the tendency to telescope events and taking into account other problems in placing events and situations in time, dating phases in a more or less continuous process are likely to be especially error prone unless records can be consulted. It would be extremely risky to estimate retrospectively in adult years knowledge or ability at an earlier age, say at age 13, unless the result of an actual test at that age was recalled; it would be so risky, indeed, that it seems out of the question. The reasonable retrospective alternative is, of course, to ask for grades as presumably relevant measures. The nonretrospective item of present ability would be a test with tasks that the respondent would try to solve, presumably exerting himself in doing so. Obviously, this is not possible retrospectively. However, the retrospective difficulty is not limited to items where a taxing test is required. Other aspects of a gradual process may be correspondingly out of reach (e.g., height and weight at age 13) again unless nonretrospective records, such as a door post with old markings, can be consulted or special measuring situations have been memorized. This may be the case fairly often for some measures of income, for example, for first jobs and when changing jobs. If not, past income in an inflationary economy has the characteristic of a difficult retrospective item. However, Ferber and Birnbaum (1979) concluded that information on past earnings was not substantially less accurate than that obtained for current salary, and that self-reported income data are somewhat unreliable whether past or present.

Earlier attitudes, if changed, would also be difficult to estimate retrospectively. In the 1972 or 1973 and the 1982 American General Social Surveys, respondents were asked about their opinions on communism, busing, and miscegenation. In 1982 they were also asked about their opinions on these matters in 1972 or 1973. The retrospective distributions of opinions in 1972 or 1973 were then compared to the contemporary 1972/73 distribution for the same cohorts. On busing, the 1972 distribution was closely reproduced, although whites tended to remember themselves somewhat more positive than they were in 1972. However, as to miscegenation, on which the cohorts had changed very little in the 10 years, whites were less positive retrospectively. On communism the discrepancies were very large. In 1973 44.2% said communism was the worst form of government, and in 1982 70.7% remembered themselves as thinking so in 1973. On all three questions there were strong differences among educational levels. Those with education beyond high school remembered themselves as more positive to busing in 1972 than they were (27.2% agaisnt 19.9%), were on the average accurate as to their past views on racial intermarriage, and were very wrong as to their views on communism, with 27.6% actually giving the most negative answer in 1973 against 64.1% believing they did so in 1982 (Smith, 1984).

Inevitably, retrospective questions are answered in hindsight, from the vantage point of present time, knowing how things turned out in later circumstances and with the contemporary-time world outlook. This may not influence answers as to simple facts, except that those that proved to be important in later life will be easier to recall than the false starts and inconsequential episodes, some of which seemed important at the time they happened. This could seem to be an advantage, because the main features of the life history would stand out better and thus be more accessible. This may be so for simple facts, but as soon as one goes beyond them, hindsight can cause complications. Summary descriptions of how things "usually were" and any description that carries an evaluative meaning can easily be colored by later experience. It is difficult to describe married life in the reference period without being influenced by its later breakdown or happy continuation, or to describe business disregarding later failure or success. Traces of what happened subsequently are easily read into the early situation. Differential recall of events according to their later meaning can give a distorted view of the actual choices available and make the life history appear unduly straight and purposeful. It is usually conceded that the interpretative light of later history means such a risk of bias in retrospective measures of attitudes and values that such measures should be avoided, whereas factual events and situations can generally be ascertained retrospectively, with recall being fairly undisturbed by later outcomes. It is, however, difficult to draw a sharp distinction here between attitudes and values on the one hand and events and actions on the other, because action is one of the conceptual dimensions of an attitude (if the other dimensions are perception, cognition, and emotion). Attitudinally relevant actions and events are thus recalled and evaluatively characterized in the light of later development and present values. Factual sex-role behavior around 1965 reported around 1988 would be a likely illustration. Voting is another.

In American surveys voting tends to be overreported. Cannell and Kahn (1968:546) quote a study in which checking against registers showed 40% overreporting of voting against 2% overreporting of the possession of a telephone. In a survey Traugott and Katosh (1979) found that 39% of respondents who had not registered said they had, and 29% even said they voted, whereas only 4% of those who had registered said they had not. Retrospective surveys tend to get election figures adjusted according to hindsight, with winners getting more and losers less. The exemplar is the 1952 questioning on the 1948 American presidential election allocating 57, 41, and 2% of the votes to Truman, Dewey, and Thurmond-Wallace against the actual results of 50, 45, and 5% (Campbell, Gurin, & Miller, 1954:218). Until the end of the 1960s, Swedish Communist voters were rarer in retrospective surveys than in the election booths, and in the radical 1970s the same held for Swedes voting on a bourgeois party.

Probably, the inevitable risk of hindsight bias on attitudes, values, and evaluated actions and events limits the usefulness of retrospective questioning as much as the difficulty of recollection. When good reasons can be given for suspecting hindsight to be a strong influence on responses, the burden of proof should be on the one who wants to use the data.

Socially undesirable behavior

The discussion has already touched upon the subject of socially undesirable behavior. Our recollections are partly molded by the relevance they have on our self-conception. Because a fair amount of social esteem is often a necessary condition of our self-respect, our opinion of the desirability of our behavior, situation, and characteristics is a powerful functional factor in what and how we recollect. In various fields tendencies are noticed to overreport socially desirable aspects, such as voting, respectable opinions, possessions, and going abroad or by air, and to underreport socially undesirable aspects, such as taking loans, being fired, smoking, and drinking alcohol. As structural factors can be assumed to weaken over time, recollection can be expected to decrease and distortions to increase. Decreasing functional importance could at least partially compensate for this as to distortion.

Various face-saving formulations are often used to diminish underreporting. Questionnaire studies avoid the embarrassing face-to-face relation of the interview (cf. Björkman, 1979; about telephone interviews, see Groves & Kahn, 1979), but tend to give high nonresponse. Anonymous questionnaires are assumed to ease the reporting of deviant or otherwise socially undesirable behavior.

Certainly, there are problems in recalling such behavior. Inconspicuous details of socially undesirable habits or gradual changes in these habits cannot be recalled any better than other routine activities. Frequent minor offenses are hard to recall as to dates, number, and details in a rather short period of time. Questions on alcohol consumption usually require very short time spans and ask about the latest drinking occasion, providing various cues; yet there is still considerable underreporting (cf. Midanik, 1982). Reasonably, more noteworthy events such as being picked up by the police or being hospitalized after an overdose (if these things do not happen too often) can be recalled longer. Delinquency self-reports seldom span more than a year and mostly focus on minor offenses, which dominate numerically (cf. Hindelang, Hirschi, & Weis, 1981; Elliot, Huizinga, & Ageton, 1985). Usually, self-reports about police or other judiciary contacts agree fairly well with official records (e.g., Farrington, 1983), which in most cases is the only check that can be made. Presumably, at least some respondents may know or suspect that this item in their records can be checked as to recent events.[9] Of course, with anonymous questionnaires nothing can be checked on an individual level. As a note of caution it can be mentioned that, for a discussion of the validity of an anonymous survey about drug use in school, Kühlhorn and Åslund (1983) instead of drug-use questions, asked about the latest marks in a class and found a considerably elevated distribution compared to what the school register said. As to the underreporting of abortions, see Mosher, 1985.

Efficient studies of socially undesirable behavior in most cases presume a rather limited time range for possible retrospective items; how short a range depends on the type of behavior studied. Yet when it comes to strongly undesirable behavior, problems of recall are not the main difficulty. They would remain even with a nonretrospective survey. When respondents feel that affirming a behavior asked about is a matter of their confessing, admitting, being exposed or unmasked, their predicament is at least as great if the question concerns present-time as if it concerns past-time behavior, which they recall fairly vividly. Now it is not a matter of recall but a question whether to answer truthfully (assuming the correct answer is positive). If anything, the dilemma of respondents' admitting they are now alcoholic or on welfare would be worse than admitting they were so some time ago. Respondents are under no obligation always to tell the truth. They are participating out of pressure, citizenship, or what they can get out of being questioned. Like most people, they prefer telling the truth as long as it is not too uncomfortable. Occasionally, they might be "helpful" by giving the answer they believe is expected of them. The interviewer is not a significant person to them, and the research is of moderate interest, so they might not care very much what the interviewer thinks of them and even less what the results of the study will be; but they might not trust the interviewer very much and might not like to have negative information on them fed into the computer.

The choice respondents make, whether to admit, to deny, or to refuse to answer, or perhaps not to recall, will, of course, depend on the question, what they have to admit, the general context, and their general values and attitudes. It will also depend on their attitude to their own behavior. There are often better ways of coping with it than not to recall it. The behavior may be undesirable in principle, but those who tend to engage in it can develop schemes of rationalizations according to which the behavior was perfectly justified (as to juvenile delinquents, see the classic paper by Sykes and Matza, 1957). It can be seen as a prank by a teenager and something to brag about. When a majority of young people report that they think they drink less than their peers, this can be interpreted (if they are honest about it) as fictitious social pressure, which may not influence their drinking (Kühlhorn & Helmersson, 1984) but still make it easier to report or even to exaggerate their drinking. The AA member is eager to define himself or herself as an alcoholic, and converted sinners excel in their past sins as contrasted with their present pure life. Aiken (1986) thinks that some drug addicts on a treatment program wanted to present themselves in a favorable light to obtain treatment (methadone), but retrospectively gave a less favorable picture of themselves (except as to trouble with the law).

In view of all this, in the field of strongly undesirable behavior one can agree with Nettler that "asking people questions about their behavior is a poor way of observing it" (Nettler, 1978:107). At least it seems fair to let the burden of proof rest on whoever wants to challenge that.

Evaluations of retrospective survey data

Most of the behavioral science literature on retrospective survey data fall into two broad categories. The first includes discussions of problems and defects of retrospective data, sometimes concluding with warnings against, or suggestions for improving, retrospective data. The other category consists of reports that retrospective data have been successfully used in a given study. Besides the tendency to protect professional investments and positions on both sides and different scientific orientations, four main reasons for this apparently contradictory situation can be conjectured.

First, it is clear that retrospective data work differently in different fields and on different problems. Second, data quality is usually most profitably seen as better or worse, rather than yes or no, and is also often evaluated against available alternatives.

Third, it is usually difficult to evaluate the validity of a retrospective item. A parallel can be drawn to the evaluation of nonresponse. We often cannot check with the factual state of affairs because we do not know it, which is precisely why we asked the retrospective question. Sometimes we can compare with other sources, nonretrospective answers, or register data, and so can find some degree of correspondence, but the criterion is only approximate and also contains some deficiencies. Often the comparisons concern net differences (i.e., distributions), but sometimes individual data can be compared.

Holland (1987) finds retrospective data on breast-feeding valid essentially because they fit a logit model very well. Akers, Massey, Clarke, and Lauer (1983:248) find evidence "that self-reports of deviant behavior in adolescent populations are usually valid," and Ben-Yehuda (1980:1269) concludes that addicts' self-reports are valid if given in a "neutral, nonthreatening, nonmanipulative situation." To Bernard, Killworth, Kronenfeld, and Sailer (1984), Akers et al. represent a minority position. Comparing with records, Marquis (1984) finds no bias in survey data on health care and undesirable behavior. Robins et al. (1985) compared interviews at age 40 with former psychiatric patients on childhood conditions with clinical records and found modest agreement. However, when answers by former patients and their siblings were compared, they exhibited somewhat better, although still modest, agreement than that between controls and their siblings. Robins et al. think this is "encouraging because it suggests that such retrospective interviews may be reasonably valid." Yarrow, Campbell, and Burton (1970) compared retrospective interviews with mothers and children on childhood development with baseline data collected during the child's years in nursery school. The results show only moderate agreement. Data "are perhaps as much the products of the informants and instruments as they are of the phenomena being investigated" (1970:36).

In 1971 Natalie Ramsöy sampled 3,472 men, 1,094 of whom were born in 1931, to be interviewed retrospectively about their life histories. She could compare the answers of 622 men in 1971 about their father's occupation when they were 14 (in 1945) with the answers they gave when interviewed by a military psychologist around 1950, when most were aged 19. Unfortunately, the retrospective interviews in 1971 did not contain a question about their father's occupation in 1950, although the comparison with the military interviews was planned. However, considering the five-year gap, the agreement is seen as "very encouraging." In a nine-category classification, almost 82% of 622 main breadwinners were classified in the same category according to both answers. When the men's own occupations at the end of 1950, according to the 1971 interviews and at the time of the military interviews, were compared for all boys not still in school, almost 77% of 477 pairs of answers were identically classified.[10] Ramsöy points out that the two sets of interviews do not refer to exactly the same time and that boys at this age often change occupations (Ramsöy, 1977:54–60).

Certainly, it would be unfair to blame the retrospective character of the questions for the total discrepancy from full agreement, even to the extent that it cannot be attributed to imprecision in the comparisons with records. Even a contemporary survey would have given differences if it had been repeated in, say, three weeks. Nevertheless, adding errors to already somewhat unreliable nonretrospective data evidently makes data even less reliable.

Furthermore, a closer scrutiny of the figures (*Ibid.*, 58f.) shows that the largest category for both fathers and sons, that is, "farming, forestry, and fishing," is significantly larger according to the contemporary military interviews than according to the retrospective life-history interviews, 45.2% against 41.5% for the fathers and 32.5% against 26.4% for the sons themselves. As the 1950 interviews generally refer to somewhat earlier dates than the 1971 interviews, some boys may have moved to town in the interval, but one would expect the category's share of fathers not to be larger in 1950 than in 1945. Nevertheless, the quality of Ramsöy's data should be evaluated in relation to the way data are used.

Thus, the fourth reason for disagreement about the value of retrospective questions is the different uses to which they are put. Although the precision of some data is too low for one kind of analysis, it may be sufficient for some other kind. Even if the consumption of alcohol, the extent of smoking, or frequency of delinquent acts is grossly underestimated in a given set of data, it can be used profitably to analyze differences among categories in alcohol consumption, smoking, or delinquency (perhaps in prevalence if not in incidence) or associations between such behavior and other variables, if errors are random or not associated with the category or the variables used. If so, differences and associations would be attenuated but would stand up, if observed. Also, bias in the opposite direction would, of course, not invalidate findings.

Systematic errors in recall can often be indicated, but differential errors afflicting some categories of respondents more than others with the same true answer to the question are more difficult to establish, although they could be expected for theoretical or technical reasons. Of course, even without differential errors, attenuation can be considerable but hard to estimate, and categories defined by retrospective question can be uncomfortably heterogeneous. It may be mentioned that with both omissions and telescoping occurring, it is those who acknowledge infrequent behavior or events that make up a heterogeneous category containing true and false positives, whereas the false negatives will make only a small percentage of the negatives.

Nonretrospective alternatives

As pointed out, in evaluating the merits of retrospective surveys alternatives should also be considered. The quality of retrospective items will not be better or worse in an absolute sense depending on the quality of possible alternatives, but evidently the research strategy in taking the risk of using less than perfect data will, here as elsewhere, appear more rational if alternative strategies of studying a subject on the whole involve greater risk; and it will appear less rational if alternative strategies with less risk are available.

Two main alternatives to the retrospective study in instant longitudinal research are immediately obvious. The first is the nonretrospective survey, or rather a series of such surveys, to produce and record the items at or near reference time. This would (almost) eliminate problems of recall and telescoping, and would make possible the recording of attitudes, values, abilities, and stages of continuous change – variables that are generally conceded highly unsuitable for retrospective recording. Although many of the difficulties in getting valid data on socially nondesirable and otherwise ego-threatening behavior would remain, nonretrospective surveys would undoubtedly give distinct advantages, especially as to attitudes, early abilities, and similar variables.

However, there are costs for this. First, of course, the study would no longer be instant but would instead drag on at least for the interval between the first survey and the end of the period under observation. This is not to say that there would be need for an uninterrupted project organization all this time. Even so, it is often asserted that the protracted longitudinal project is necessarily substantially more expensive than the instant variant. Of course, the strong difference in time-cost is definitional. A series of nonretrospective surveys would probably be more expensive than a comprehensive retrospective survey, but some circumstances may make the difference less than sometimes seems to be assumed. In the last 30 years or so the cost of fieldwork has increased to reach exorbitant levels. Furthermore, for a school-age cohort one may arrange to have questionnaires filled out in school with much reduced cost and nonresponse. On the other hand, if small problem categories can be identified in drawing a retrospective sample, a much smaller sample of control cases is necessary. This, however, will not do for general life-history studies (e.g., of social mobility) and only to a limited extent for studies of several problem categories, each in need of its own control sample.

A well-known problem often afflicting protracted longitudinal studies is case attrition, whereas the instant variety loses only deceased cases, out-migrants (replaced by in-migrants), and nonresponse cases. However, some longitudinal projects show that attrition can be kept within reasonable limits by frequent contacts and when good population bookkeeping is available (cf. Farrington's chapter on case attrition).

Finally, a more basic disadvantage of the longitudinal study of long duration would be the risk of data's fading relevance (Janson, 1978:39–43). In 20 years, for example, there can be considerable development in research technique, statistical models, and theory. Data collected with contemporary statistical procedures in mind to test specified hypotheses from then-current theories can be less suited to fashionable procedures at the end of the observed period, and the original hypotheses as well as the theories they were derived from can be of less interest as new theoretical questions come into focus.

Such fading can certainly be dangerous to all protracted research when the research is neither brilliant nor lucky. If research were as cumulative as it should be, the danger would probably be greater than it is with theoretical and analytical fashions coming and going. However, some strategies make fading less likely than otherwise. What is claimed here is that the lag between the time of recording and the time of analysis is also of some importance to the quality of the data. On closer inspection it is rather the lag between the time or times at which the characteristics of data are settled on the one hand (phases c and d) and the times of the analysis and reporting on the other hand (phase e) that matters. Contrary to what is usually prescribed in sociological teachings on methods, a rule for good planning here as elsewhere appears to be keeping alternatives open as long as feasible. In this case decisions on data specifications can be taken at stage d (making data ready for analysis) and this stage placed close to the final stage of analysis and interpretation of results, thus making the lag between crucial decisions and analysis as small as possible. This will do when relevant events or situations have been recorded and the current value of data is a question of aspects. For instance, occupation is likely to retain its relevance in studies of social stratification and social mobility, whereas preferred classifications according to social classes or strata may change with time. Keeping recorded occupations in text *en clair* or in a detailed classification will make it possible to adapt to several class or stratification models. A broad approach to data will increase the chance that relevant data have been collected. Narrowly restricting data to what is relevant in terms of a courageously unestablished and highly specified model obviously increases the risk of missing data relevant in terms of other models.

A second alternative to the retrospective survey is to use nonretrospective documents, particularly governmental microdata from administrative registers and files. If a register is cumulative and unpruned, the excerpts to be recorded can be made as close to the analytical phase as in a retrospective survey. It is often pointed out that documentary data are not themselves free of errors and cannot be used without reservation as criteria for the validity of survey data. On the other hand, sociologists generally seem to consider the extracting of files as tedious but unproblematic. As secondary data, governmental microdata are often considered to be second-rate data. Undoubtedly they have limitations. The first has to do with what has been produced, preserved, and is now available. Second, what is available for extracting is almost exclusively factual and often decidedly "etic" information with other data missing. As generally agreed, however, it also holds for long-term retrospective surveys that they cannot usually provide valid attitudinal and early ability data. It should also be pointed out that governmental microdata are of many kinds: government surveys such as censuses of population and taxation registers; reports on tests, inspections, investigations, or proceedings; minutes of decisions by agencies; lists of school grades, and so forth. The critical but open mind of the historian would be desirable.

A factor strongly in favor of good governmental microdata as compared with surveys is the low rate of missing values, which can often rather easily be brought down to a few percent before one is giving up on cases demanding a disproportional amount of work. In surveys the nonresponse rate is seldom much below 10% and sometimes well above 20%. Possibly selective nonresponse of that order is difficult to handle, at least in the absence of extensive supplementary information from other sources. Just giving the nonresponse figures, showing a few tables on sampling categories such as sex and race, adjusting weights on categories, and then proceeding is not always an acceptable solution. Take as an illustration of survey nonresponse the central study of modern criminology, Travis Hirschi's *Causes of Delinquency* (1969). Among non-Negro boys the nonresponse at the high school survey varies from table to table from 28% and up. For example, in Table 2 (Ibid:43) it is 37%.[11] There one can calculate the corresponding figure for non-Negro boys known to the police for at least three offenses to be at least 70%.

It is clearly possible to make a meaningful instant longitudinal study based on nonretrospective governmental microdata if one can dispense with attitudinal and original ability data. Gunnar Boalt's study (1947) of the selection to higher education within a Stockholm cohort born around 1925 is an example. The analyses are based on parental occupation, assessed income, and dependency according to population registers, and the cohort members' gender, marks, and educational careers according to school records. Subsequently, register data were added for studies of the male cohort members' social mobility (1954): mental test scores at military enlistment and occupations according to a population register.

The clearest advantage in using documentary data probably relates to studies of socially undesirable situations and behavior, for some deviant behavior in studies focusing on prevalence rather than incidence. Most likely, most researchers find it more reassuring to know from the records of the relevant social-welfare agency that a given family was not on welfare in a given period than to hear the head of the family claim that the family was not. The amount of economic support received may also be more validly found with the agency than from the family head, although errors in records should not be ruled out.

Conclusions

In longitudinal studies, with their focus on differential processes, some information is risky to obtain through retrospective surveys. This holds true for attitudes and opinions and generally for behavior containing important evaluative elements as well as for abilities and some gradual changes. Here the nonretrospective, contemporary survey can provide more valid information. However, in the case of undesirable behavior and threatening events, such a survey may reduce problems of recall but still has to solve the main problem of getting the respondents to tell what they recall. If focus is mainly on prevalence rather than on incidence, governmental microdata may help out here. Finally, hindsight may distort reporting in retrospective surveys.

Excluding the types of information mentioned above and with some other general limitations as to data, instant longitudinal surveys are feasible and may be supplemented to good effect in some substantive areas by nonretrospective register data. In fact, instant longitudinal studies can be built exclusively on nonretrospective governmental microdata, although this puts severe restrictions on aspects to be included in the study.

Considering time and money factors, the instant longitudinal variety is probably bound to be the most popular or at least the most frequent version. However, it is imperative that analyses of theoretically crucial questions can be based also on nonretrospective data, when retrospective data are likely to be deficient in relevant aspects or as long as serious doubts on their validity remain. Since registers can provide only certain types of data, this means that the protracted longitudinal study still has an important part to play.

Notes

1 By "longitudinal studies" is meant "cohort studies and other long-term studies of micro-units, individually compared over time, and with observations covering a period, either by a series of cross-sections or by more or less continuous records or both" (Janson, 1984:5).

2 If the study deals with a series of points in time rather than with a period, the necessary adequate modifications of definitions and comments are obvious. Thus, the end of the period will correspond to the latest point in time, and the beginning of the period to the earliest point.

3 As the discussion here concerns longitudinal studies as defined above, it can be limited to large-scale statistical studies.

4 By definition, if the purpose of asking a question about past circumstances is to find out the respondent's present view on these circumstances, the question is not retrospective. Its time of reference coincides with the time the question is answered, that is, "produced."

5 If A denotes the original experience, a its recall, and B the occurrence of an interfering experience, the interference is proactive if the time sequence is $B\ A\ a$ and retroactive if the sequence is $A\ B\ a$. In a series of similar events or situations, the recall of early events can be retroactively interfered by later events and the latest events proactively interfered by earlier events. Within the series, the items in the middle would be subjected to both proactive and retroactive interferences and thus would be difficult to recall, whereas the first items would be interfered with only retroactively and would be somewhat more easily recalled (primacy effect); and the latest items, because subjected only to proactive interference, also would be better recalled (recency effect). Interference could also originate in other series of events (Cf. diagrams for learned material in Murdock, 1973:536, and Baddeley, 1986:155–157.)

6 Sudman and Bradburn (1973) suggest that the rate of recalled events within time t varies according to the formula

$$r(t) = ae^{-b_1 t}\left[1 + \frac{\log b_2 t}{t} \right]$$

where the second term refers to telescoping.

7 For another example of comparing retrospective data with contemporary data from a longitudinal study, see Cherry and Rodgers (1979).

8 This item was really not of the have-you-ever type, because it was "Can you file a complaint to a governmental agency?"

9 If records are pruned to underline rehabilitation, as in the Swedish National Police Register, the possibility to check is limited to a few years.

10 In the first cross-tabulation, the largest three categories contained about 81% of the fathers, and in the second table they held about 89% of the boys.

11 Note that Hirschi's sample consists of school children, caught in school, whereas the instant longitudinal sample is one of adult persons to be contacted individually. If the school register misses some drop outs, the nonresponse rate will be even higher.

References

Aiken, L. S. (1986). Retrospective self-reports by clients differ from original reports. *International Journal of the Addictions, 21*(7), 767–788.

Akers, R. L., Massey, J., Clarke, W., & Lauer, R. M. (1983). Are self-reports of adolescent deviance valid? *Social Forces, 62,* 234–251.

Bachman, J. G., & O'Malley, P. M. (1981). When four months equal a year. *Public Opinion Quarterly, 45,* 536–548.

Baddeley, A. (1979). The limitations of human memory. In Moss & Goldstein, 1979:13–27.

Baddeley, A. (1986). *Working memory.* Oxford: Clarendon Press.

Baddeley, A., Lewis, V., Eldridge, M., & Thomsen, N. (1985). Attention and retrieval from long-term memory." *Journal of Experimental Psychology, 9*(113), 518–540.

Bartlett, F. C. (1932). *Remembering.* Cambridge: Cambridge University Press.

Ben-Yehuda, N. (1980). Are addicts' self-reports to be trusted? *International Journal of the Addictions, 15,* 1265–1270.

Bernard, H. R., Killworth, P., Kronenfeld, D., & Sailer, L. (1984). The problem of informant accuracy. *Annual Review of Anthropology 13,* 495–517.

Björkman, N.-M. (1979). *Social önskvärdhet som felkälla i frågeundersökningar.* Stockholm: Department of Sociology.

Boalt, G. (1947). *Skolutbildning och skolresultat.* Stockholm: Norstedts.

Boalt, G. (1954). Social mobility in Stockholm. *Transactions of the Second World Congress of Sociology* (Vol. 2).

Bradburn, N. M. (1983). Response effects. In P. H. Rossi, J. D. Wright, & A. B. Anderson (Eds.), *Handbook of survey research* (pp. 289–328). New York: Academic Press.

Bradburn, N. M., Rips, L. J., & Shevell, S. K. (1987). Answering autobiographical questions. *Science, 236,* 157–161.

Brown, N. R., Rips, L. J., & Shevell, S. K. (1985). The subjective dates of natural events in very-long-term memory. *Cognitive Psychology, 17,* 139–177.

Campbell, A., Gurin, G., & Miller, W. E. (1954). *The voter decides.* New York: Harper & Brothers.

Cannell, C. F., & Kahn, R. L. (1968). Interviewing. In G. Lindzey & E. Aronson (Eds.), *The handbook of social psychology* (Vol. 2, pp. 526–595). Reading, MA: Addison-Wesley.

Carlsson, G. (1954). *Socialpsykologisk metod.* Stockholm: Svenska bokförlaget.

Carroll, G. R., & Mayer, K. V. (1986). Job-shift patterns in the Federal Republic of Germany. *American Sociological Review 51*(3), 323–341.

Cherry, N., & Rodgers, B. (1979). Using a longitudinal study to assess the quality of retrospective data. In Moss & Goldstein, 1979:31–42.

Conway, M. A., & Bekerian, D. A. (1987). Organization in autobiographical memory. *Memory and Cognition, 15*(2), 119–132.

Crowder, R. G. (1976). *Principles of learning and memory.* New York: Wiley.

Elliot, D. S., Huizinga, D., & Ageton, S. (1985). *Explaining delinquency and drug use.* Beverly Hills, CA: Sage.

Farrington, D. P. (1983). Offending from 10 to 25 years of age. In K. T. Van Dusen & S. A. Mednick (Eds.), *Prospective studies of crime and delinquency* (pp. 17–37). Boston: Kluwer-Nijhoff.

Ferber, M. A., & Birnbaum, B. G. (1979). Retrospective earning data. *Public Opinion Quarterly, 43,* 112–118.

Gray, P. G. (1955). The memory factor in social surveys. *Journal of the American Statistical Association, 50,* 344–363.

Groves, R. M., & Kahn, R. L. (1979). *Surveys by telephone.* New York: Academic Press.

Gruneberg, M. M., & Morris, P. (Eds.), (1978). *Aspects of memory.* London: Methuen.

Harris, M. (1980). *Cultural materialism.* New York: Random House.

Hindelang, M. J., Hirschi, T., & Weis, J. G. (1981). *Measuring delinquency.* Beverly Hills, CA: Sage.

Hirschi, T. (1969). *Causes of delinquency.* Berkeley: University of California Press, 1969.

Holland, B. (1987). The validity of retrospective breast-feeding duration data. *Human Biology, 59*(3), 477–487.

Hunter, I. M. L. (1964). *Memory.* Middlesex: Penguin.

Jabine, T. B., Straf, M. L., Tanur, J. M., & Tourangean, R. (Eds.). (1984). *Cognitive aspects of survey methodology.* Washington, DC: National Academy Press.

Janson, C.-G. (1978). *The longitudinal approach.* Research Report No. 9. Stockholm: Project Metropolitan. Also in Schulsinger, F., Mednick, S. A., & Knop, J. (Eds.) (1981). *Longitudinal research* (pp. 19–55). Boston: Martinus Nijhoff.

Janson, C.-G. (1984). *Project metropolitan: A presentation and progress report.* Research Report No. 21. Stockholm: Project Metropolitan.

Kühlhorn, E., & Åslund, P. (1983). Skolöverstyrelsens frekvensundersökningar och verkligheten. In A. Solarz (Ed.), *Narkotikautvecklingen.* Report No. 6. Stockholm: Crime Prevention Council.

Kühlhorn, E., & Helmersson, K. (1984). Fiktivt socialt tryck och majoritetsmissförståndet. *Alkohol och narkotika 7,* 8–12.

Marquis, K. (1984). Record checks for sample surveys. In Jabine et al., 1984:130–147.

Midanik, L. (1982). The validity of self-reported alcohol consumption and alcohol problems. *British Journal of Addiction, 77,* 357–382.

Miller, A. R. (1976). Retrospective data on work status in the 1970 census of population. *Journal of the American Statistical Association, 71*(354), 286–292.

Morgenstern, R. D., & Barrett, N. S. (1974). The retrospective bias in unemployment reporting by sex, race and age. *Journal of the American Statistical Association, 69*(346), 355–357.

Morris, P. (1978). Encoding and retrieval. In Gruneberg & Morris, 1978:61–83.

Mosher, W. D. (1985). Reproductive impairments in the United States. *Demography, 22,* 415–430.

Moss, L. (1979). Overview. In Moss & Goldstein, 1979:159–169.

Moss, L., & Goldstein, H. (Eds.) (1979). *The recall method in social surveys.* London: University of London.

Murdock, B. B. (1973). Remembering and forgetting. In B. B. Wolman (Ed.), *Handbook of general psychology* (pp. 530–543). Englewood Cliffs, NJ: Prentice-Hall.

Nettler, G. (1978). *Explaining crime* (2nd ed.). New York: McGraw-Hill.

Norlén, U. (1977). Response errors in the answers to retrospective questions. *Statistisk Tidskrift 4,* 331–341.

Postman, L. (1951). Toward a general theory of cognition. In J. Rohrer & M. Sherif (Eds.), *Social psychology at the crossroads* (pp. 248–265). New York: Harper & Brothers.

Ramsöy, N. R. (1977). *Sosial Mobilitet i Norge*. Oslo: Tiden Norsk Forlag.

Reiser, B. J., Black, J. B., & Abelson, R. P. (1985). Knowledge structures in the organization and retrieval of autobiographical memories. *Cognitive Psychology, 17*(1), 89–137.

Robbins, L. C. (1963). The accuracy of parental recall of aspects of child development and of child-rearing practices. *Journal of Abnormal and Social Psychology, 66*, 261–270.

Robins, L. N., Schoenberg, S. P., Holmes, S. J., Ratcliff, K. S., Benham, A., & Workes, J. (1985). Early home-environment and retrospective recall. *American Journal of Orthopsychiatry, 55*(1), 27–41.

Rubin, D. C. (1986). *Autobiographical memory*. Cambridge: Cambridge University Press.

Schyberger, B. W. (1965). *Methods of readership research*. Lund: Gleerup.

Shweder, R. A., & D'Andrade, R. G. (1980). The systematic distortion hypothesis. *New directions for the methodology of behavioral science 4*, 37–58, as quoted by Bernard et al., 1984.

Sikkel, D. (1985). Models for memory effects. *Journal of American Statistical Association, 80*(392), 835–840.

Smith, T. (1984). Recalling attitudes. *Public Opinion Quarterly, 48*(3), 639–649.

Stunkard, A., Foster, G., Glassman, J., & Rosato, E. (1985). Retrospective exaggeration of symptoms. *Psychosomatic Medicine, 47*(2), 150–155.

Sudman, S., & Bradburn, N. M. (1973). Effects of time and memory factors on response in surveys. *Journal of the American Statistical Association, 68*, 344, Appl. Sec., 805–815.

Sudman, S., & Bradburn, N. M. (1983). *Asking questions*. San Francisco: Jossey-Bass.

Sykes, G. M., & Matza, D. (1957). Techniques of neutralization. *American Sociological Review, 22*, 664–670.

Torstensson, M. (1987). *Drug-abusers in a metropolitan cohort*. Research Report No. 25. Stockholm: Project Metropolitan.

Traugott, M. W., & Katosh, J. P. (1979). Response validity in surveys of voting behavior. *Public Opinion Quarterly, 43*, 359–377.

Wagenaar, W. A. (1986). My Memory. *Cognitive Psychology, 18*(2), 225–252.

Yarrow, M. R., Campbell, J. D., & Burton, R. V. (1970). Recollections of Childhood. *Monographs of the Society for Research in Child Development, 35*(5), Serial No. 138).

7   Minimizing attrition in
     longitudinal research:
     Methods of tracing and securing
     cooperation in a 24-year follow-up study

DAVID P. FARRINGTON, BERNARD GALLAGHER,
LYNDA MORLEY, RAYMOND J. St. LEDGER, AND
DONALD J. WEST

Introduction

Attrition refers to the loss of subjects from a survey. In a survey based on searches of records, for example, it is often true that not all the target sample can be found in the records. Similarly, in a survey based on interviewing, the actual number of persons interviewed is almost invariably less than the target sample ideally to be interviewed. The focus of interest in this paper is on surveys that involve face-to-face personal interviews. Of concern for researchers, refusal rates in social surveys have increased considerably since the 1950s (Steeh, 1981).

Attrition can be a problem in cross-sectional research, but it is potentially a much greater problem in longitudinal surveys because longitudinal researchers need to contact specified persons repeatedly. In a one-off cross-sectional survey it may not matter who is contacted, so long as the sample interviewed is representative of the population.

For example, in attempting to interview a representative sample of persons aged 16 or over in England and Wales about crimes committed against them, Hough and Mayhew (1983) began by selecting persons listed on the electoral registers. It is known that about 96% of addresses of private households are listed on these registers. When an interviewer called at each address, he or she first enquired about all persons aged 16 or over living there. If the persons living there exactly matched those on the electoral register, an interview was sought with the selected person. If not, the interviewer enumerated all persons in the household aged 16 and over and selected one for interview according to a random number grid.

It should be noted that, in this cross-sectional survey, an attempt was not made to interview specified persons listed on the electoral registers. This would have created difficulties, because the labor force survey shows that 11% of adults move during the currency of any electoral register. Hence, an attempt to interview specified persons would inevitably have involved attempts to trace the movers. Even without this complication, interviews were not achieved at 20% of selected households (in addition to the 4% that were found to be vacant or derelict).

There are many reasons for attrition. For example, Farrington and Dowds (1985) provided detailed attrition figures for a similar cross-sectional victim survey in three English counties. Out of 3,990 addresses selected, 142 (3.6%) were vacant or derelict. Of the remainder, it was not possible to contact anyone at 99 addresses (2.6%), and there was complete refusal of information at a further 123 (3.2%). The selected person refused in 296 cases (7.7%), there were 107 refusals on behalf of the selected person (2.8%), the selected person broke an appointment in 25 cases (0.6%), and the selected person was always out in 48 cases (1.2%). Other reasons for attrition were that the selected person was away or in the hospital (36 cases, or 0.9%), senile or ill (66 cases, or 1.7%), or spoke inadequate English (18 cases, or 0.5%), and there were 8 other miscellaneous reasons (0.2%). The total attrition rate was 826 out of 3,848 addresses not vacant or derelict, or 21.5%; this was rather similar to the British Crime Survey figure of 20.4% (Hough & Mayhew, 1983).

We believe that it is important for researchers to report detailed attrition figures. It is distressing to read that the "majority of research reports published in the major international psychiatric journals fail to state explicitly what proportion of subjects approached declined to participate. Instead, a variety of literary devices are used to convey the impression that the sample is representative of the group under study" (Condon, 1986:87).

Unlike cross-sectional reseachers, longitudinal researchers do not have the luxury of selecting a random person at an address. The focus in longitudinal research on change and continuity means that specified persons have to be interviewed at every data collection point. Missing persons cannot be replaced. Because longitudinal researchers have to interview specified persons, this raises the major problem of tracing subjects. Longitudinal researchers also have to contend with death and emigration as reasons for attrition. Hence, it might be expected that attrition rates would be greater in longitudinal surveys than in cross-sectional ones and that they would increase with the length of the follow-up, because problems of tracing, death, and emigration are likely to increase over time.

Cordray and Polk (1983) reviewed attrition rates in longitudinal surveys of crime and delinquency, and concluded that they varied widely, from 5% to 60%. Famous pioneers such as the Gluecks (1940), Robins (1966), and McCord (1978) were able to locate and interview high proportions of their samples over follow-up periods of 15 years or more. Robins, West, and Herjanic (1975), for example, located and interviewed 223 out of 235 black males identified in records in St. Louis 20 years before. More recently, Cairns and Cairns (1987) traced all except 4 out of nearly 700 schoolchildren over a 5-year period, and reinterviewed 97%.

Attrition rates, however, have been very high in some longitudinal surveys. Capaldi and Patterson (1987) found that the average attrition rate in major American surveys with follow-up periods of 4–10 years was 47%. In the classic Philadelphia cohort study of Wolfgang, Thornberry, and Figlio (1987), they were able to interview only 567 of their target sample of 975 males at age 26 (58%). The major problem was that many could not be located, despite three years of diligent searching, using the Selective Service address file, motor vehicle registrations, post office assistance, the social service exchange, and other agencies. Locating subjects is less of a problem in the Scandinavian countries, because each person has a unique identification number based on his or her date of birth and because of the ease of linking up all computerized records.

Effects of attrition

The major problem with attrition is that those who are lost are usually not representative of all subjects. On the contrary, they often include a disproportionate number of the more antisocial and criminal people who are the most interesting to researchers in criminology and psychopathology. In their Philadelphia survey, Wolfgang et al. (1987) found that the missing subjects were disproportionately nonwhite, of low socioeconomic status, and officially delinquent. Hence, conclusions drawn from surveys with high attrition rates may be seriously in error, for example, in underestimating the true prevalence of antisocial and criminal behavior.

An advantage of a longitudinal (as opposed to a cross-sectional) survey is that many characteristics of missing subjects may be known from earlier interviews, thereby permitting an estimate of the maximum error caused by attrition. For example, Eron, Huesmann, Dubow, Romanoff, and Yarmel (1987) reported that the males who were missing in their follow-up at age 30 tended to have had high aggressiveness and low intelligence at age 8. (For examples of other research on the characteristics of elusive and refusing subjects, see Bebbington, 1970; Cottler, Zipp, Robins, & Spitznagel, 1987; Crider & Willits, 1973; Fitzgerald & Fuller, 1982; Friday & Sonnad, 1979; Paikin et al., 1974).

In earlier work on the longitudinal survey to be described in this chapter, West and Farrington (1973) reported that parents who were uncooperative (5%) or reluctant (5%) to participate in the survey when their boys were aged 8 were significantly likely to have boys who were later convicted as juveniles. About 40% of these boys became juvenile delinquents, in comparison with only 18% of those who had cooperative parents at age 8. Similarly, when the boys were aged 18, West and Farrington (1977) showed that 36% of the one-fifth of the sample who were the most difficult to interview were convicted, in comparison with only 22% of the majority who were interviewed more easily, a statistically significant difference.

In this survey, we have been unusually successful in tracing over 400 men and in securing their cooperation over a 24-year time period, from age 8 to age 32. For example, 10 years after the survey began, when the men were aged 18, we traced all except one and interviewed 95%. For our most recent interview at age 32, every man was eventually traced, and 94% were interviewed or completed questionnaires. The aim of this paper is to describe and analyze the methods of tracing and securing cooperation used at age 32, and to study the factors that are related to elusiveness and uncooperativeness.

There are many interesting craft reports on tracing and securing cooperation in the literature (e.g., Call, Otto, & Spenner, 1982; Campbell, 1965; Eckland, 1968; Freedman, Thornton, & Camburn, 1980; Hewitt, 1984; Hoinville & Jowell, 1978; McAllister, Butler, & Goe, 1973; Rogers, 1986). However, there is a lack of systematic empirical research on tracing and securing cooperation in longitudinal surveys, in contrast to the well-designed studies, sometimes using randomized experiments, of other methodological issues in survey research (e.g., Dohrenwend, 1970; Schuman & Presser, 1981; Singer, 1978). The most relevant tracing study may be the early comparison of letters, telephone calls, community visits, and public records by Crider, Willits, and Bealer (1971). Our chapter is a small attempt to fill this obvious gap in the literature.

The Cambridge Study in Delinquent Development

This is a prospective longitudinal study of 411 males. At the time they were first contacted in 1961–1962, they were all living in a working class area of London, England. The vast majority of the sample was chosen by taking all the boys who were then aged 8–9 and on the registers of six state primary schools within a one-mile radius of our research office. In addition to 399 boys from these six schools, 12 boys from a local school for the educationally subnormal were included in the sample, to make it more representative of the population of boys living in the area. The boys were overwhelmingly white, working class, and of British origin. Some of the past results of this survey have been published in four books (West, 1969, 1982; West & Farrington, 1973, 1977), and a concise summary has been produced by Farrington and West (1981).

The aim in this survey was to measure as many factors as possible that were alleged to be causes or correlates of offending. The boys were interviewed or tested in their schools when they were aged about 8, 10, and 14, and they were interviewed in our research office at about ages 16 and 18. At each of these ages, all or nearly all of the boys were interviewed. For example, at age 16, only 12 were missing, and at age 18 only 22 (6 abroad, 1 dead, 1 untraceable, and 14 refusers). Interviews were carried out with subsamples at ages 21 ($N = 218$) and 25 ($N = 85$).

Information has also been obtained in this survey from many other sources. The boys' parents were interviewed in their homes about once a year from when the boys were aged 8 until they were aged 14–15 and in their last year of compulsory education. The boys' teachers completed questionnaires when the boys were aged about 8, 10, 12, and 14. Peer ratings were obtained for the boys at ages 8 and 10. In addition, repeated searches have been made in the central Criminal Record Office in London to try to locate findings of guilt sustained by the boys, by their parents, by their brothers and sisters, and (in recent years) by their wives and cohabitees.

More recently (December 1984–November 1986), a further attempt was made to interview the whole sample at age 32, in their homes. Up to this age, 8 men had died, and 20 had emigrated permanently. All the men who were still alive were eventually traced and contacted. Of the 383 who were in the United Kingdom, 360 were interviewed personally (94.0%). Of the remaining 23, 19 refused (5%), and the remaining 4 (1.0%) could not be seen personally but did not respond positively to interview invitations passed on to them by relatives.

Seven of the emigrated men were also interviewed, either abroad or during a temporary return visit that they made to the United Kingdom, giving a total number interviewed of 367. In addition, 9 emigrated men filled in self-completion questionnaires, and 2 cooperative wives of refusers filled in questionnaires on behalf of their husbands, in at least one case with the husband's collaboration and assistance. Therefore, interviews or questionnaires were obtained for 378 of the 403 men still alive (93.8%).

For the interviews at age 32 (as in earlier years), a research office was established in the area from which the sample was originally drawn. Each man was randomly allocated to one of two male interviewers (B. G. and R. S.), so that it would be possible to investigate interviewer effects. The two interviewers were responsible for tracing and obtaining the cooperation of the men as well as for carrying out the interviews. There are advantages in having the same person tracing, securing cooperation, and interviewing, because information obtained during the tracing process may prove helpful in securing cooperation or in interviewing.

The interviewers were given freedom to select what they considered to be the best methods of tracing and securing cooperation, although guidelines were developed in collaboration with other members of the research team. No time limit was set on the tracing process, other than the two-year interviewing period, and this undoubtedly increased the number of men traced. Since the two interviewers had previous interviewing experience, they did not need extensive training. However, they had detailed discussions with past and present researchers on this project, which helped them to develop relevant skills and, of more importance, to avoid mistakes.

As in earlier years of this study, the interviewers were not part-time employees paid for each completed interview, which might have encouraged them to concentrate on the easier cases. They were full-time employees and fully involved as collaborators in the research enterprise. They participated in all aspects of the project, including designing and piloting the interview schedule; coding, computerizing, and checking data; and analyzing and writing material for progress reports. They had a great stake in the success of the study, were convinced of its importance, and were highly motivated, committed, and enthusiastic. Hence, they worked exceptionally hard, endured unsocial hours and difficult working conditions, and showed great persistence in the face of the inevitable setbacks. Other researchers (e.g., Thornton, Freedman, & Camburn, 1982) have discussed the advantages that can accrue when interviewers are involved as research collaborators.

The study men became eligible for interview in order of birth. They were allocated to an interviewer in batches of 25 at a time, a number less daunting and more manageable than the whole caseload of over 200. Since they were originally drawn from two school years, most were born between September 1952 and August 1953 ($N = 229$) or between September 1953 and August 1954 ($N = 159$). The second age cohort was smaller than the first because of the omission of two schools. There were also 23 boys in the study, originally regarded as a pilot group, who were born between September 1951 and August 1952, and drawn from one class in one school. Because the interviewing period was from December 1984 to November 1986, and because most of the men were born between September 1952 and August 1954, it was not surprising to find that the median age at interview was 32 years 3 months.

When each man became eligible for interview, a pre-interview sheet was completed for him. This listed the man's full name, date of birth, last known address, the date and place of his last interview, whether the man or his parents were thought to be hostile or uncooperative, whether he was illiterate, whether he was convicted, the name of his wife (if applicable), the type of his last known employment, and the schools he attended. It also included impressionistic details from earlier interviews that might be helpful (e.g., the man's attitude to being paid for his interview). This information was used by the interviewer in tracing and securing cooperation.

Methods of tracing

All attempts to trace and contact the man (together with dates and times) were recorded on the pre-interview sheet, and, after the interviewing was completed, they were coded and computerized. While the interviewing was in progress, it was not anticipated that these pre-interview sheets would be coded. Table 7.1 shows the tracing methods used. For example, a telephone call to a man's presumed address, a letter to a man, and a visit to a man's presumed address would all count as attempts to trace.

Only one attempt of any given type was counted on one day; for example, several visits to a man's house on one day were counted as only one attempt using this method. Hence, this coding system underestimates the amount of effort expended by interviewers in tracing the men. The same method used on different days was counted as more than one attempt, and different methods used on the same day were also counted as more than one attempt. Methods were sometimes used in conjunction, but they were coded according to the order in which they were used. It was uncommon for the same method to be used on more than one day with a man. Most attempts were completed in one day, but some (e.g., searching the National Health Service central register) could take months to complete. In such long-drawn-out cases, the order of the attempt was determined by the first day on which it was initiated.

Each attempt was counted as a success attempt if, in retrospect, it had contributed to tracing the man (e.g., if it had yielded accurate and useful information or if it helped to narrow down the possibilities for the man's address). Other attempts were counted as failure attempts. Typically, a man's pre-interview sheet would begin with a chain of failure attempts and end with a chain of success attempts. In some cases, the initial chain of failure attempts would be followed by a few alternating success and failure attempts until the final chain of success attempts began. The tracing

Table 7.1. *Tracing methods.*

	All			First 3			First S (5F)		
	T	S	%	T	S	%	T	S	%
All telephone attempts	608	(258)	42	105	(55)	52	160	(16)	10
Man's address	164	(128)	78	37	(30)	81	8	(2)	25
Family address	97	(61)	63	18	(12)	67	16	(5)	31
Others	20	(6)	30	0	(0)	0	10	(1)	10
Man's workplace	99	(24)	24	12	(2)	17	44	(8)	18
Exploratory: Man	127	(18)	14	33	(6)	18	40	(0)	0
Exploratory: Other	101	(21)	21	5	(5)	100	42	(0)	0
All letters	38	(21)	55	9	(3)	33	6	(0)	0
Man's address	16	(9)	56	7	(3)	43	2	(0)	0
Family address	13	(10)	77	1	(0)	0	1	(0)	0
Man's workplace	9	(2)	22	1	(0)	0	3	(0)	0
All visits	839	(427)	51	215	(117)	54	138	(26)	19
Man's address	352	(204)	58	127	(76)	60	44	(11)	25
Family address	163	(94)	58	21	(14)	67	24	(9)	38
Others	89	(32)	36	11	(5)	45	35	(4)	11
Man's workplace	35	(24)	69	4	(2)	50	5	(1)	20
Exploratory	200	(73)	37	52	(20)	38	30	(1)	3
All other attempts	1430	(477)	33	824	(307)	37	260	(59)	23
Local electoral register	356	(137)	38	255	(107)	42	37	(9)	24
Other electoral register	289	(80)	28	130	(35)	27	57	(8)	14
Telephone directory: Man	323	(56)	17	208	(38)	18	45	(3)	7
Telephone directory: Family	179	(71)	40	86	(46)	53	40	(7)	18
Criminal Record Office	78	(46)	59	60	(35)	58	10	(9)	90
National Health Service	26	(17)	65	6	(5)	83	15	(10)	67
DHSS	4	(0)	0	0	(0)	0	2	(0)	0
Local Housing Department	12	(3)	25	0	(0)	0	4	(0)	0
Leads from other men	101	(52)	51	51	(30)	59	29	(12)	41
Marriage certificates	19	(4)	21	9	(3)	33	9	(1)	11
Other	43	(11)	26	19	(8)	42	12	(0)	0
Total	2915	(1183)	41	1153	(482)	42	564	(101)	18

Notes:

DHSS = Department of Health and Social Security

T = Total attempts

S = Success attempts

5F = After 5 or more failure attempts

process was defined as ending when the man was first contacted personally (or when he was known to have received a message). At that point, attempts to gain an interview with the man began.

Table 7.1 shows that it required a total of 2,915 attempts to trace the 403 men, or an average of 7.2 attempts each. Of these, 1,183 were success attempts (an average of 2.9 each), and the remaining 1,732 were failure attempts (an average of 4.3 each). Overall, 41% of tracing attempts were successful.

The attempts were classified into telephone calls (608), letters (38), visits (839), and other (1,430). Letters were not often written to the men or their families because of our past experiences showing that they rarely elicited replies. They were used primarily when we had some prior reason to think that they might be useful. Similarly, the man or his family were telephoned primarily when it was believed that they would be cooperative. Exploratory calls and visits were those made when the interviewer was uncertain whether the person answering was the one with whom he wanted to talk. They were made in the hope of discovering relevant addresses or other information (e.g., about the man's workplace). Personal visits were usually made to a present or past address of the man (352 attempts) or of another family member (163 attempts). Neighbors and current occupants of past addresses often provided helpful information.

In order to obtain valid information from a personal visit, it is necessary for the potential informant to cooperate with someone who, until a few moments ago, was an unidentified stranger. It is interesting to note that only two people out of the many who were contacted ever asked the interviewers for proof of their identity. However, many of the men, their families, and other useful informants were living on densely populated inner-city housing estates and, with some justification, were suspicious of a stranger on their doorstep. Debt collectors, welfare benefit inspectors from the Department of Health and Social Security, potential thieves or assailants, police officers, and insurance salesmen posing as market research interviewers were only some of the types of visitors that people often wished to avoid. The presence of spy-holes in front doors on such estates enabled occupants to hear, see, and (if they chose) ignore a stranger without being detected themselves. It was sometimes difficult to distinguish between a recently vacated property and one with uncooperative occupants.

Both the men and members of their families sometimes told deliberate lies to our interviewers. For example, two men denied their own identity when first approached. On one visit to a man's family home, his brother said that our man (case 393) was working abroad and that there had been no contact with him for the last few years. On a later visit his mother was seen, and she readily provided the man's address, which was less than two miles away.

The most common tracing method used (356 attempts) was to consult the local electoral register. Fortunately, the borough in which our men originally lived compiled an alphabetical index by surname of their electoral register, and this facilitated searching. Electoral registers for other areas were also searched (289 attempts) to see if our man was still registered at his last known address. Electoral registers for earlier years were also searched to see approximately when our man moved, who he was living with at that time, changes in surnames or Christian names, and to identify long-standing local residents who might provide useful information. For example, the surname recorded on an old electoral register for case 732 corresponded to his second Christian name in our records. This discovery made it possible for us to trace him through a telephone directory search using this different surname.

The absence of a man's name on the electoral register for a particular address did not necessarily mean that he did not live there. Several of our men, contrary to legal requirements, either neglected or chose not to fill in the form for the electoral register. For example, case 603 had not registered for the last five years, even though he had a relatively stable life-style, living with a long-standing cohabitee and their child. Similarly, the absence of an entry for an address did not necessarily mean that it was unoccupied.

The presence of a man's name on the electoral register for a particular address did not necessarily mean that he lived there at the time of registration. Some boroughs simply duplicated the last entry on the register if no new information was forthcoming. Even in areas where this was not done, new occupants might illegally reenter the names of previous occupants. For example, the name of case 801 was still on the electoral register for an address more than two years after he had left. Another problem was that the information on the electoral register rapidly became out of date, as people moved. The form is completed in October, and the electoral register is then current from the following February until the February afterwards, 16 months later.

The prevalence of telephone ownership has greatly increased in England in the past 20 years. Telephone directories for the area including the last known address of the man (323 attempts) or other members of his family (179 attempts) were often searched. Such searches were easier to carry out if the target person had an uncommon surname and several Christian names. Quite a few of our men had no telephone or an exdirectory number. As with electoral registers, the information in telephone directories soon becomes out of date, because they are updated (at least in London) only about every 18 months.

In the case of men who had been convicted recently, the last known addresses provided by the Criminal Record Office were often useful. Similarly, marriage certificates sometimes provided helpful addresses. Through the Institute of Psychiatry, we were able to search the National Health Service central register to obtain the last known general practitioner with whom a man had been registered. This doctor would sometimes give us the man's latest address. This method tended to be used when other methods had failed and, as mentioned earlier, often took a long time to yield results. It might have been more useful if we had started with it at an earlier stage. The records branch of the Department of Health and Social Security would not provide us with addresses but agreed to forward letters to men. We used this sparingly because of our previous experience that it was not productive, and Table 7.1 shows that none of the four attempts we made at age 32 was successful.

The local Housing Department also agreed to forward letters for us to anyone whose address they held. This included anyone who was currently living in, or had recently moved out of, local council accommodation. However, this tracing method was also rather unproductive. At least one man (case 260) denied that he had ever received a letter that had allegedly been forwarded to him. Leads from other men were more useful. Every man who was interviewed was given a list of other men from his primary school class (and also of Study men who happened to be in his secondary school class) and was asked if he knew the current whereabouts of any of them. Over half (55%) could provide the address of at least one other man in his primary school class. Finally, a number of other methods were used, including obtaining information from a local newspaper, a local hospital, and trade unions. For example, an electrician, a printer, and a teacher were all traced using records specific to their occupations.

Evaluating different tracing methods

Table 7.1 shows the percentage of attempts that ultimately led to successful tracing. This percentage was highest for telephoning the man's address (78%), sending a letter to the family (77%), visiting the man's workplace (69%), searching National Health Service records (65%), and telephoning the family (63%). (Family members included parents, siblings, wives, aunts, uncles, and grandparents.) However, it does not necessarily follow that these were the most successful tracing methods, because they may have been used relatively late in the tracing process, after other methods had enabled some progress to be made.

Because we were concerned to maximize the number of persons traced rather than to evaluate the relative efficacy of different tracing methods, we did not randomly allocate persons to methods, but rather tailored the methods to fit what we knew about the persons. Consequently, it is difficult to determine the precise effect on tracing of any given method. However, we can get some idea about the relative usefulness of different methods by studying the less and more elusive men separately.

In general, the quicker methods – such as searches of electoral registers and telephone directories – tended to be used first, and the more time-consuming ones – such as personal visits – later. This could be demonstrated by calculating the mean serial position of each attempt or by using transition matrices showing the probability of one tracing method following another. Table 7.1 demonstrates it more simply by showing the methods used in the first three tracing attempts. It can be seen that most searches of the local electoral register (255 out of 356) and in the telephone directory (208 out of 323) came in the first three attempts, in comparison with only 127 of the 352 visits to the man's presumed address and only 21 of the 163 visits to a family address.

Searching the local electoral register (107), visiting the man's presumed address (76), searching for the family in the telephone directory (46), searching for the man in the telephone directory (38), searching the Criminal Record Office (35), searching other electoral registers (35), eliciting leads from other men (30), and telephoning the man's presumed address (30) yielded the most success on the first three attempts. In general, these were also the methods that led to the first success attempt. They were quite useful in finding the men who were not particularly elusive.

However, it is perhaps most important to determine which method led to the first success attempt for the more elusive men. The length of the initial failure chain varied from 0 to 36 attempts. As many as 167 men had no failure attempts before their first success attempt and hence were relatively easy to find. In contrast, 101 men had 5 or more failure attempts before their first success attempt, and so were relatively elusive.

Table 7.1 shows the methods used with these 101 more elusive men and their likelihood of leading to the first success attempt. A total of 564 tracing attempts were made after at least 5 failure attempts; 101 of these led to the first success, and the other 463 were failures. (Success and failure attempts after the first success attempt were not included in this analysis.) Some men, of course, contributed disproportionately to the total. For example, the man with 36 failure attempts contributed 31 failure attempts (after the first 5) and 1 success attempt.

It can be seen that the methods that proved to be successful with the more elusive men were remarkably variable. The most common methods were eliciting leads from other men (12), visiting the man's address (11), searching National Health Service records (10), visiting the family address (9), searching the local electoral register (9), searching the Criminal Record Office (9), telephoning the man's workplace (8), searching another electoral register (8), and searching for the family in the telephone directory (7). The methods with the highest probability of being successful were searching the Criminal Record Office (90%), searching National Health Service records (67%), eliciting leads from other men (41%), visiting the family address (38%), and telephoning the family address (31%). Methods that were numerically rather unimportant overall – such as searching National Health Service records, searching the Criminal Record Office, telephoning the man's workplace, and eliciting leads from other men – proved to be relatively important in breaking the failure chain for these elusive men.

Table 7.2 shows, for each of the first 20 attempts, the number of methods that were successful and the number that were failures. It is remarkable that the percentage of methods that were successful remained fairly constant at about 40%, at least up to the fifteenth method used. It is equally remarkable that the percentage of men who were finally traced on each attempt (out of all those not traced up to that point) stayed fairly constant at 16–20% from the third to the thirteenth attempt. The cumulative percentage of men traced increased after each attempt, of course, being 51% after the fifth attempt and 81% after the tenth. The consistency of the percentage of methods successful and of the percentage of men traced suggests that the best advice to give tracers may be just to keep trying.

The average number of tracing attempts was 7.2 per man, as already mentioned, but this number varied widely, from 1 to 39. The median was 5, and the interquartile range was from 3 to 9. The most elusive men were the 50 who required 13 or more attempts and the 41 who required between 10 and 12 attempts. It took almost as many attempts to trace the most elusive 91 men as the remaining 312

Table 7.2. *Success of consecutive tracing attempts.*

Attempt	Success	Failure	%S	Trace	Not	%T	Cumulative Traced	%
1	167	236	41	7	396	2	7	2
2	163	233	41	42	354	11	49	12
3	148	206	42	58	296	16	107	27
4	130	166	44	56	240	19	163	40
5	90	150	38	41	199	17	204	51
6	87	112	44	38	161	19	242	60
7	70	91	43	32	129	20	274	68
8	48	81	37	19	110	15	293	73
9	43	67	39	19	91	17	312	77
10	40	51	44	15	76	16	327	81
11	32	44	42	16	60	21	343	85
12	21	39	35	10	50	17	353	88
13	18	32	36	8	42	16	361	90
14	19	23	45	3	39	7	364	90
15	15	24	38	8	31	21	372	92
16	10	21	32	1	30	3	373	93
17	10	20	33	5	25	17	378	94
18	10	15	40	5	20	20	383	95
19	5	15	25	3	17	15	386	96
20	6	11	35	1	16	6	387	96

(1,446 as opposed to 1,469). The 50 extremely elusive men required a total of exactly 1,000 attempts, or an average of 20 each. The number of failure attempts also varied widely, from 0 to 36. However, the number of success attempts only varied from 1 to 9; 304 men required between 1 and 3 success attempts before they were traced, and 99 required between 4 and 9.

The number of days taken to trace a man varied from 1 to 605. Nearly a quarter of the men (90) were traced in the first day, whereas at the other extreme 50 men took between 33 and 80 days, and 52 took more than 80 days. The average number of days taken to trace a man was 36, but this figure is a little misleading because of the highly skewed distribution. The median was 8, and the interquartile range was from 2 to 32. Hence, a quarter of the sample would not have been traced if the maximum number of days allowed to trace each man had been set at 32. Clarridge, Sheehy, and Hauser (1977) also showed how the average time to trace people increased with each successive decile of a survey.

Several possible measures of difficulty of tracing were investigated, and all had highly skewed distributions. In order to calculate product–moment correlations, each measure was transformed by taking its natural logarithm (see Cottler et al., 1987, for the use of a similar transformation with similar data). This transformation was made because skewed distributions contravene an underlying statistical assumption of the product—moment correlation, but in fact the results without the transformation were quite similar to the results with it.

The number of days taken to trace a man was highly correlated with the number of attempts ($r = .64$, $p < .001$; two-tailed significance tests are used throughout). Both were highly correlated with the number of failure attempts ($r = .62$ with days to trace and .93 with number of attempts) and with the length of the initial failure chain ($r = .50$ and .78 respectively). They were less strongly, but still significantly, correlated with the number of success attempts ($r = .24$ and .46 respectively). The number of success attempts was significantly correlated with the number of failure attempts ($r = .17$, $p < .001$), suggesting that both reflected elusiveness. The length of the final success chain was not at all related to either the number of attempts ($r = .05$) or to the number of days to trace ($r = -.08$). The number of days taken to trace a man is used here as the best summary measure of difficulty of tracing.

Securing cooperation

Methods of securing cooperation could not be studied in as much detail as methods of tracing, because the precise methods used in approaching each man were not recorded sufficiently fully. This would have required the interviewer to tape-record and transcribe every conversation he had with a man or with a man's friends or relatives, which was impractical. (The interviews themselves were fully tape-recorded and transcribed.)

In approaching each man, the interviewer explained that he was from Cambridge University and that he was involved in a social survey, following up those who went to the man's primary school to see how well the men were getting on now. He stressed how helpful most people had been, the consequent value of the study, the importance of each man's individual participation, and the fact that the man could not be replaced by anyone else. Most of the men remembered the study and had positive feelings towards it. We were also helped a little by the fact that some of the men had recently seen a television program entitled "28 up" that followed up 14 people at ages 7, 14, 21, and 28. Because they had found this program very interesting, they could see some value in following up people throughout their lives.

The interviewer adopted a very pleasant and friendly approach, and stressed how much he personally would appreciate the man's assistance. The man was assured that the interview would be completely confidential and that no one outside the research team would see his interview schedule, which would only be identified by a code number. He was also told that the interview would not take long (about an hour) and that it could be completed at any time and day convenient to him – in his home or elsewhere if he preferred.

The man was paid a small fee (£10) for his time in being interviewed, but this was usually mentioned only casually (or not at all) by the interviewer. This was partly because the small amount of money provided an easy excuse for refusal (it was often insignificant in comparison with the man's current income) and partly because the interviewer liked to keep the fee as an added incentive to be introduced later in the discussion if necessary. In a few cases, an increased fee (up to £20) was offered, if the interviewer felt that this might be a factor in securing cooperation.

Visits to the man's presumed place of residence were usually made between 5:30 p.m. and 8:30 p.m., when it was hoped that he would have returned from work but not yet gone out for the evening. There is some empirical evidence that the probability of finding someone at home is greatest during these hours (Weeks, Jones, Folsom, & Benrud, 1980). If someone other than the man was encountered – usually a wife or other family member – the interviewer would try to establish when the man would return and would then revisit as soon as possible. Many visits were made without prior warning, because the men's surprise at being unexpectedly recontacted after so many (7–14) years seemed to make them more willing to agree to an interview. Efforts were made to ensure that, as far as possible, the man first heard about our desire to reinterview him in a face-to-face meeting with an interviewer, although some men had to be telephoned or sent letters.

The interviewers were similar to the men in age and social background, and were sometimes assumed to be friends of the men by their family members. They dressed informally but not too casually, and sometimes varied their dress according to the circumstances. For example, the interviewer dressed smartly to see a man who was a successful stockbroker (case 071) in a wine bar close to his workplace. Conversely, the interviewer's scruffy dress helped him gain entry to a house where one man (case 103) was squatting. The man said to the interviewer, "Your face must fit." He explained that he was trying to avoid payment of a fine and had expected his friend, who granted admission, to be more wary of strangers.

The interviewer addressed the man with as much familiarity as seemed appropriate or feasible. In order to foster a feeling of intimacy, he might refer casually to friends or family members with whom he had previously established some degree of rapport. The interviewer would use nicknames or other informal variations on a man's Christian name if these were known from earlier interviews. A failure to do this caused one man (case 012) to comment that "only my bank manager calls me that."

If the man was reluctant to be interviewed, the interviewer would try to discover any reasons for reluctance and to assuage them (e.g., concerns about confidentiality or about the purpose of the study). If the man firmly refused to be interviewed, the interviewer would try to leave on good terms with him and to persuade him to allow a further visit at some specified time in the future. In most cases, we did not give up after a man refused once, because our experience was that some refusals were situationally influenced, occurring because the man was too busy or not in the right mood at that particular time. After a refusal, the interviewer usually revisited the man a few months later to give him another opportunity to agree to an interview. The man was then asked to consider additional factors, such as the recent interview of an old friend or acquaintance, or the fact that he was the last remaining man to be interviewed from his primary school class. The subsequent visit also showed the man the importance that we placed on his involvement. If the man gave a second refusal, he was not normally contacted again.

About three-quarters of the men (306, or 75.9%) agreed fairly readily to be interviewed as a result of only one contact (visit, telephone call, or letter) with them. Of the remaining 97, 59 were reluctant or resistant but did not give a firm refusal, 11 refused but were subsequently interviewed, and 27 refused and were not interviewed (although in two cases, as mentioned, their wives filled in a questionnaire). It was interesting to note that over a quarter of the initial refusals (11 out of 38) were nevertheless followed by interviews. The corresponding figure at age 18 was over one-third (8 out of 22). Similar results were reported by Robins (1963).

The number of days taken to interview a man after he had been contacted varied from 0 to 529, with an average of 16.5. The median was 4, and the interquartile range was from 2 to 9. Apart from the 27 men not interviewed, the men who were the most difficult to interview were the 51 who took 18 days or more and the 57 who took 8–17 days. The number of days to interview a man was significantly correlated with the number of days required to trace him ($r = .19$, $p < .001$, after logarithmic transformation) and almost significantly related to the number of tracing methods used ($r = .09$, $p = .059$).

Excluding the 27 men not interviewed, the 70 men who were the most resistant overlapped significantly with the 108 men who took the most days to interview (54.3% of 70 as opposed to 22.9% of 306, excluding the two "wife questionnaire" cases: $\chi^2 = 25.94$, $p < .001$). The most uncooperative (most difficult to interview) men are defined here as the 70 who were the most reluctant and the 27 who refused.

Case histories

Case histories can be useful in showing how specific men were traced and how their cooperation was achieved. The following four case histories show the tracing of two quite elusive men (cases 651 and 481) and attempts to secure cooperation from one man who was resistant (case 093) and one who refused (case 011):

Case 651 (48 days to trace):

There was only one entry in the London telephone directory that could have been this man, but a visit to the address eliminated this possibility. The man's last known address was then visited. The building was now operating as a shoe shop, and the manager knew nothing of the man. The interviewer then went to the man's address at the time of his marriage (an old address), but enquiries among neighbors yielded nothing.

At the time of his last interview the man had expressed an intention of entering the shoe repair business. By chance, the interviewer heard of a shoe repair shop near the research office trading under the man's surname. However, a visit to this shop yielded nothing. Exploratory telephone calls were made on the basis of searches in the London directory, and then surrounding areas, for the man and members of his family, but these yielded nothing.

The search then focused on the man's parents, and this proved to be the first step towards tracing him. When he had been last interviewed, his father had been the caretaker of a primary school. On telephoning the school, the interviewer discovered that the father had retired, and the teaching staff recommended contacting the current caretaker. This man was visited, and he told the interviewer that the parents had moved to Kent. He did, however, know that our man's brother was in the Metropolitan Police.

The interviewer then contacted Scotland Yard, who agreed to pass on a message to the brother if he was still a serving police officer. The following day, the brother contacted the research office and made enquiries about the study. After having had the project explained to him, he agreed to contact his brother. That evening our man telephoned the interviewer and a meeting was arranged.

Case 481 (37 days to trace)

The last known address for this man was 14 years old. A check of the electoral register indicated that the whole family had moved. Neither a search of this register nor exploratory telephone calls based on the London directory produced any leads. The man's father had a printing business in the Midlands prior to the family's moving to London, and it was thought worthwhile to direct the search to this area. Both private and trade directories were searched for the entire East Midlands, but again no leads could be found. A search of North Wales telephone directories – where the man's mother had moved after separation from her husband – was equally fruitless.

Two visits were then made to the man's previous address to speak to the current occupants and neighbors. The family were remembered quite well, but nobody had any idea where they had moved. Earlier interview schedules indicated that our man hoped to study printing at a local college. The records department of the college was contacted, but they could find no trace of the man.

A short time later a former friend of the man was interviewed, and he provided the interviewer with a more recent address for the man. The electoral register was then searched to find the precise dates when our man was at this address and to discover the names of the house-sharers and neighbors at that time. None of these persons were currently living in the street, and no trace of them could be found in the London telephone directories. The interviewer visited this street and spoke to the current occupants of the address, but without success.

The interviewer then wondered if our man had died and so contacted the local registrar of deaths and the local hospital, but neither had any record of our man's death. Both the man and his father had been in the printing trade, and so the main print unions were contacted. They had computerized records for all current and past members, but this search yielded no useful information.

The interviewer then searched telephone directories for counties surrounding London, and national trade directories. In desperation, the interviewer studied the criminal record of the man's family and found that one of his brothers had been convicted in Cambridgeshire several years ago. The telephone directory for this area was searched, and the man's father was found. He agreed to pass on a message to his son. Minutes later, the man telephoned and agreed to be interviewed.

Case 093 (resistant):

This man was traced easily, because his current address was provided by a friend who was also in the study. After two unsuccessful visits to this address the interviewer finally met the man's wife. She was hospitable and positively disposed towards the study, but told the interviewer that the man had not yet returned from work. The interviewer left a written message for the man and said that he would be in touch.

The following day, the man telephoned the interviewer. He was pleasant but said that he did not want to be interviewed. The interviewer explained how flexible he was about timing, how short the interview was, and emphasized its confidentiality. However, these arguments had little effect. The interviewer then tried to find out if the man had any specific worries about the study and discovered that he was concerned about the contents of the interview schedule. The interviewer then suggested that he visit the man at his home and show him the interview schedule, and the man agreed to this.

On arrival at the man's home, the interviewer was invited in, which was thought to be an optimistic sign. Once the interviewer had run through the schedule with the man, the man appeared quite content and agreed to be interviewed then and there.

Case 011 (refuser):

This man was at the same address as that of his previous interview 13 years before. He was therefore traced and contacted in the same day. However, when he opened the front door, he kept most of his body behind it, simply poking out his head to talk to the interviewer. He refused to be interviewed, and no amount of persuasion could change his mind.

On reflection, the interviewer concluded that the conditions of the first meeting (a cold, wet, and dark winter's evening, quite late at night) were rather unfavorable. He therefore made a second visit on a warm spring day. The man was a little more cooperative and talked more, but he would not change his mind.

The interviewer thought that, with time, the man might change his mind, and so visited him again. However, the man was pleasant but steadfast in his refusal. He would not even consider completing a shortened questionnaire. This man was therefore abandoned.

Elusiveness and uncooperativeness

The main measure of elusiveness developed at age 32 was the number of days taken to trace a man, whereas the main measure of uncooperativeness was the man's reluctance or refusal to be interviewed. The most elusive men were the 102 who took 33 or more days to trace, whereas the most uncooperative ones were the 97 who were reluctant or who refused. In comparing elusiveness and uncooperativeness with other factors, all variables were dichotomized into (as far as possible) the "worst" quarter versus the remaining three-quarters, and 2 × 2 tables were calculated. The use of this method facilitated the understandable presentation of results and meant that all variables could be compared directly. Also, in investigating attrition, one of the most important questions centers on the effects on conclusions of missing out the more elusive or uncooperative people, and some idea of this could be obtained easily by inspecting 2 × 2 tables.

Table 7.3 investigates some possible predictors and correlates of elusiveness and uncooperativeness. For example, 41 of the men had uncooperative parents when they were aged 8, and 18 of these (43.9%) were among the most elusive at age 32. In contrast, only 23.2% of 362 men with cooperative parents at age 8 were elusive, a statistically significant difference ($\chi^2 = 7.29$, corrected for continuity, 1 df, $p = .007$, two-tailed; all statistical tests in this section are of this type).

The more elusive men at age 32 tended to have been uncooperative at age 18, and also rated uncooperative at some time before the 32 year interview. (Fewer men were rated as previously uncooperative than as cooperative at 18, because the previous rating required active uncooperativeness whereas the 18 year rating merely required lack of active cooperativeness.) The men who had moved from their last known address and those whose parents had moved also tended to be among the more elusive. Also, those who lived outside London and the Home Counties (i.e., the counties surrounding London) and those who lived 25 or more miles away from our research office proved more difficult to trace. Elusiveness was not significantly related to the length of time since a man had been interviewed, to the age of his or his parents' last known address, or to the commonness of his surname (coded according to the number of column inches occupied by each surname in the London telephone directories).

The more uncooperative men at age 32 tended to have had uncooperative parents at ages 8 and 14, or at some time previous to age 32, and to have been uncooperative themselves at age 18 or at some time previous to age 32. Hence, there seemed to be remarkable continuity in uncooperativeness, from the parents when the man was aged 8 and 14, to the man himself at ages 18 and 32. Of the nonsignificant relationships, it was noteworthy that the length of time since a man was last interviewed was not related to uncooperativeness.

Problems of interpretation arise from the fact that elusiveness and uncooperativeness varied somewhat with the interviewer. Interviewer 1 was originally allocated (at random) 204 men to trace, whereas interviewer 2 was allocated 199. However, when

Table 7.3. *Predictors and correlates of elusiveness and uncooperativeness.*

Variable (N)	% Elusive	(Sig.)	% Uncooperative	(Sig.)
Uncooperative parents at 8 (41)	43.9	(.007)	46.3	(.001)
Not uncooperative (362)	23.2		21.5	
Uncooperative parents at 14 (54)	33.3	(N.S.)	42.6	(.001)
Not uncooperative (345)	23.8		21.4	
Uncooperative man at 18 (79)	36.7	(.014)	46.8	(.001)
Not uncooperative (320)	22.5		18.4	
Last interview 18 or before (163)	28.2	(N.S.)	26.4	(N.S.)
Last interview 21 or 25 (240)	23.3		22.5	
Man's last address 12+ years old (99)	30.3	(N.S.)	28.3	(N.S.)
More recent address (303)	23.4		22.4	
Man has moved from last address (330)	29.1	(.001)	22.7	(N.S.)
Man still at same address (72)	8.3		30.6	
Man previously uncooperative (72)	34.7	(.060)	54.2	(.001)
Not uncooperative (327)	23.2		17.4	
Parental last address 14+ years old (87)	26.4	(N.S.)	27.6	(N.S.)
More recent parental address (312)	24.7		22.4	
Parents moved from last address (124)	39.5	(.001)	28.2	(N.S.)
Parents still at same address (149)	16.8		24.2	
Parents previously uncooperative (63)	36.5	(N.S.)	39.7	(.002)
Parents not uncooperative (253)	25.3		20.2	
Man not living with parents (352)	26.7	(N.S.)	23.0	(N.S.)
Man living with parents (51)	15.7		31.4	
Man has common surname (102)	31.4	(N.S.)	24.5	(N.S.)
Man has less common surname (301)	23.3		23.9	
Man lives outside home counties (57)	47.4	(.001)	19.3	(N.S.)
Man in London or home counties (342)	21.3		24.3	
Man lives 25+ miles away (107)	35.5	(.005)	20.6	(N.S.)
Man lives less than 25 miles away (292)	21.2		24.7	
Interviewer 1 (204–209)[a]	28.9	(N.S.)	19.6	(.040)
Interviewer 2 (199–194)	21.6		28.9	

Notes:

Sig. = Significant

N.S. = Not significant

[a]Interviewer 1 was allocated 204 to trace but 209 to interview; see text.

interviewer 2 left the study, his five outstanding cases (two not traced and three traced but not interviewed) were reallocated to interviewer 1. Therefore, the interviewer coding on elusiveness in tracing (204 men for interviewer 1 and 199 for interviewer 2) differed in five cases from the interviewer coding on uncooperativeness in interviewing (209 men for interviewer 1 and 194 for interviewer 2). As Table 7.3 shows, interviewer 1 had slightly more elusive men (28.9%, as opposed to 21.6% for interviewer 2; $\chi^2 = 2.48$, N.S.), while interviewer 2 had significantly more unco-operative men (28.9%, as opposed to 19.6% for interviewer 1; $\chi^2 = 4.22$, $p = .040$).

It is possible that interviewer 1 may have tried to trace men a little differently than interviewer 2, taking a little longer in the process. However, it was noticeable that interviewer 1 was significantly more likely to learn that the man's parents had moved from their last address (51.9%, as opposed to 39.3% for interviewer 2; $\chi^2 = 3.87$, $p = .049$). As Table 7.3 shows, the men whose parents had moved tended to be more elusive. Also, interviewer 1's men were significantly more likely to have common names (30.9%, as opposed to 19.6% for interviewer 2; $\chi^2 = 6.20$, $p = .013$), and this was also associated with somewhat greater difficulty in tracing. The slightly greater elusiveness of interviewer 1's men could well be explained on the basis of differences in the mobility of their parents and in the commonness of their names, rather than differences in interviewer behavior.

It is also possible that an interviewer's prior knowledge about a man and his family, listed on the pre-interview sheet, affected his methods of tracing and securing cooperation. If the interviewer knew that the man or his family had previously been uncooperative, he made a special effort to ensure that his first contact with the man was face to face, whereas if the interviewer knew that the man and his family had previously been cooperative he would be more willing to make telephone calls or write letters. The interviewer's prior knowledge would have had less influence on the rating of the man's cooperativeness, because this was more dependent on the man's own behavior and because the interviewers tried hard to develop explicit and consis-tent coding standards on this (as on everything else).

Conceivably, interviewer 2 may have been a little more willing to classify men as reluctant or resistant. However, it was noticeable that significantly more of inter-viewer 2's men had parents who were previously uncooperative (26.0%, as opposed to 14.7% for interviewer 1; $\chi^2 = 5.62$, $p = .018$). As Table 7.3 shows, the men whose parents had previously been uncooperative were significantly more likely to be uncooperative themselves. The slightly greater uncooperativeness of interviewer 2's men could well be explained on the basis of differences in their parents' previous uncooperativeness rather than being ascribed to interviewer bias.

If any interviewer bias exists, its extent is likely to differ between the two interviewers. In investigating this, all significant relationships in Table 7.3 were studied separately for the two interviewers. One relationship that differed markedly was between elusiveness and the distance of a man's residence from the research office. This was highly significant for interviewer 1 ($p = .003$) but not for inter-viewer 2. Hence, interviewer 1 took longer to trace the men who lived farther away. (Because of the state of the traffic in London, it might take two hours to drive 25 miles from the research office.) Another different relationship was between elusive-ness and the uncooperativeness of the man at age 18, which was also significant for interviewer 1 ($p = .012$) but not for interviewer 2. Third, the relationship between the uncooperativeness of the man at age 32 and the uncooperativeness of his parents when he was age 8 was highly significant for interviewer 1 ($p = .001$) but not for interviewer 2.

With these three exceptions, the significant relationships were of comparable strength for the two interviewers. Taking all factors into account, it seems unlikely that the results in Table 7.3 are caused by interviewer bias. In the most extreme example, for interviewer 1, 10 of the 18 men with uncooperative parents at age 8 were rated uncooperative at age 32, in comparison with 16.2% of the other 191 men. For interviewer 2, 9 of the 23 men with uncooperative parents at age 8 were rated uncooperative at age 32, in comparison with 27.5% of the other 171 men. Hence, the difference between the two interviewers could have reflected the fact that interviewer 2 had more uncooperative men rather than that interviewer 1 was particularly likely to rate men with uncooperative parents as uncooperative themselves.

Table 7.4 shows some characteristics of elusive and uncooperative men, percentaging in the opposite direction from Table 7.3. For example, 30.9% of 97 uncooperative men had been convicted after their twenty-first birthdays, in comparison with 19.3% of 306 cooperative men, a statistically significant difference ($\chi^2 = 5.15$, $p = .023$). Hence, if only the cooperative men had been interviewed, there would have been a significant underrepresentation of men with adult convictions. When all convictions (including juvenile and young adult ones up to age 20) were included, the relationship with uncooperativeness was in the expected direction but not significant.

Table 7.4 shows that the more elusive men were significantly likely to report in the interview that they had lived at four or more addresses in the last five years, and they were significantly less likely to know the current whereabouts of some other man from their primary school class. The uncooperative men were especially likely to have no wife or cohabitee, to have been involved in fights (where blows were struck) in the last five years, to be tenants rather than homeowners, and to be relatively heavy smokers (20 cigarettes per day or more). In addition, of those who had children, more of the uncooperative men had difficulties with their children (i.e., two or more of the following: a child living elsewhere, a real problem with a child, or disagreement with their wife or cohabitee about child rearing; for more details of all these codings, see Farrington, Gallagher, Morley, St. Ledger, & West, 1988).

An important question is the extent to which men who are reluctant to be interviewed might provide less valid information in the interview. Table 7.4 shows that the uncooperative men were significantly likely to be rated as possibly not truthful and not fully cooperative in the interview. In both cases, there were marked interviewer differences, with the relationship much stronger for interviewer 1. Hence, the association between uncooperativeness in being interviewed and in the interview itself could have been mediated by the expectations of the interviewer. Interviewer effects are less likely with other variables shown in Table 7.4, which

Table 7.4 *Characteristics of elusive and uncooperative men.*

Variable (%)	% of less Elusive	% of more Elusive	% of Coop.	% of Uncoop.
Convicted (36.2)	34.9	40.2	34.3	42.3
(Sig.)		(N.S.)		(N.S.)
Convicted after 21 (22.1)	21.3	24.5	19.3	30.9
(Sig.)		(N.S.)		(.023)
Convicted in last 5 years (11.2)	11.0	11.8	10.5	13.4
(Sig.)		(N.S.)		(N.S.)
Four or more addresses[a] (13.3)	11.1	20.2	13.4	12.5
(Sig.)		(.042)		(N.S.)
Four or more evenings out p.w. (17.2)	17.8	15.1	15.5	24.3
(Sig.)		(N.S.)		(N.S.)
Not home owner (51.6)	50.9	53.9	49.0	62.5
(Sig.)		(N.S.)		(.054)
No wife or cohabitee (23.5)	24.2	21.3	20.6	36.1
(Sig.)		(N.S.)		(.008)
Divorced or separated (19.6)	20.1	18.0	19.0	22.2
(Sig.)		(N.S.)		(N.S.)
Difficulties with children (23.6)	23.7	23.1	20.7	37.0
(Sig.)		(N.S.)		(.030)
Not currently employed (11.9)	11.8	12.4	11.4	14.1
(Sig.)		(N.S.)		(N.S.)
Self-reported offender[a] (22.2)	23.5	18.0	21.2	26.4
(Sig.)		(N.S.)		(N.S.)
Involved in fights[a] (37.1)	36.8	38.2	34.3	49.3
(Sig.)		(N.S.)		(.027)
Heavy smoker (27.2)	27.0	27.9	24.9	37.1
(Sig.)		(N.S.)		(.055)
Heavy drinker (19.7)	18.5	23.9	18.1	26.8
(Sig.)		(N.S.)		(N.S.)
Taken drug except marijuana[a] (9.5)	9.0	11.2	9.8	8.5
(Sig.)		(N.S.)		(N.S.)
Knows man from primary school (55.3)	59.1	43.0	56.9	48.6
(Sig.)		(.013)		(N.S.)
Possibly not truthful in int. (15.0)	12.1	24.4	10.1	35.7
(Sig.)		(.009)		(.001)
Not fully cooperative in int. (8.4)	7.1	12.8	4.7	24.3
(Sig.)		(N.S.)		(.001)

Notes:
Uncoop. = Uncooperative
Sig. = Significant
N.S. = Not significant
p.w. = per week
Coop. = Cooperative
Int. = Interview

derived from the man's answers to direct questions in a highly structured interview. Interviewer bias seems most likely to affect interviewer ratings.

Conclusions

Attrition rates in longitudinal surveys are not always high. They were very low in the Cambridge Study in Delinquent Development, a prospective longitudinal study of over 400 males from age 8 to age 32. This paper has described the methods of tracing and securing cooperation used in this survey. In general, success in tracing was achieved by persistence and by using a wide variety of methods. No one method was frequently successful in breaking the initial chain of failure attempts that sometimes occurred in trying to trace a man. On the contrary, every succeeding method had a roughly constant probability of contributing to the final successful tracing.

This research indicates that searching for the man in electoral registers and telephone directories and visits to the man's presumed address were the most successful tracing methods for the men who were not particularly elusive. Searches in the Criminal Record Office, National Health Service records, and leads from other men were the most useful for the more elusive men.

The more elusive and uncooperative men at age 32 tended to have uncooperative parents at age 8 and to have been uncooperative themselves at age 18. Hence, this paper provides evidence of continuity in uncooperativeness from one generation to the next and from youth to adulthood. The more elusive men were more mobile in changing addresses more frequently, lived farther away from the research office, and had less contact with other study men. The more uncooperative men tended to be adult offenders, living without a wife or cohabitee, having difficulties with their children, involved in fights, tenants rather than home owners, and heavy smokers. There were some slight interviewer differences in the frequency of elusive and uncooperative men, but it is unlikely that any of the findings were caused by interviewer bias. There was some indication that a minority of the men who were reluctant to be interviewed might have given less valid answers.

Methods of tracing and securing cooperation inevitably raise ethical issues, especially in regard to privacy. Some researchers may feel that we should not have searched for the men so remorselessly, that we should have obtained written consent in all cases, and that we should not have returned to the men after they had refused once. Ethical codes promulgated by professional bodies usually emphasize some form of weighing social benefits against social costs in reaching ethical decisions (see, e.g., Diener & Crandall, 1978). We believe that the social benefits of our methods were considerable, in maximizing the number of men traced and interviewed. Conclusions would have been different – and indeed mistaken – if the uncooperative men had not been interviewed. All researchers have an ethical responsibility to reach only honest and correct conclusions.

The social costs of our methods seem minimal, for example, in giving the men an opportunity to reconsider a refusal. We have been very careful to ensure that no participants in our research would suffer any negative consequences as a result. We are, of course, extremely grateful to the men and their families for their valuable help over the years. If our research leads to an advance in knowledge about the causes of offending or of desistance from offending, this may eventually contribute to a decrease in crime, which would be a very great social benefit. The social costs of a minor invasion of privacy seem small in comparison with the social costs of robbery, burglary, or forcible rape.

Random assignment experiments should be carried out to investigate the relative efficacy (perhaps in relation to cost) of different methods of tracing and securing cooperation. Such experiments should be linked to theories of how interviewer behavior interacts with interviewee characteristics in producing success or failure in tracing and securing cooperation. For example, whether a person agreed to be interviewed might depend on the balance of perceived costs and benefits.

We hope that this paper will be especially useful to researchers in Great Britain and North America, where problems of tracing and securing cooperation in longitudinal projects seem particularly acute. It would be interesting to study how far difficulties in tracing and securing cooperation vary with the country, with the area (e.g., urban versus rural), with the nature of the sample (e.g., male vs. female, national vs. local, old vs. young), with the main purpose of the research, and with the design of the study (e.g., longitudinal vs. cross-sectional, the number and frequency of contacts with the subjects, the variety of data sources used). It would also be interesting to investigate what steps could be taken early in a longitudinal study to facilitate lasting contact and cooperation.

It is ironic that more books and articles have been written about technical problems such as sampling, research design, and statistical analysis than about practical problems that may be more difficult to solve and more important in their consequences for the validity of conclusions, such as tracing and securing cooperation. We hope that this chapter will help to redress that imbalance.

References

Bebbington, A. C. (1970). The effect of non-response in the sample survey with an example. *Human Relations, 23,* 169–180.

Cairns, R. B., & Cairns, B. D. (1987). *Child aggression and adolescent survival.* Chapel Hill, NC: University of North Carolina Department of Psychology.

Call, V. R. A., Otto, L. B., & Spenner, K. I. (1982). *Tracking respondents.* Lexington, MA: Heath.

Campbell, D. P. (1965). *The results of counseling.* Philadelphia: Saunders.

Capaldi, D., & Patterson, G. R. (1987). An approach to the problem of recruitment and retention rates for longitudinal research. *Behavioral Assessment, 9,* 169–177.

Clarridge, B. R., Sheehy, L. L., & Hauser, T. S. (1977). Tracing members of a panel: A 17-year follow-up. In K. F. Schuessler (Ed.), *Sociological Methodology 1978* (pp. 185–203). San Francisco: Jossey-Bass.

Condon, J. T. (1986). The "unresearched" – Those who decline to participate. *Australian and New Zealand Journal of Psychiatry, 20,* 87–89.

Cordray, S., & Polk, K. (1983). The implications of respondent loss in panel studies of deviant behavior. *Journal of Research in Crime and Delinquency, 20,* 214–242.

Cottler, L. B., Zipp, J. F., Robins, L. N., & Spitznagel, E. L. (1987). Difficult-to-recruit respondents and their effect on prevalence estimates in an epidemiologic survey. *American Journal of Epidemiology, 125,* 329–339.

Crider, D. M., & Willits, F. K. (1973). Respondent retrieval bias in a longitudinal survey. *Sociology and Social Research, 58,* 56–65.

Crider, D. M., Willits, F. K., & Bealer, R. C. (1971). Tracking respondents in longitudinal surveys. *Public Opinion Quarterly, 35,* 613–620.

Diener, E., & Crandall, R. (1978). *Ethics in social and behavioral research.* Chicago: University of Chicago Press.

Dohrenwend, B. S. (1970). An experimental study of payments to respondents. *Public Opinion Quarterly, 34,* 621–624.

Eckland, B. K. (1968). Retrieving mobile cases in longitudinal surveys. *Public Opinion Quarterly, 32,* 51–64.

Eron, L. D., Huesmann, L. R., Dubow, E., Romanoff, R., & Yarmel, P. W. (1987). Aggression and its correlates over 22 years. In D. H. Crowell, I. M. Evans, and C. R. O'Donnell (Eds.), *Childhood aggression and violence* (pp. 249–262). New York: Plenum Press.

Farrington, D. P., & Dowds, E. A. (1985). Disentangling criminal behavior and police reaction. In D. P. Farrington & J. Gunn (Eds.), *Reactions to crime* (pp. 41–72). Chichester: Wiley.

Farrington, D. P., Gallagher, B., Morley, L., St. Ledger, R. J., & West, D. J. (1988). A 24-year follow-up of men from vulnerable backgrounds. In R. L. Jenkins and W. K. Brown (Eds.), *The abandonment of delinquent behavior* (pp. 155–173). New York: Praeger.

Farrington, D. P., & West, D. J. (1981). The Cambridge Study in Delinquent Development. In S. A. Mednick & A. E. Baert (Eds.), *Prospective longitudinal research* (pp. 137–145). Oxford: Oxford University Press.

Fitzgerald, R., & Fuller, L. (1982). I hear you knocking but you can't come in: The effects of reluctant respondents and refusers on sample survey estimates. *Sociological Methods and Research, 11,* 3–32.

Freedman, D. S., Thornton, A., & Camburn, D. (1980). Maintaining response rates in longitudinal studies. *Sociological Methods and Research, 9,* 87–98.

Friday, P. C., & Sonnad, S. R. (1979). Respondents and non-respondents in survey research: The offender sample. *International Journal of Comparative and Applied Criminal Justice, 3,* 35–42.

Glueck, S., & Glueck, E. (1940). *Juvenile delinquents grown up.* New York: Commonwealth Fund.

Hewitt, A. (1984). The follow-up study: Tracing and interviewing the children. In R. Illsley & R. G. Mitchell (Eds.), *Low birth weight* (pp. 105–132). Chichester: Wiley.

Hoinville, G., & Jowell, R. (1978). *Survey research practice.* London: Heinemann.

Hough, M., & Mayhew, P. (1983). *The British crime survey.* London: Her Majesty's Stationery Office.

McAllister, R. J., Butler, E. W., & Goe, S. J. (1973). Evolution of a strategy for the retrieval of cases in longitudinal survey research. *Sociology and Social Research, 58,* 37–47.

McCord, J. (1978). A thirty-year follow-up of treatment effects. *American Psychologist, 33,* 284–289.

Paikin, H., Jacobsen, B., Schulsinger, F., Godtfredson, K., Rosenthal, D., Wender, P., & Kety, S. S. (1974). Characteristics of people who refused to participate in a social and psychopathological study. In S. A. Mednick, F. Schulsinger, J. Higgins, & B. Bell (Eds.), *Genetics, environment and psychopathology* (pp. 293–322). Amsterdam: North-Holland.

Robins, L. N. (1963). The reluctant respondent. *Public Opinion Quarterly, 27,* 276–286.

Robins, L. N. (1966). *Deviant children grown up.* Baltimore, MD: Williams & Wilkins.

Robins, L. N., West, P. A., & Herjanic, B. L. (1975). Arrests and delinquency in two generations. *Journal of Child Psychology and Psychiatry, 16,* 125–140.

Rogers, C. D. (1986). *Tracing missing persons.* Manchester: Manchester University Press.

Schuman, H., & Presser, S. (1981). *Questions and answers in attitude surveys.* New York: Academic Press.

Singer, E. (1978). Informed consent: Consequences for response rate and response quality in social surveys. *American Sociological Review, 43,* 144–162.

Steeh, C. G. (1981). Trends in nonresponse rates, 1952–1979. *Public Opinion Quarterly, 45,* 40–57.

Thornton, A., Freedman, D. S., & Camburn, D. (1982). Obtaining respondent cooperation in family panel studies. *Sociological Methods and Research, 11,* 33–51.

Weeks, M. F., Jones, B. L., Folsom, R. E., & Benrud, C. H. (1980). Optimal times to contact sample households. *Public Opinion Quarterly, 44,* 101–114.

West, D. J. (1969). *Present conduct and future delinquency.* London: Heinemann.

West, D. J. (1982). *Delinquency: Its roots, careers and prospects.* London: Heinemann.

West, D. J., & Farrington, D. P. (1973). *Who becomes delinquent?* London: Heinemann.

West, D. J. & Farrington, D. P. (1977). *The delinquent way of life.* London: Heinemann.

Wolfgang, M. E., Thornberry, T. P., & Figlio, R. M. (1987). *From boy to man, from delinquency to crime.* Chicago: University of Chicago Press.

8   Minimizing attrition in longitudinal studies: Means or end?

MICHAEL MURPHY

Introduction

The objectives of any particular piece of research, such as a social survey, are often difficult to set down clearly. This is particularly true for longitudinal studies where the uses to which data collected in an earlier sweep will be put are often very unclear. For example, two of the major British birth cohort studies, the 1946 National Survey of Health and Development (NSHD) (Douglas & Blomfield, 1958) and the 1958 National Child Development Study (NCDS) (Fox & Fogelman, see ch. 13) were originally undertaken as single-round perinatal studies and only later became longitudinal studies. In some cases, the objective of a longitudinal study may be unique and clear, as in the case of many epidemiological studies where the criteria for sample selection and conduct of the study are well established.

In many surveys, a major objective is to obtain the maximum amount of useful information for a given cost. If problems such as nonresponse and inaccurate answers are disregarded, the problem is often considered to be one of choosing a suitable, stratified, multistage design in order to maximize the information collected, usually measured by the standard errors of the estimates that are obtained (see, for example, Moser & Kalton, 1971; Kish, 1965).

The problems associated with nonresponse usually receive less attention for a number of reasons, which include the following:

1. Methods of dealing with nonresponse are often specific to a particular survey design, and it is difficult to generalize.

2. The suggestions that are frequently made appear to be obvious and common-sense ones.

3. The problem is seen as essentially practical rather than theoretical, and practical problems have lower prestige among academic researchers.

4. The subject is slightly embarrassing, because we often seem to be attempting to

This chapter was prepared while I was at the Demography Section of the University of Stockholm. Grateful thanks are due to Professor Jan Hoem and his colleagues for their hospitality and to the Tercentenary Foundation of the Royal Bank of Sweden for financial assistance.

obtain information from at least a small fraction of the population who are somewhat reluctant to participate.

A number of articles and books have been written on this topic (Dijkstra & van der Zouwern, 1982; Goyder, 1987; Panel on Incomplete Data, 1983; Sudman & Bradburn, 1974). This chapter will discuss in more detail nonresponse in longitudinal studies, especially the problem of attrition in multiround surveys, and the special considerations that apply to such studies. A number of examples will be drawn from one of the best-documented studies of attrition, that of Farrington, Gallagher, Morley, St. Ledger, and West, which forms chapter 7 of this volume.

Response rates in surveys: General considerations

Samples for surveys may be drawn in a number of scientific (probability) or nonscientific (nonprobability) ways. The benefit of a scientific sample is that results from such a sample can be confidently generalized to the universe from which that sample is drawn. However, longitudinal studies may often have constraints imposed upon them, such as ease of tracing or matching individuals, or minimizing certain aspects of variability between sample members (such as social class or neighborhood factors) so as to concentrate on other differences between them. Indeed, unless the results found in the sample can be generalized to a wider population, either formally or informally, there is little benefit in undertaking most studies, a point emphasized by Sudman's construction of a "credibility scale" for scoring different sample types (Rossi, Wright, & Anderson, 1983, ch. 5).

However, it is usually assumed that the closer response is to 100%, the more representative the sample results will be; but in this context, the question arises as to what are good, acceptable, and unacceptable levels of response. In surveys in the Third World, such as the World Fertility Survey, response rates of well over 95% have been reported; although other evidence, such as an unexpected excess of women reported as being in the 50–54 age group when the survey cutoff age was 49, suggests that such high figures may be misleading. Nevertheless, response rates are usually high. In developed countries, on the other hand, response rates of approximately 70–85% are common. For example, a British Fertility Survey in 1976 obtained a response rate of 85% for a sample of women aged 16–49, and a Swedish Fertility Survey in 1981 obtained a response rate of 87% for women aged 20–44 (Dunnell, 1979; World Fertility Survey, 1984).

There is clear evidence that response rates in surveys have been falling in developed countries in recent decades. In some cases the authors have concluded that the decline was substantial, but the decline recently may have stopped (Goyder, 1987, ch. 4; American Statistical Association, 1974; Panel on Incomplete Data, 1983, vol. 1, ch. 2). Another conclusion is that even where total nonresponse has been kept relatively constant, the proportion of nonresponse accounted for by refusals has increased substantially. For example, in the United States Current Population Survey, the proportion of nonresponse accounted for by refusals rose from about 40% in the late 1960s to about

Table 8.1. *Response and attrition at various ages: National Survey of Health and Development and Farrington et al. Study.*

| Age | Number known to be alive and nonmigrant | | | | | |
| | NSHD | | | Farrington et al. | | |
	(a)	(b)	(c)	(a)	(b)	(c)
0	5362					
8				411		
16	4720	88	(97)	399	97	(100)
32	4587	86	73	383	88	94

Notes:

(a) = Number of people

(b) = Eligible numbers as percent of original sample

(c) = Percentage of eligibles interviewed

60% a decade later. The reason for this increase in refusals is likely to be associated at least in part with concerns about privacy and confidentiality.

In most studies of nonresponse, a distinction is made between *item nonresponse*, where the chosen sample member gives some information, and *unit nonresponse*, where all the information from a particular unit is missing or unusable. The third form of nonresponse is *undercoverage*, in which certain eligible units are not included in the sample frame. For longitudinal studies, a unique and major problem is one aspect of nonresponse, namely, *attrition*, loss to the study of an eligible survey member. The calculation of attrition may be difficult in some cases, depending on the definition of the universe. Thus, if a study includes all those born on a particular date living within the country, then emigrants should be excluded and immigrants included. However, data on migration are frequently of low reliability even in countries with otherwise well-developed population data systems that are able to provide accurate information about deaths to sample members in the geographic area of study.

A good review of the characteristics of those most likely to be lost to longitudinal studies by attrition has recently been undertaken by Waterton and Lievesley (1987), and this topic will not be discussed in further detail here. Information from the NSHD and the study by Farrington et al. are shown in Table 8.1.

The NSHD uses conventional methods of keeping contact, including the sending out of regular birthday cards in order to maintain interest among survey members and to keep up-to-date addresses, together with tracing via the health registration data contained in the National Health Service Central Register (NHSCR). The Farrington et al. study used a much larger number of tracing methods, described in more detail in chapter 7; and it is based on a much smaller, geographically concentrated and interlinked group. The high response rates show the sorts of levels that may be obtained by highly motivated and competent research teams in countries without centralized population registers. The proportions of the eligible sample that were finally interviewed, therefore, is similar to that of major cross-sectional surveys (the response rate in the U.S. Current Population Survey is about 96%, and the British General Household Survey, about 83%), but longitudinal studies have had the additional problem of tracing eligible members rather than simply interviewing at a number of sampled addresses. Evidence from other major longitudinal studies, such as the 1958 National Child Development Study (Fox & Fogelman, ch. 13), the Panel Study on Income Dynamics (Duncan & Morgan, 1985:54), and the 1972 National Longitudinal Study (Haseeb Rizvi, 1983) show acceptably high levels of response compared with conventional cross-sectional studies.

Factors potentially related to attrition

A number of factors that are likely to be associated with attrition can be readily identified, but others that might be expected to be important turn out not to be so. Among both types of items are the following:

Sample characteristics. Some populations – for example, schoolchildren – will be easier to keep track of because of special characteristics and also because access to them may be easier through their schools. (This is a different problem from differential attrition, and its implication within a particular sample will be considered later.)

Sponsors. Most informants are relatively unconcerned about the sponsoring organization. Cannell (1985:16) reports that in a survey conducted by the U.S. Bureau of the Census, only 11% actually knew what organization was conducting the survey, even though the respondents had received an elaborate information brochure and interviewers had emphasized the Bureau's role. In addition, the organization undertaking the survey will often be doing so on behalf of some other agency. It is considered good ethical practice to inform sample members of the identity of the sponsor.

Survey organization. Training, motivation, and competence of interviewers are important; in addition, response is likely to be improved if there is a permanent central body to maintain records and contact with the survey members.

Content. Ignoring item nonresponse, the content of a particular sweep is likely to affect the willingness of survey members to take part in subsequent sweeps and, perhaps, surveys in general.

Confidentiality. Longitudinal data are frequently much more sensitive than cross-sectional data. There are three aspects of confidentiality that need to be considered: the first is release of individual-level data to third parties; the second is linkage of interview data to other records; and the third is the methods used to contact individuals. Although these are important issues that will be discussed in more detail later, they do not seem to be of major concern to informants in longitudinal studies.

Use of data. Informants often have no interest in why a particular study is undertaken (Cannell, 1985:16), even though the information may be used for policy purposes that are not in their best interests or may lead to negative stereotyping. This is one aspect of the principle of informed consent discussed by Jowell (1986).

Interviewer. Interviewer effects are important for two reasons. The first is that high-quality staff will tend to achieve higher response rates than will less-qualified interviewers. The second is that there is also a well-established body of evidence for the existence of interviewer effects; that is, respondents will often amend their replies according to the characteristics of the interviewer.

Frequency. Too-frequent interviewing will lead to respondent fatigue, but too-infrequent interviewing may lead to reduced identification with the survey and also to more difficulty in tracing the addresses of movers. Of course, because such surveys will also frequently collect retrospective information, there is also the question of memory lapse (Moss & Goldstein, 1979).

A cost-benefit approach to reducing attrition

It is usually assumed that minimizing attrition is desirable in itself. However, it would be rare for maximized response to be a final objective of a survey, because there are also a number of costs as well as benefits associated with this, as set out in Table 8.2.

If we have a scientifically drawn sample and attrition is random (i.e., missing cases are no different on average from those interviewed), then the lower the attrition, the higher the achieved sample size and the lower the standard error. If attrition were to be reduced by a given percentage of the initial sample, standard errors would be reduced by about half of this percentage. Because the scope for reduction of attrition is usually limited, the benefit of reduced standard errors is slight and could be gained by increasing the initial sample size in many cases.

However, if the characteristics of difficult-to-contact cases are different from those of the contacted group, they may substantially influence the results obtained. The difference in characteristics of those interviewed after different numbers of attempts at contact have been known for half a century (see, e.g., Clausen & Ford, 1947). In the context of longitudinal studies, Farrington et al. (ch. 7) find that those in the "difficult-to-contact" group are substantially different from the rest, but Fox and Fogelman (ch. 13) conclude that such factors are relatively unimportant for at least some of the uses to which the NCDS will be put.

One reason for minimizing loss in any particular sweep is that loss is likely to be cumulative, because a person who was uncontactable or refused in a given sweep

Table 8.2. *Cost and benefits of reduced attrition.*

Benefits	Costs
Lower sampling errors	Survey costs:
	Money
Possible lower nonsampling errors	Time
Cumulative loss in successive sweeps is reduced	Public acceptability
Prestige of survey researchers	Accuracy of marginal responses

would be less likely to participate in later ones also. For example, if there were 10% loss per sweep, after 10 rounds only one-third of the original sample would remain.

The standing of a survey and its impact are likely to be associated with response rates. If rates are too low the results may not even be disseminated (as essentially happened with the income follow-up survey to the 1971 Census of Great Britain, which achieved only a 50% response). Within the survey organization itself, the standing of individual interviewers is also likely to be closely associated with one of the main indicators of success, a high response rate.

On the other hand, the marginal cost of an interview is likely to rise as the response rate rises. This could be shown graphically by means of a Gini curve. There is clearly a trade-off between cost and improvements to accuracy. Closely related to the financial cost of reducing attrition are costs in time. Farrington et al. had one case where it took 605 days to obtain an interview, or nearly two years. Only in rare circumstances would a survey organization be able to work to such an unpredictable schedule in terms of fieldwork, administration, processing, and so forth. Furthermore, if the survey is undertaken in order for policy or other decision-making reasons, the more out-of-date the information is, the less likely it is that it will be useful.

In general, the majority of respondents report themselves as enjoying taking part in surveys, but often a minority of potential subjects are unwilling to participate. In the Farrington et al. study, 59 (15%) subjects were classified as "resistant but did not refuse," and of the 37 who initially refused, 10 (27%) were later interviewed. The process of obtaining an interview from a resistant subject is a sensitive one. Interviewers are articulate, trained, and motivated to achieve an interview. Potential respondents may be less articulate and have vague but real objections. Ideally, these informants should have time to consider their reactions, but that could cause difficulties for those who wish to maximize response. "Many visits were made without prior warning, because the men's surprise at being unexpectedly recontacted after so many (7–14) years seemed to make them more willing to agree to an interview" (Farrington et al., ch. 7).

Other organizations adopt a more measured approach to making contact. The

General Household Survey, the main British official multipurpose household survey, sends a letter in advance to selected sample members so that they can form their opinions on participation. Social and Community Planning Research, a major survey organization, gives a written declaration to respondents, that states, among other information, "Your participation is entirely voluntary. Once you have agreed to take part you may still change your mind during the interview and withdraw information you have already given. Also, if you prefer not to answer any question, you may simply decline to do so" (Jowell, 1986:230).

One potential problem in maximizing response is the quality of data obtained from reluctant respondents. The evidence that the characteristics of those interviewed at first contact differ from those interviewed later and from those who do not respond at all is clear-cut and overwhelming (although Fox and Fogelman appear to find it relatively unimportant for some of the NCDS analyses). What is not established is how far the *quality* of data obtained from reluctant informants differs from that of more willing participants, although it would be expected to be of lower quality.

In general, informants who are of lower social status are less likely to refuse to be interviewed, compared with those of higher status who have formed a view about whether to participate or not. Lower status informants are more used to various agencies such as housing, social services, and social security officials seeking information from them; and they frequently lack interest in the content, the purpose, and the characteristics of the agency involved.

If attrition is to be reduced and conventional methods of tracing eligible subjects fail, then unconventional ones may have to be employed. In the study of Farrington et al. (ch. 7), the following methods were used:

> Electoral register
> Telephone directory
> Letter
> Criminal Records Office
> National Health Service Central Register/family doctor
> Department of Health and Social Security (by forwarded letter)
> Local authority housing records (by forwarded letter)
> School classmates/neighbor contacts
> Local newspapers
> Local hospitals
> Trade union lists
> Workplace visits

For elusive men in particular, certain methods including health service and criminal records, telephoning the subject's workplace, and leads from other men turned out to be very important. All of these raise more substantial problems of privacy than do some of the other methods employed. The UN Declaration on Human Rights states that people should not be subject to arbitrary interference with their privacy, and they should have the right to the protection of the law against such interference.

Clearly, attitudes about what represents an intrusion of privacy will be a matter of personal judgment; in my view some of these methods are questionable. However, evaluation of the costs and benefits of any act can be particularly difficult when the costs and benefits accrue to different individuals or groups; indeed, in many cases the beneficiary will be society itself, and this long-standing debate is well outside the bounds of this paper.

General survey practice recommends that the conditions for a set of interviews be as similar as possible. Different interviewers are likely to elicit different responses – the well-known "interviewer effect"; but also the place where the interview takes place, the presence of other people, and so forth, may affect the answers that are obtained. Furthermore, there is a problem in that some techniques used to minimize attrition may tend to maximize heterogeneity of interviewing context. For example, in the Farrington et al. study, the interviewer sometimes deliberately changed his appearance in order to obtain the interview. Although the same interviewer may be used, such changes are likely to lead to similar (but in this case unmeasurable) effects as those that are part of the conventional interviewer effect.

Confidentiality of dissemination

Longitudinal data are usually much more sensitive than data obtained from single-round studies for a number of reasons:

1. The sorts of topics investigated by the more precise instrument of longitudinal studies, such as psychological precursors of crime and deviance, are inherently sensitive.

2. The form of sample designs necessary for tracing individuals frequently makes it much easier for membership of the sample to be deduced; for example, the NCDS is based on all births in one week in March 1958.

3. The volume of data collected, in conjunction with the sample design, makes the identification of a particular individual relatively straightforward.

4. Because tracing will often require the linkage of records and because there is a need for a unique personal identifier, linkage of records to other registers will often be relatively easy.

These considerations relate both to the use that is made of the survey itself by the organizers and sponsors, and to access to the survey by outside researchers via public access data archives. This problem is exacerbated, because at the start of an investigation the uses to which the data will be put are often unclear.

Conclusions

Any particular round of interviewing in a longitudinal study is not an isolated event; it is influenced by previous rounds, and it is likely to effect what happens in any later rounds. Moreover, it will both be affected by and potentially affect the conduct of other past and future surveys. Reduction of attrition is desirable as one means toward the end of obtaining as truly representative a sample as possible. Surveys with low response rates, even given representative samples, are likely to be discounted by both public and professionals; but very high response rates may frequently be obtained only at a disproportionate cost in terms of time, money, and acceptability. It is therefore clear that the optimal level of response lies between 0 and 100%, and that the optimal value will differ with the survey objectives. In practice, it will be impossible to establish this level precisely. Rather, it serves to emphasize that achieving a particular level of attrition is not damaging to a survey but constitutes a means to achieving its true objectives.

References

American Statistical Association. (1974). Report on the ASA conference on surveys of human populations. *American Statistician, 28,* 30–34.

Cannell, C. F. (1985). Overview: Response bias and interviewer variability in surveys. In T. W. Beed & R. J. Stimson, *Survey interviewing: Theory and techniques* (pp. 1–23). Sydney: George Allen & Unwin.

Clausen, J. A., & Ford, R. N. (1947). Controlling bias in mail questionnaires. *Journal of the American Statistical Association, 42* 497–511.

Dijkstra, W., & van der Zouwen, J. (Eds.) (1982). *Response behaviour in the survey interview.* London: Academic Press.

Douglas, J. W. B., & Blomfield, J. M. (1958). *Children under five.* London: George Allen & Unwin.

Duncan, G. J., & Morgan, J. N. (1985). The panel study of income dynamics. In G. H. Elder (Ed.), *Life course dynamics: Trajectories and transitions, 1968–80* (pp. 50–71). Ithaca: Cornell University Press.

Dunnell, K. (1979). *Family formation 1976.* London: Her Majesty's Stationery Office.

Goyder, J. (1987). *The silent minority: Nonrespondents on sample surveys.* Cambridge: Polity Press.

Haseeb Rizvi, M. (1983). An empirical investigation of some item nonresponse adjustment procedures. In Panel on Incomplete Data, *Incomplete data in sample surveys* (Vol. 1: *Report and Case Studies,* pp. 299–366). New York: Academic Press.

Jowell, R. (1986). The codification of statistical ethics. *Journal of Official Statistics, 2,* 217–253.

Kish, L. (1965). *Survey sampling.* New York: Wiley.

Moser, C. A., & Kalton, G. (1971). *Survey methods in social investigation.* London: Heinemann.

Moss, L., & Goldstein, H. (Eds.) (1979). *The Recall Method in Social Surveys.* London: University of London Institute of Education.

Panel on Incomplete Data. (1983). *Incomplete data in sample surveys* (3 vols.). New York: Academic Press.

Rossi, P. H., Wright, J. D., & Anderson, A. B. (1983). *Handbook of Survey Research.* New York: Academic Press.

Sudman, S., & Bradburn, N. M. (1974). *Response effects in surveys: A review and synthesis.* Chicago: Aldine.

Waterton, J., & Lievesley, D. (1987). Attrition in a panel study of attitudes. *Journal of Official Statistics 3,* 267–282.

World Fertility Survey. (1984). *Fertility Survey in Sweden, 1981: A summary of findings.* London: World Fertility Survey.

9   N's, times, and number of variables in longitudinal research

GEORG RUDINGER AND PHILLIP KARL WOOD

Introduction

Issues of subject selection, timing, and number of variables, as well as the appropriate selection of variables are topics often discussed within psychology in general as well as in developmental psychology (e.g., Buss, 1979).

Taxonomies employing categories of "N's (Persons) × Times (Occasions) × Variables" are well known since Cattell's presentation of his "covariation chart" (Cattell, 1946), which served as a framework for defining six primary factor analytic techiques. Cattell's generalization of this covariation chart – the Basic Data Relation Matrix (BDRM) – extends the three-dimensional box to a ten-dimensional one and allows for derivation of many more covariation techniques based on combinations of the 10 dimensions (see also Cattell 1988) Within developmental psychology, Coan (1966) has defined twenty-four covariation techniques in terms of four design components, facets, or dimensions, namely, external stimuli, person variables, occasions, and subjects.

Because the focus of this chapter is on the role of these factors in the design of longitudinal assessments, we will not take up all methodological points made in these previous discussions (see for this, e.g., Baltes, Reese, & Nesselroade, 1977; Nesselroade & Baltes, 1979; Nesselroade & von Eye, 1985; Rudinger, 1979).

Longitudinal design orientation

"Developmental psychology concerns itself with the description, explanation and modification of interindividual differences (and similarities) in intraindividual change" (Baltes, Reese, & Nesselroade, 1977:7). In order to provide an understanding of intraindividual changes and changes across individual differences in development, this task involves identifying the form, sequence, and patterning of behavioral development as well as searching for underlying mechanisms and causes of development.

This assumption implies an often-overlooked crucial requirement for developmental research: The entity the researcher is interested in must be observed repeatedly as it exists and evolves over time (McCall, 1977). Consequently, repeated measurement of a given entity and variation of time are essential to developmental research. Baltes

& Nesselroade (1979) speak of the longitudinal method as a broad concept that might be better called a design orientation rather than a specific method per se. In terms of our taxonomy, a longitudinal design situation contains at least two measurement points over time: $T(=times) \geq 2$.

Because techniques of data analysis, however, are not the subject of this book, we will discuss only the framework of three facets (N, times, variables) as they relate to design methodology for longitudinal research and to a conceptualization of testable models reflecting central conceptual issues of developmental research.

One important commonality of these three characteristics is how they are used to define and estimate errors of measurement (in a broad sense) within a given developmental study. Researchers from various perspectives within developmental psychology use these three dimensions differentially to conceptualize error.

Many researchers involved in experimental design sample across several individuals in order to come up with an estimate of the error of measurement (Cronbach, 1957, 1975; Lord & Novick, 1968). This approach assumes that individuals differ only by a linear function of one underlying construct as measured by the items of the instrument.

Increasingly, developmental researchers have become aware that this approach to estimating error and relationships between variables may severely limit the validity of inferences drawn from a study. Recently, an increasing number of researchers (Nesselroade, 1987) and statisticians (Molenaar, 1987) have concentrated on the development of repeated assessments of single individuals or small numbers of individuals over many points in time in order to arrive at an estimate of errors of measurement associated with a given variable across people. Some approaches have taken an independent and stochastic view of the individual across time, whereas recent developments in time series and frequency analysis have investigated the extent to which variables measured at different points in time (immediately, recently, etc.) influence subsequent performance. Longitudinal methodology does not specify in a prospective manner the span of time included in a study. Frequency of assessment must be considered as a design feature as it relates to the phenomenon under investigation and the researchers' assumptions about the change process.

Other researchers, most notably those from a classical psychometric background, employ several (assumed to be equivalent) variables that purportedly measure the same construct. In this context, research in classical test theory is similar to research adapting a uni- or multidimensional scaling approach (Roskam, in press).

Within developmental psychology, all three approaches have been employed to assess change and the degree to which change is systematic across the life span. These three fundamental approaches to design empirical research all share a further similarity in that they explore the existence of relationships or compare relationships among variables (Coombs, 1964). In one sense, developmental researchers who are "only interested in changes over time" can be thought of as assessing relationships as well, in that they examine the relationship of time with the substantive variables under study. The manner in which these relationships are defined varies depending on assumed processes of developmental change and level of measurement assumed, and varies from methodological approach to approach.

Although we will not discuss a technical treatment of methodological aspects of *N*'s or time, we will discuss how conceptual assumptions of the researcher regarding the underlying processes at work (including error processes) as well as types or relationships between constructs under study involve a delicate balance of tradeoffs in assessing different *N*'s, times, and numbers of variables. The term *error* in this paper will be used to describe the general phenomenon "empirical misclassification." As such, this error concept is broader than the term as it is used in many methodological discussions. For example, to refer to the latter concept, error, as defined within much of classical test theory, is a continuous quantity affecting observed variables to the same degree as at all levels of the latent variable. Error, however, can also apply to a nominal variable and in this case means a classification error in assigning an individual to a given category compared with a "true" latent class (Rindskopf, 1987).

To demonstrate the tradeoffs involved, we will discuss simple representative experimental designs often found in developmental psychology. For the more elementary designs presented, alternate explanations for observed findings (such as differential reliability) are not estimable. More elaborate designs, however, allow estimation of the presence of these alternate measurement models. Although problems of reliability, stability, invariance of constructs, measurement error, and misclassification or misspecification have been often discussed in data analytic discussions (Nesselroade & Baltes, 1979), determination and interpretation of these are conceptual issues central to the formulation and testing of hypotheses for a construct. As such, these issues constitute a list of "bold conjectures" that the researcher must make about the activity and presence of the construct prior to conducting a study or beginning an analysis. Construct definition is open for operationalization in a number of ways, depending on developmental metatheories (mechanistic, organismic), theories (trait, state, process, stage-theory), and types of variables (quantitative, qualitative) and populations (individuals, subclasses, or normative groups) to which the researcher wishes to generalize.

Longitudinal observations: Multimodal selections

Referring to the taxonomy "Subjects $\times$ Times $\times$ Variables" ($N \times T \times M$), the hypothetical universe from which the observation is drawn is composed of "scores" for every possible person at each and every possible occasion of measurement on all possible variables (Cattell, 1966; Cronbach, Gleser, Nanda, & Rajaratnam, 1972).

The procedures and methods by which one collects a specific set of observations can be thought of as selection operations (Nesselroade, 1987) that produce *selection effects*. These selection effects as a rule jeopardize the generalizations that the researcher wants to make to a broader universe of persons, times, or variables. As such, generalizations from this research may be incomplete or even biased. Even if one considers each mode separately for expository purposes, it is important to realize that a set of data represents a selected subset with respect to the remaining modes; that is, it is still a sample drawn from a universe of potential observations simultaneously defined by the person, occasion, and variable modes.

Person mode

The person mode is most generally taken up in discussions of selection and its effects in terms of its generalizability to population. In most cases it is the mode most explicitly considered in designing longitudinal study. For our purposes we can differentiate two classes of selection: "$N = 1$" and samples of more than 1 person, "$N > 1$." Of course, the labels "$N > 1$" or "$N = 1$" say nothing about the quality of selection or the heterogeneity of the person sample with respect to organismic variables and/or response variables. The person "selection effect" affects assessment of relations between variables under study as well as generalizations of a subject to a population universe.

Variable mode

Selection effects on variables are less frequently recognized than person selection effects. The problems can be phrased as: Is Variable $Y1$ or $Y2$ the more valid indicator for concept Q? How does one make the choice of which manifest variables to include in a given study? What are the consequences of one's choice of variables to represent a given concept?

Problems of construct validity or variable validity are discussed as "cause construct validity" and "effect construct validity" by Cook and Campbell (1976, 1979) and have become increasingly relevant in order to identify latent variables by means of manifest variables (indicators or markers) under various scaling procedures (e.g., Scalogram-, Rasch-, IRT-modeling).

For the purposes of our discussion, two broad classes of variable (M) selection exist: $M = 1$, that is, just one variable is chosen for study; and, second, a larger sample of variables, ($M > 1$) is drawn. The case $M > 1$ needs further differentiation by introducing some more facets for the variable domain. In the context of differential longitudinal designs, at most four types of variables exist:

      Independent (manipulated) variables X
      Dependent (observed, measured) variables Y
      Person or organismic variables (like age): W
      Background variables (like cohort): Z

Organismic variables (W) and background variables (Z) can play different roles in various designs as concomitant variables, moderator variables, grouping variables, or "quasi"-independent variables by theoretical declaration. This can happen jointly together with introduction of an experimental treatment or intervention (X) or without explicit treatment (i.e., in case of nonexperimental studies).

In this context, additional features of variables must also be considered. Depending on theoretical knowledge about development or metatheoretical assumptions, variables can be defined and conceptualized as qualitative (e.g., nominal, ordinally scaled) or quantitative (e.g., interval, ratio scaled) ones.

Reaction time, for example, since physical time is taken, seems self-evidently to be measured on ratio-scale level. If, however, the model of cognitive structures or processes that is going to be tested by these data is a qualitative one (e.g., mental network described by relative distances between nodes, i.e., concepts), these highly precise measures can provide only ordinality information, and every statistical model appropriate for this ratio-scale-level not represented by theory yields a surplus or even misleading information. Data is always an operationalization of researchers' theory of behavior.

Data. The term *data* is quite often used very loosely. We will briefly mention the understanding of data from the point of view of pscyhologists inclined to a tradition established by researchers such as Coombs, Dawes, and Tversky (1970), and Roskam (1983).

Naive (psychological) observations are interpretations or attributions; that is, one infers someone's mood from his or her behavior. Of course, these interpretations and attributions can become the subject of research, but this is another point beyond the discussion of the nature of data. Objective observation is needed in categories like acceptance versus rejection, agreement versus disagreement, correctness versus incorrectness, or in terms of preferences. Primary data (the so-called raw data) are always the recording of single behavioral events, like the correctness of a response, the endorsement of an opinion, and so forth, condensed in an observation matrix; but these observations are not yet data. There is a popular psychological belief that measurements are data and that data are measurements. Neither is true because psychological phenomena do not carry numbers. Measurement depends on theory and implies modeling about reality. If something is measured (or rather, if the value of a theoretical latent variable or construct is estimated), these measures can be input for higher order theorizing and on that level can be considered as data. The term *construct* denotes a contrived or invented notion, with the purpose of explaining a phenomenon (MacCorquodale & Meehl, 1948). Theoretical constructs refer to a lawful relation, pattern, or structure in the data of observation, and they are defined through the theory about those phenomena. A theoretical construct explains that certain behaviors occur and others don't, and from this follows a definite data structure. The crucial point is the appropriate mapping of theoretical structures into designs and data structures on the one hand and model structures on the other hand. This is formally represented by the theoretical hypothesis that the data are constrained to be what they are, and that this constraint satisfies a rule, principle, or law. The empirical world and the theoretical world touch each other just by comparing data structures (such as patterns in frequency matrices or order relations in covariance matrices) with model structures (e.g., defined by parameters) derived from theory. This is consentaneous with Guttman's (1977) view that a theory is a rationale for a hypothesis of a correspondence between a definitional system for a universe of observations and an aspect of the empirical structure of those observationos. A theory that is not stated in terms of the data analysis to be used cannot be tested.

To take another example, consider the assumption that there is a linear rise in intelligence up to adulthood (30 years) and, afterwards, a slight but steady decline of 5% in every decade. In order to test this theory, one has to test hypotheses about ratios of differences; in this case, at least interval-scaled latent variables are necessary in order to test these assumptions.

Given the view that development is qualitative structural change of the psychic system as opposed to continuous change (development vs. growth; see Overton & Reese, 1973; Wohlwill, 1973), hypotheses to be tested have to be formulated in terms of order relations and variables have to be defined at least as ordinal ones. Inferences must refer to statements about order and change of order relations instead of numerical differences. It is easy to see that selection of an appropriateness scaling model or statistical technique are primarily not empirical questions, but must be theory guided. This statement is also valid for another additional classification of variables, namely, with regard to absence or presence of measurement error (strong or weak measurement). Measurement error can be conceptualized within every scaling model and for every scale type of measurement as response uncertainty, misclassification, or random disturbances, as was mentioned earlier.

Time mode

The notion of selection and selection effects also has important implications for the occasion/time mode. This mode is obviously a key one for developmentalists or any researcher concerned with change. Time is that variable through which the trajectories of development are projected. Decisions about how to sample time within developmental study cannot be left to the chance requirements for a preferred statistical technique, nor is this decision an arbitrary one.

Time, as we use the term here, is an independent design variable, for as such it can also be conceptualized as a continuous variable (as is evident in developmental assessments that employ frequency analysis [Molenaar, 1987] or time series designs), discrete (ANOVA), or ordinal (as in the case of analyses of sequentiality of events). This decision represents conceptual assumptions about how "time" affects the processes under study and the time duration of the processes under study. The degree to which manifest time affects aging or developmental processes of the organism is a conceptual assumption (Riegel, 1972, 1977; Sterns & Alexander, 1977). Mayer and Huinink (see ch. 12) have examined inherent problems of the conceptual identification of time as they relate to the familiar concepts of age, cohort, and period. One has to differentiate the logical, conceptual "confounding" of these classical design concepts (Schaie, 1965; Baltes, 1968; Schaie & Baltes, 1975) from effect confounding (Mason, Mason, Winsborough, & Poole, 1973; Horn & McArdle, 1980) in longitudinal designs. Some experimental designs allow the researcher to disentangle the influences of time, age, and cohort design effects within the framework of a three-factorial design (e.g., Erdfelder, 1987).

The relation of time to a given variable or variables under study is a central issue of developmental psychology called "change." Whether from a developmental perspective this change is also to be termed *development* is a conceptual issue. By relationship here, developmentalists do not necessarily mean just a correlation coefficient (Wohlwill, 1980); there are distinct classes of types of relationship defined as

- Relations between *distributions* of one variable ($M = 1$; $N > 1$) and time ($T > 2$).
- Relations between a linking function of two (or more) variables ($M > 2$; $N > 1$) and time ($T > 2$); for example, constancy or change in a relation between variables across time (Runkel & McGrath, 1972).

Types and shapes of relationships between variables in general (i.e., also between psychological variables and nonpsychological variables as "time") depend again on theoretical status of these variables in the researcher's theory.

Thus, measurement decisions determine the nature of the state space (finite, countably infinite, continuous), the number of variables (univariate, multivariate), and the presence or absence of measurement error (weak or strong measurement). Most longitudinal research conducted in psychology involves discrete time sampling. Decisions concerning the frequency of observations in time and extent of the series are important in determining the characteristic of the series (e.g., probability structure) in terms of transition matrices. Infrequent time sampling will document long-term changes in a behavior trait. Too-frequent time sampling may fail to detect longer-term developmental changes. For example, suppose one wants to study a process that changes rapidly, or one for which the relationships between variables across time are immediately antecedent. It is then inappropriate to design a study with infrequent testing over a longitudinal period.

Another problem connected with timing of observations (i.e., spacing, frequency, duration) is called "causal lag". Historical causation, with its emphasis on distal causes, requires explanatory constructions with conceptions of causal lag. Concrete examples are frequent in the medical sciences, where several diseases exist that have a symptomatology at points in time many years removed from the onset of the disorder. Causal lag requires special consideration in longitudinal research design. Heise (1975), for example, has argued that a theory of causal lag is necessary and must be available in order to decide the duration and spacing of longitudinal observations (see also Singer & Spilerman, 1979).

Equal-interval spacing of observations is not necessarily an optimal solution, although it appears to be routinely practiced. Departure from equal-interval spacing is likely to become more frequent as theoretical knowledge of causal processes increases.

Table 9.1. *Data-gathering strategies for interindividual differences, intraindividual differences, and intraindividual changes.*

	Dimension 1: sample across	Dimension 2: compare on	Dimension 3: sample through	Type
	Individuals	No	No	Inter-ID
	Variables	No	No	Intra-ID
	Occasions	No	No	Intra-IC
(1)	Variables	Individuals	No	Inter-ID in intra-ID
(2)	Individuals	Variables	No	Inter-VD in inter-ID
(3)	Variables	Occasions	No	Inter-OD in intra-ID
*(4)	Occasions	Variables	No	Inter-VD in intra-IC
*(5)	Occasions	Individuals	No	Inter-ID in intra-IC
(6)	Individuals	Occasions	No	Inter-OD in inter-ID
(1')	Variables	Individuals	Occasions	Inter-OD in inter-ID in intra-ID
(2')	Individuals	Variables	Occasions	Inter-OD in inter-VD in inter-ID
(3')	Variables	Occasions	Individuals	Inter-ID in inter-OD in intra-ID
*(4')	Occasions	Variables	Individuals	Inter-ID in inter-VD in intra-IC
*(5')	Occasions	Individuals	Variables	Inter-VD in inter-ID in intra-IC
(6')	Individuals	Occasions	Variables	Inter-VD in inter-OD in inter-ID

Notes:
ID = Individual differences
IC = Individual changes
VD = Variable differences
OD = Occasion differences
(1) . . . (6) number referred to in the text
*Dealing with intraindividual changes

A taxonomy of change: The Buss model

From the viewpoint of a psychometrician and already in line with the multimodal selection idea, Buss (1974, 1979) developed a unified conceptual framework of change and stability. This approach is not identical with developmental designs (Schaie, 1965, 1977; Baltes, 1968), but is based on Cattell's (1966) three-dimensional "Person × Variable × Occasion Box." The taxonomy orders and defines different types of change as well as their relationships and is, in Buss's view, restricted to quantitative concepts of change. After slight modification, however, it serves here to structure types of change in general. The modal selection procedure applied across the three facets of the N-Times-Variables-Box results in 15 methods of data collection for interindividual differences, intraindividual differences, and intraindividual changes. The first three consider only one dimension at a time. The next six work with two dimensions. In the last six, all three dimensions are compared in a three-step process (Table 9.1.).

The three steps mentioned are the following. First, Buss starts with the sample case, where the datum in each cell of the $N \times T \times M$-box is an individual's score on a variable at a particular occasion. Interindividual differences are defined by sampling across individuals for each variable at one occasion; intraindividual differences are defined by sampling across variables for each individual at one occasion; and, finally, intraindividual changes are specified by sampling across occasions for each variable for one individual.

In a second step, the concepts of interindividual differences, intraindividual differences, and intraindividual changes are enlarged by considering the six possible ways of comparative sampling across each of the three dimensions.

Comparing each of these dimensions to the other two results in six cases. Two examples are presented:

4. "Intervariable" differences (or intraindividual differences) in intraindividual change. Variables are compared for all occasions of one individual.
5. Interindividual differences in intraindividual change. Individuals are compared for all occasions in one variable.

Each of these six data-gathering strategies is defined by what is compared (which gives the first aspect or the interindividual differences, intervariable differences, or interoccasion differences part) and in terms of what set is sampled across (which gives the second part of interindividual differences, intraindividual differences, or intraindividual changes aspect).

In each case, the dimension mentioned first is the point of interest and is compared through samples taken from elements of the second dimension.

In a third step, it would, of course, be possible to expand each of the six methods of data collection. So, for purposes of comparison, a sample would also be taken from the third dimension, which, up to now, has remained constant.

A still more general case would involve successful samplng of entire matrices through the third dimension. Two examples out of the six three-step cases are given:

Case 3′. Interindividual differences in interoccasion differences (changes) in intraindividual differences, in which the variances reflecting the extent of intraindividuala differences for each occasion for an individual are compared for occasions through the individual dimension.

Case 4′. Interindividual differences in intervariable differences (intraindividual differences) in intraindividual changes, in which variable scores across occasions for an individual are compared for variables through individual dimension.

According to Buss (1979) limitations of this general conceptual framework include the following:

- The taxonomy and the concepts of IC, ID, VD, OD rest upon the assumption that the meaning of the constructs that the variables are measuring remains invariant across the facets of persons and/or times.
- The model is not equipped to deal in an analytic way with interbehavioral change (patterns and structures). But, in our opinion, this is not a major limitation. One

can derive further concepts within the framework of this taxonomy that take into account relations between persons and/or times and/or variables.

Structure and sequences

As already mentioned, qualitative approaches face design problems similar to those of the psychometric paradigm in measuring and structuring change. We will demonstrate this with reference to the concepts of structure and sequence (van den Daele, 1969; Wohlwill, 1973; Aebli, 1978; Fisher, 1980; Coombs & Smith, 1973).

A developmental sequence can be defined as an ontogenetic series of states of the psychic system that occurs with a theoretically predicted regularity in all observed individuals (i.e., with interindividual uniformity). Regularity is assumed if there is a high probability that the states are concantenated with each other in the theoretically postulated order. It is difficult, however, even in the case of simple, unitary sequences to demonstrate such a regularity indicated by high probability.

For example, also for qualitative concepts from a cross-sectional design, it is possible only to infer change (i.e., a developmental sequence). Based on aggregated data of many individuals gathered at one measurement occasion, the inference of change is drawn from the configuration of variables in relation to a theoretical developmental process. This procedure leads to acceptable results only under the strong assumption that the underlying developmental process is cumulative in character. In a longitudinal design, the sequence can be directly observed, loosely speaking. Only in a longitudinal design is the researcher in the position to compare, in a manner analogous to the psychometric approach, different types of changes such as intraindividual change and interindividual differences in intraindividual changes (Henning & Rudinger, 1985).

For a long time the assumption of universal, invariant sequences generalizable over people, time, cultures, and social classes was of special theoretical interest. Empirical research, however, failed to establish the types of developmental sequence as predominantly valid developmental patterns. Empirical and some critical theoretical analyses (e.g., Broughton, 1977; Phillips & Kelly, 1975; Rest, 1979) of hierarchical theories of development (e.g., the Piagetian invariance approach) led to the conclusion that the development of cognitive structures is not acccurately represented by strict sequences in the structure of concrete operations (e.g., Quantity→Weight→Volume; Shepard, 1978). As a result, hypotheses emerged that cognitive structure is more differentiated and more complex than a unidimensional "Guttman-like" simple order. Developmental sequences and structures can be designated either in the "logical Piagetian structure" of a unidimensional hierarchy or as multiple/multidimensional patterns if partial orders, tree-structure, bi- or multiform scales are adopted (see also Bart & Airasian, 1974; Krus, 1977).

The well-known Guttman-scalogram-structure forms a sequence of simple ordinal character. This scale was termed by Goodman (1978) a "uniform scale". It is assumed that most of the subjects can be classified or scaled by the true score pattern of that scale form; that is, there exist no interindividual differences.

A "biform scale" may be the result of different substantial strategies being used to establish a definite pattern of behavior, developmental stage, or task. For instance, on the one hand, a biform-scale can be the representation of a cognitive process reaching the highest level by two alternative ways. On the other hand, however, a biform-scale gives evidence of the existence of two different classes of subjects in the population of interest (Dayton & Macready, 1980; Rindskopf, 1987). Each of these classes fits a uniform scale, but they differ from each other in one or more response patterns. The combined uniform scales comprise the biform scale. These scale types give an alternative representation of unilineal progressions – with stage skipping or regression processes to an earlier level of development – to that presented in the dynamic models of Singer and Spilerman (1979); that is, there exist interindividual differences. Multiform scales are an extension of biform scales that represent divergent or convergent progression (van den Daele, 1969), another class of interindividual differences (Rudinger, 1987).

Selected longitudinal designs

Combination of the above-mentioned classes of selection procedures outlined by Cattell, Buss, and Nesselroade for N: ($N = 1$ or $N > 1$) and of the classes of selection procedures for M: ($M = 1$ or $M > 1$) as well as for independent, dependent, person or background variables; that is: $X = (0, 1, >1)$, $Y = (1, >1)$, $W = (0, 1, >1)$, or $Z = (0, 1, >1)$, as well as the two facets of the time concept (discrete or continuous) leads to an insurmountable variety of designs impossible to discuss within this work. In order to outline the central conceptual issues of longitudinal research, we will now discuss elementary examples representing approaches in much current developmental research.

Situation: $N > 2$, $M = 1$, ($Y = 1$), $T = 2$

Consider the simple case of a study that consists of longitudinal testing, employing only one dependent variable (Y), across many individuals ($N > 2$). For our first discussion, let Y be a continuous variable. This is the basic design of a simple longitudinal study involving a pretest–posttest arrangement with a minimum of two occasions of measurement. In a nonexperimental situation, some specific interval of time is the intervening "treatment" variable, such as a difference in chronological age.

From this type of studies, representative of many approaches, two basic types of relations with time can be analyzed: We can examine patterns of means across individuals over time, and/or patterns of variability across individuals over time. Many conceptual problems, however, arise from interpretation of patterns and relations so revealed. It is precisely these interpretation problems that provided the impetus for development of the more comprehensive research designs outlined below. For example, given an increasing pattern of variation and increasing means across time, differential reliability of Y could act to produce a false pattern of increasing spread (Wood, in press a). Differential trajectories of learning could also account for this pattern.

This simple longitudinal scheme is included in what Campbell and Stanley (1963) labeled preexperimental design. It is well known that such designs are afflicted with many confounds and potential sources of error that severely jeopardize both internal and external validity. A simple inspection of Campbell and Stanley's (1963) design framework (see also Cook & Campbell, 1976, 1979) shows the extent of the problem, involving such sources of error as sampling, history, maturation, testing, instrumentation, statistical regression, experimental mortality.

Although these counterarguments to account for such a pattern are well known in the methodological literature, similar arguments are not so often advanced for studies that are but minor adaptations of such a design. Instead of a continuous dependent variable, consider a nominal variable, Y, over time. Errors of measurement still exist for such a situation but are represented by errors of classification. As an example, consider a task where adolescents are asked what social environment they prefer (e.g., movies, disco, working at home, or shopping mall) at 15 years of age and again at 16 years of age. To the extent that an adolescent might falsely report that they prefer to work at home when in fact they actually prefer to go to a movie, an error of classification will result for this individual. These errors of classification lead to a biased or distorted estimate of conditional probabilities or transition probabilities. The theoretically unspecified change model as presently stated is insufficiently sophisticated to account for this source of error in the data (cf. Coleman, 1964).

Similar difficulties of interpretation exist for studies that employ two ordinal variables like position in a stage variable. Whether this measurement error results from a false classification of the individual at time 1 or at time 2 or both cannot be determined from such a study. In those cases, however, where a strong conceptual rationale for the processes of development (e.g., strong ordinal progression over time) exists, a precise model of error rates can be formulated and tested (Dayton & Macready, 1983; Rudinger, Chaselon, Zimmermann, & Henning, 1985). Apparent regressions in performance over time are consequently assumed due to the operation of measurement error ordinally related to the categories under study. However, lack of such sophisticated models of error classification characterize many developmental models currently employed in developmental psychology.

Another limitation in available developmental-research designs is due to the fact that some of the sources of error listed in the classical design framework of Campbell and Stanley (1963) are important theoretical or process variables in developmental research. For example, history and maturation are both sources of error in classical nondevelopmental research design. For developmentalists, however, some processes associated with history (e.g., cohort) and maturation are important ingredients in the theory of development and thereby attain the status of relevant explanatory variables rather than error. Another example is that of mortality. Experimental and biological mortality is a source of error in nondevelopmental research. But in the study of life-span development, changes in the composition of a given birth cohort

Table 9.2. *Classifications of quasi-experimental designs (see Campbell & Stanley, 1963; Cook & Campbell, 1976) in terms of familiar developmental paradigms (abridged from Schaie, 1977).*

	Quasi-experimental design	Equivalent developmental paradigm
1.	Time series	Single cohort longitudinal
2.	Equivalent time samples	None
3.	Equivalent material samples	Single cohort longitudinal with alternate forms for each measurement
4.	Nonequivalent control group design	Time sequential
5.	Counterbalanced designs	None
6.	Separate sample	Cross-sectional
	a. Controlled for history	Cohort-sequential with independent samples
	b. Controlled for trends	Cross-sequential with repeated measurement
7.	Separate sample pretest–posttest design control group design	Cross-sequential with independent samples
8.	Multiple time series	Cohort-sequential with repeated measurement
9.	Institutional cycle design	Time-lag or time sequential
10.	Regression discontinuity	Functional age analysis

associated with increasing age and reflecting differences in length of life provide important information about life-span development and are not at all a source of error but a facet of external validity.

Thus, to elevate simple longitudinal research to the level of quasi-experimental and experimental designs is not always desirable or possible in the study of development. As already discussed by Wohlwill (1973), some aspects of development are not fully manipulable for theoretical reasons. If chronological age, for example, is an important component of developmental theory or a defining characteristic of developmental-change functions, full experimentation is not possible. Because of the preponderance of such situations in developmental research, an alternative strategy of simulating developmental processes was introduced (Baltes & Goulet, 1971; Baltes, Nesselroade, & Cornelius, 1978).

Taking these arguments into account, longitudinal research can be moved from the status of preexperimental designs in the direction of quasi-experimental designs by (1) including control groups; (2) including treatment groups via random assignment; and (3) extending the number of occasions across the sequence of longitudinal observations. Thus, the improvement of design characteristics refers to introducing X-Variables, W- and/or Z-Variables and/or additional Y-variables, and extending $T = 2$ to $T >> 2$ (see Table 9.2, taken in an abridged form from Schaie, 1977).

Situation: $N > 1$, $M = 1$, $(Y = 1)$, $T >> 2$

With the extension from $T = 2$ to $T >> 2$ we enter the domain of time-series designs. In single-group descriptive research the primary interest is in the characteristic of the growth process in a single group. At first we consider a study composed of several testings over time ($T > 2$) of a group of individuals ($N > 1$) on a single variable ($M = 1$). An example of such a study could be the repeated administration of an intelligence test over several years.

Stability for the latent traits and differential or invariant reliability across testings as postulated by the researcher can be defined and tested under this design (Rudinger, 1986). This is a significant advantage of this study over the single repeated testing described in the example above. Such a design also enables the researcher to state the hypothesis of more complex underlying processes of development, such as differential latent growth (McArdle & Epstein, 1987), Markovian or autoregressive models of different orders (Rudinger & Rietz, 1987) or metameters that explain systematic interindividual differences (McArdle, 1988). In other words, this design enables the researcher to examine more complex developmental (i.e., substantive) models and to test corresponding hypotheses; this is the conceptual advantage of this design.

In multiple-group studies, interest centers in the differences between natural stratified groups (by introducing W- or Z-variables) in their developmental characteristics. Equivalent groups are constructed by random sampling from a single population with random assignment. Equivalent groups might be studied in a descriptive study if the principal interest were in the generalizability of the characteristics of a time series. However, most research employing equivalent groups is experimental, involving the introduction of an intervention (X) to one or more of the groups.

In time-series experiments, in which an intervention can be applied at different times in a series, design of an intervention plan involves decisions concerning the time, duration, and pattern of interventions as well as their number and type. In general, five design dimensions may be used to specify an intervention plan in time-series experiments: (1) the number and types of interventions; (2) the time at which an intervention occurs in a series; (3) the duration of the intervention; (4) the number of repetitions of an intervention; and (5) the sequence of different types of interventions in designs involving the application of more than one type of intervention to a group.

Situation: $N = 1$, $M = 1$, $T >> 2$

Similar advantages apply to studies that involve measuring a single individual ($N = 1$) in one variable ($M = 1$) across several times ($T >> 2$). Such a study might be the examination of a given individual's blood pressure over several days. Naturally, the researcher, in conducting this study, is assuming that this individual's intraindividual performance is somehow representative of some groups of individuals and as such is a facet of the selection of individuals that the researcher makes in designing the study. The example, however, is useful for again highlighting the role of appropriate choice of a time measure for the study. For example, if the researcher believes that there exist short-term dependencies in the blood pressure of a previous day as they relate to present blood pressure, then the study must either incorporate daily testing or block randomization.

Situation: $N = 1, M > 1, T >> 2$

Further conceptual inferences can be made from studies that involve the examination of several variables ($M > 2$) over time ($T >> 2$) for one individual ($N = 1$). These studies enable the examination of whether, for example, a previous day's mood has any influence on the current day's blood pressure. There can be made several competing (and testable) assumptions by the researcher either that there are minimal or nonexistent time-bound relationships among the variables or localized time-bound effects attain between the variables. Dependent on these assumptions are definitions of systematic and "noise" variations. These, in turn, affect the choice of data analytic method. Cyclic effects across such time series await development of appropriate analytic techniques. The logical extension of this model to a research situation in which several individuals on repeated testings with several variables are sampled and later on aggregated (Buss's case 3′) is one that awaits development of a fully articulated methodological model.

Situation: $N > 1, M > 1, T > 2$

Finally, we turn to models with many dependent variables (Y) with many individuals ($N > 1$) over many times ($T > 2$). This model enables the examination of many types of changes. Changes in variability and level, as in previous models, can be examined here as well, but the new feature is that the research can, on the one hand, now focus on changes in relationships between variables, and examine, on the other hand, how these relationships change over time. This family of changes over time has been referred to as the "structuring of change," as opposed to just "measuring change" (Nesselroade, 1973). The heart of this distinction is whether change should be cast in terms of a single measurement variable ($M = 1$; $Y = 1$) or in terms of one or more composite variables reflecting patterns of interrelationship among several measurement variables. As we have seen in the previous paragraphs, change in a single dependent variable ($Y = 1$) can be studied either descriptively, as a function of age or time, or in a traditional experimental design as a function of one or more manipulated independent variables (X).

Through the use of multiple measures (more than one variable; $M > 1$) it is possible to combine inductive quasi-experiments and manipulative (deductive) experiments. In the context of multiple measures, the developmentalist is in the position to study both inter- and intraindividual differences (see Buss's model), and move to a more abstract higher order type of change concepts – changes in patterns of interrelationships among all kinds of variables employed in a study (Y, X, W, Z).

Theory measurement interplay

To discuss these points more explicitly, consider a study that examines the relation between two variables and how this relation changes over time (e.g., the relationship between moral reasoning and empathy might be weak for young children but stronger for the same children at an older age). Although it is possible to examine how the strength of this relationship might change over time, testing whether this relationship does in fact change involves a postulation of an explicit model of measurement error as applied to repeated measurements (Wood, in press; Brabeck & Wood, in press). It is necessary to distinguish between the reliability of the measurement process and stability of the phenomenon being measured (see the section on $N > 1$, $M = 1$, $T >> 2$).

Even with such a simple example as we have chosen, alternate explanations for a difference in the magnitude of observed relationships exist. These include the presence of differential reliability, ceiling or floor effects (i.e., measurement error) and, in the case of continuous measurement assuming linear relationships, presence of a global curvilinear relationship between the two measures or departures from multivariate normality (i.e., specification error). All of these alternate explanations can be (mis)used to preserve (or to reject the) hypothesis of the same degree of relationship over time.

We can learn again from this example that change implies some type of comparison across time. These comparisons can refer to different features of psychological measures: the observed means, variances, distributions, relations (as associations or differences), patterns, and/or the latent counterparts of all of them. A necessary precondition for such a comparison implies the correct identity of the concept under study.

The distinction between (observed) measures and (theoretical) concepts leads to a corresponding distinction between theoretical models and measurement models. Theoretical models specify structural relations hypothesized to be present in a set of theoretical constructs. Measurement models denote the relation of these concepts to a set of observed variables. This is the theoretical distinction we have in mind throughout the chapter when talking about testable models for these two sets of relations. Inferences about structural relations cannot be made without either implicit or (better) explicit assumptions about one's measures and the concept of interest (Labouvie, 1980). There is need for considerable interplay between theoretical notions of change and the development and refinement of measurement devices. This is not primarily a matter of data analysis. With the guideline of this theoretical thinking, one can turn to a large variety of statistical models in order to establish the identity of constructs across subjects and/or times and other facets of the data box included in a study (Wohlwill, 1973). For reaching this aim, developmentalists can be encouraged by advances in measurement and scaling theory (Henning & Rudinger, 1985), multivariate reliability and validity conceptualizations (Wittmann, 1987), and mathematical-statistical modeling in general (Jöreskog, 1979; Bentler, 1980; Rogosa, 1979).

Types of relations

Developmental psychologists frequently summarize relationships between more than two variables as a system of relationships, as is the case of linear structural modeling. A system of such relationships might change in several ways.

One case is that the ordering of relationships between variables might remain the same over time, but increase or decrease in absolute magnitude. Such a pattern of relationships remains the same; that is, the same order of relationships over time is preserved.

A second type of change involves the preservation of the overall structure of relationships (e.g., an overall circumplex might still be an adequate model of the general family of relationships under study over time), but the relative ordering of the variables within the model is changed from time to time. This might occur within developmental psychology when the relative importance of variables as markers of the construct changes over time.

The final type of change in relationships that can be modeled involves the documentation of an essentially different type of structure. One such example of structural change in the overall structure is the process of differentation/integration in intelligence tasks. The postulate of such a fundamental change in overall structure as well as of all types of changes already mentioned is a theoretical assumption and not an empirical conclusion.

Invariance of constructs

One topic frequently addressed by developmental psychologists involves assessment of invariance of constructs over time, or the invariance of developmental dimensions, or the problem of the validity of using a measurement instrument for all age groups, cohorts, and points of measurement. From a classical perspective, the invariance definition of constructs over time is synonymous with definitions of factorial invariance. This involves the same relative magnitude of factor loadings of variables on factors as well as the same degree of relation between the factors. The three models of change of structures outlined above provide several possible operationalizations of what such variance or systematic invariance might be. Emergence of "qualitatively" new structures could emphasize the differential relative salience of a variable to a factor at a given time, or could postulate a change in the degree to which the postulated latent structures correlate.

Systematic changes in the relationships between variables thought to measure the same construct are an often unstated focus also of Piagetian inquiry. Very often, differences in the relationships of indicators of Piagetian operations are observed. In order to retain the hypotehsis of the *structure d'ensemble,* these are assumed to be systematic in that the variables differ according to decalage. Decalage is frequently discussed as the "Piagetian" equivalent of measurement error. In order to disentangle this concept from measurement error traditionally defined, one needs to have an explicit theory of how types of decalage can be detected and accounted for. Systematic differences between Piagetian tasks, for example, can be thought of as a content dimension along which the individual systematically varies. Measurement error that does not systematically vary by task can be considered merely a disturbance decalage more closely related to the traditional definition of error with respect to misclassification or unappropriate ranking (Rudinger, 1987).

Stability

In addition to change and variability, stability has also proved to be a central concept in the description of development. According to Buss, the multivariate developmental situation can mean stability or differences either betewen or within subjects over time. An excellent discussion of the various meanings of stability can be found in Wohlwill (1973); for example, stability as predictability, as invariance, as regularity, as consensus, as the constancy of the relative position within a group, and as the preservation of individual differences. The numerous attempts to establish developmental functions and growth curves, especially in the area of cognitive functions (stability as regularity and predictability) make clear the dominance of this concept.

This seems to be an anomaly in the study of behavioral change over time in that in many instances the orientation, development, and use of measuring instruments have emphasized stability rather than lability as a target concern (Nesselroade, 1973).

The orientation, however, depends on your theoretical standpoint. For example, if, as a consequence of a strict and classical trait-oriented perspective, one has to assume that change is just of quantitative kind, change can occur only with respect to the level of the traits, that is with respect to the means of the latent variables. In order to determine this hypothetical "locus of change" in a precise manner, one has to make a nondevelopmental stand for invariance and stability of the other elements of the relational system under study, that is, in the structural areas of the theoretical presuppositions concerning the given constructs. The researcher must clearly and distinctively separate the different sources of developmental change and various facets of invariance and stability that have to be assumed from several theoretical viewpoints. This turns the focus to stability of interindividual differences, the only admissible variability in this context, and not at all to intraindividual changes and/or differences.

If one takes another perspective, for example, that of a "state" theoretician, alternate conclusions and assumptions about the relational system under study have to be brought up (Hertzog & Nesselroade, 1987). The crucial point, in any case, is the appropriate mapping of theoretical structures into design and model structures.

Types of change

The gist of methodological considerations presented may be summarized in the following programmatic way: The psychometric approach in perhaps its most advanced form of structural equation models distinguishes different levels and types of change. There can be change in (1) the number of latent constructs; (2) the "factor" loadings (reliability of the observed variables as indices of the latent process under study); (3) the errors of measurement in the observed variables; (4) the relation between the latent constructs; and (5) the means of the constructs (Labouvie, 1980). These facets of change can be combined in a variety of approaches (Rudinger, 1985a, b).

There are some parallels between these quantitative-structural concerns and aspects of qualitative-structural analysis. There exists also a large variety of qualitative developmental models such as synchronous progression, horizontal decalage, vertical decalage, reciprocal interaction, divergent or convergent progressions (van den Daele, 1969). Analogous to the quantitative-structural changes just listed in the qualitative domain are changes in levels of hierarchies, speed, spacing, loops, relation, and concatenation between the qualitative features of developmental processes. These relations can be disjunctive, conjunctive, or compensatory ones. However, it is important to note that, without substantial developmental theory, neither qualitative nor psychometric approaches can provide a general rule of designing and defining change and separating it from error. The researcher has to define explicitly his or her concrete conception of change, that is, which levels, aspects, and facets are involved. For a lot of developmental conceptions, methodological solutions can be offered. Thus, in the way that a psychometrically oriented researcher investigates differences among and within persons, the qualitative researcher is in a similar position in the case of multiple and cumulative sequences.

Conclusions

From even the simple examples provided above, it should be obvious that researchers employing longitudinal assessments of growth and change should make their theoretical and measurement models explicit a priori, and not await the development of statistical methodology to determine the appropriate error model and identify the testable relationships of interest. Explicit developmental models lead to assumptions about specification and measurement error. Both conceptual and measurement models guide selection of research design and are not merely a useful byproduct of statistical techniques. A strong specification of measurement error is the converse of a strong specification of developmental processes and latent variables. The stronger the theoretical specification of the developmental processes under study, the more powerful and explicit the error model.

The hierarchical progression of designs given in the examples in this chapter reflects the fact that simpler designs do not allow tests of competing alternate models of measurement error that could also account for observed differences. More elaborate models allow for both estimation of such structural differences as well as sources of measurement error.

This is not to say that more elaborate models are always more appropriate than the simpler models in psychological research. For some psychological processes, day-to-day variation has little, if any, conceptual meaning (e.g., in ego development or academic aptitude testing). For reasons of practical utility, conceptual clarity, or in situations where more subtle types of measurement error are not thought to occur, simpler designs can still be used. Some designs are appropriate for assessment of psychological states; others are appropriate for psychological traits.

In order to explain the observed changes, research designs considered in this chapter have dealt only with dependent variables and not with other aspects of the Cattelian BDRM model, such as organismic, background, or treatment variables. Selection of individuals by background variable or assignment of individuals to treatment groups involves either the explicit assumption that individuals come from a common population (as in the case in a normative study of development) or the selection of individuals in separate categories in a stratified fashion (creating several "mini-studies" that can then be later collapsed or aggregated).

Even within the psychometric approach, a satisfying answer to the question of how to establish relations between nested systems of different levels of aggregation as the macro-, meso-, microsystem does not exist. Changes in the macro-system include, for example, change from an industrial society with steadily accelerated economic growth to the state of zero growth, or change in a society from socioliberal attitudes to more conservative ones. Examples of changes in the meso-system are changes in the school system from planned curricula to maximum freedom of content choice by the student, changing proportion of female and male teachers (feminization of the teacher role), or the initiation or removal of television shows such as "Sesame Street." Changes in the micro-system (family systems or individuals) include loss of spouse, birth of a child, changed style of communication between parents and children. Multilevel-analysis from sociology may offer some promise, but, in general, the state of affairs is as disappointing for the methodologist as for the substantive researcher interested in cause–effect, interaction, and reciprocity relations between the elements of this system.

It is easy to imagine how to introduce these variables into a study, and discussions of how such variables afffect interpretation within developmental psychology are discussed elsewhere (Schaie & Baltes, 1975; Nesselroade & von Eye, 1985). Full explication of how introduction of error of measurement in organismic, background, and treatment variables affects developmental description and explanation should be the focus of future methodological developments.

References

Aebli, H. (1978). A dual model of cognitive development. *International Journal of Behavioral Development*, 3, 221–229.

Baltes, P. B. (1968). Longitudinal and cross-sectional sequences in the study of age and generation effects. *Human Development, 11,* 145–171.

Baltes, P. B., & Goulet, L. R. (1971). Exploration of development variables by simulation and manipulation of age differences in behavior. *Human Development, 14,* 149–170.

Baltes, P. B., & Nesselroade, J. R. (1979). History and rationale of longitudinal research. In J. R. Nesselroade & P. B. Baltes (Eds.), *Longitudinal research in the study of behavior and development.* New York: Academic Press.

Baltes, P. B., Nesselroade, J. R., & Cornelius, S. W. (1978). Multivariate antecedents of structural change in development: A simulation of cumulative environmental patterns. *Multivariate Behavioral Research, 13,* 127–152.

Baltes, P. B., Reese, H. W., & Nesselroade, J. R. (1977). *Life-span developmental psychology: Introduction to research methods.* Monterey, CA: Brooks/Cole.

Bart, W. M., & Airasian, P. W. (1974). Determination of the ordering among seven Piagetian tasks by an ordering-theoretical method. *Journal of Educational Psychology, 66,* 277–284.

Bentler, P. M. (1980). Multivariate analysis with latent variables: Causal models. *Annual Review of Psychology, 31,* 419–456.

Brabeck, M., & Wood, P. K. (in press). Reflective judgement and critical thinking: How strong is the longitudinal evidence. In M. Commons, F. Richards, & J. Sinnot (Eds.), *Adult intellectual development.* New York: Praeger.

Broughton, J. (1977). Beyond formal operations: Theoretical thought in adolescence and early adulthood. *Teachers College Record, 79,* 88–97.

Buss, A. R. (1974). A general developmental model for interindividual differences, intraindividual differences, and intraindividual changes. *Developmental Psychology, 19,* 70–78.

Buss, A. R. (1979). Toward a unified framework for psychometric concepts in the multivariate developmental situation: Intraindividual change and inter- and intraindividual differences. In J. R. Nesselroade and P. B. Baltes (Eds.), *Longitudinal research in the study of behavior and development.* New York and London: Academic Press.

Campbell, D. T., & Stanley, J. C. (1963). Experimental and quasi-experimental designs for research in teaching. In N. L. Gage (Ed.), *Handbook of research on teaching.* Chicago: Rand-McNally.

Cattell, R. B. (1946). *The description and measurement of personality.* Yonkers, NY: World Book.

Cattell, R. B. (1966). The data box: Its ordering of total resources in terms of possible relational systems. In R. B. Cattell (Ed.), *Handbook of multivariate experimental psychology.* Chicago: Rand-McNally.

Cattell, R. B. (1988). The data box: Its ordering of total resouces in terms of possible relational systems. In J. R. Nesselroade & R. B. Cattell (Eds.), *Handbook of multivariate experimental psychology.* New York, London: Plenum.

Coan, R. W. (1966). Child personality and developmental psychology. In R. B. Cattell (Ed.), *Handbook of multivariate experimental psychology.* Chicago: Rand-McNally.

Coleman, J. S. (1964). Introduction to mathematical sociology. New York: The Free Press.

Cook, T. D., & Campbell, D. T. (1976). The design and conduct of quasi-experiments and true experiments in field settings. In M. O. Dunnette (Ed.), *Handbook of industrial and organizational psychology.* Chicago: Rand-McNally.

Cook, T. D., & Campbell, D. T. (1979). *Quasi-experimentation: Design and analysis issues for field settings.* New York: Rand-McNally.

Coombs, C. H. (1964). *A theory of data.* New York: Wiley.

Coombs, C. H., & Smith, E. K. (1973). On the detection of structure in attitudes and developmental processes, *Psychological Review, 80,* 337–351.

Coombs, C. H., Dawes, R. M., & Tversky, A. (1970). *Mathematical psychology.* Englewood Cliffs, NJ: Prentice-Hall.

Cronbach, L. J. (1957). The two disciplines of scientific psychology. *American Psychologist, 12,* 671–684.

Cronbach, L. J. (1975). Beyond the two disciplines of scientific psychology. *American Psychologist, 30,* 116–127.

Cronbach, L. J., Gleser, G. C., Nanda, H., & Rajaratnam, N. (1972). *The dependability of behavioral measurements.* New York: Wiley.

Dayton, C. M., & Macready, G. B. (1980). A scaling model with response errors and intrinsically unscalable respondents. *Psychometrika, 45,* 343–356.

Dayton, C. M., & Macready, G. B. (1983). Latent structure and analysis of repeated classifications with dichotomous data. *British Journal of Mathematical and Statistical Psychology, 36,* 189–201.

Erdfelder, E. (1987). *Die Entwicklung psychometrischer Intelligenz.* Frankfurt: Peter Lang.

Fisher, K. W. (1980). A theory of cognitive development: The control and construction of hierarchies of skills. *Psychological Review, 87,* 477–531.

Goodman, L. A. (1978). *Analyzing qualitative/categorical data.* London: Addison-Wesley.

Guttman, L. (1977). What is not what in statistics. *Statistician, 26,* 81–107.

Heise, D. R. (1975). *Causal analysis.* New York: Wiley.

Henning, H. J., & Rudinger, G. (1985). Analysis of quantitative data in developmental psychology. In J. R. Nesselroade & A. von Eye (Eds.), *Individual development and social change.* Orlando: Academic Press.

Hertzog, C., & Nesselroade, J. R. (1987). Beyond autoregressive models: Some implications of the trait-state distinction for the structural modeling of developmental change. *Child Development, 58,* 93–109.

Horn, J. L., & McArdle, J. J. (1980). Perspectives on mathematical/statistical model building (MASMOB) in research on aging. In L. W. Poon (Ed.), *Aging in the 1980s.* Washington, DC: American Psychological Association.

Jöreskog, K. G. (1979). Statistical estimation of structural models in longitudinal-development investigation. In J. R. Nesselroade & P. B. Baltes (Ed.), *Longitudinal research in the study of behavior and development.* New York and London: Academic Press.

Krus, D. J. (1977). Order analysis: An inferential model of dimensional analysis and scaling. *Educational and Psychological Measurement, 37,* 587–601.

Labouvie, E. W. (1980). Identity versus equivalence of psychological measures and constructs. In L. W. Poon (Ed.), *Aging in the 1980s.* Washington, DC: American Psychological Association.

Lord, F. M., & Novick, M. R. (1968). *Statistical theories of mental test scores.* Reading, MA: Addison-Wesley.

MacCorquodale, K., & Meehl, P. E. (1948). On a distinction between hypothetical constructs and intervening variables. *Psychological Review, 55,* 95–107.

McArdle, J. J. (1988). Dynamic but structural equation modeling of repeated measurement data. In J. R. Nesselroade & R. B. Cattell (Eds.), *Handbook of multivariate experimental psychology.* New York and London: Plenum.

McArdle, J. J., & Epstein, D. (1987). Latent growth curves within developmental structural equation models. *Child Development, 58,* 110–133.

McCall, R. B. (1977). Challenges to a science of developmental psychology. *Child Development, 48,* 333–344.

Mason, K. O., Mason, W. M., Winsborough, H. H., & Poole, W. K. (1973). Some methodological issues in cohort analysis of archival data. *American Sociological Review, 38,* 242–258.

Molenaar, P. C. M. (1987). Dynamic factor analysis in the frequency domain: Causal modeling of multivariate psychophysical time series. *Multivariate Behavioral Research, 22,* 329–353.

Nesselroade, J. R. (1973). Faktorenanalyse von Kreuzprodukten zur Beschreibung von Veränderungsphänomen (change). *Zeitschrift für experimentelle und angewandte Psychologie, 20,* 92–106.

Nesselroade, J. R. (1987). *Multi-modal selection effects in single subject research.* Paper presented at the Biennial meeting of the International Society for the Study of Behavioral Development, Tokyo.

Nesselroade, J. R., & Baltes, P. B. (Eds.) (1979). *Longitudinal research in the study of behavior and development.* New York: Academic Press.

Nesselroade, J. R., & von Eye, A. (Eds.) (1985). *Individual development and social change: Explanatory analysis.* Orlando: Academic Press.

Overton, W. F., & Reese, H. W. (1973). Models of development: Methodological implications. In J. R. Nesselroade & H. W. Reese (Eds.), *Life-span developmental psychology: Methodological issues.* New York: Academic Press.

Phillips, D. C., & Kelly, M. E. (1975). Hierarchical theories of development in education and psychology. *Harvard Educational Review, 45,* 351–375.

Rest, J. R. (1979). *Development in judging moral issues.* Minneapolis, MN: University of Minnesota Press.

Riegel, K. F. (1972). Time and change in the development of the individual and society. In H. W. Reese (Ed.), *Advances in child development and behavior.* New York and London: Academic Press.

Riegel, K. F. (1977). The dialectics of time. In N. Datan & H. W. Reese (Eds.), *Life-span developmental psychology.* New York: Academic Press.

Rindskopf, D. (1987). Using latent class analysis to test developmental models. *Developmental Review, 7,* 66–85.

Rogosa, D. (1979). Causal models of longitudinal research: Rationale, formulation, and interpretation. In J. R. Nesselroade & P. B. Baltes (Eds.), *Longitudinal research in the study of behavior and development.* New York: Academic Press.

Roskam, E. E. (1983). Allgemeine Datentheorie. In H. Feger & J. Bredenkamp (Eds.), *Encyclopädie der Psychologie, Serie 1, Band 3: Messen und Testen.* Göttingen: Hogrefe.

Roskam, E. E. (in press). "Latent trait" Modelle. In G. Rudinger & R. Mausfeld (Eds.), *Psychologische Methoden: Handbuch in Schlüsselbegriffen.* München: Urban & Schwarzenberg.

Rudinger, G. (1979). Erfassung von Entwicklungsverläufen im Lebenslauf. In H. Rauh (Ed.), *Jahrbuch für Entwicklungspsychologie.* Stuttgart: Klett-Cotta.

Rudinger, G. (1985a). Struktur-Analysen. In T. Herrmann & E.-D. Lantermann (Eds.), *Persönlichkeitspsychologie: Ein Handbuch in Schlüsselbegriffen.* München: Urban & Schwarzenberg.

Rudinger, G. (1985b). Prozeß-Analysen. In T. Herrmann & E.-D. Lantermann (Eds.), *Persönlichkeitspsychologie: Ein Handbuch in Schlüsselbegriffen.* München: Urban & Schwarzenberg.

Rudinger, G. (1986). *Structure of change and changes of structure in longitudinal design.* Paper presented at International Conference on Longitudinal Methodology, Budapest.

Rudinger, G. (1987). *Analysis of developmental patterns and sequences in cognitive development.* Paper presented at the ninth advanced course of the Jean Piaget Archives Foundation: Universals and Individuals, Genf.

Rudinger, G., & Rietz, C. E. V. K. (1987). *Intelligenzentwicklung über einen Zeitraum von 35 Jahren.* Paper presented at "8: Deutsch Tagung für Entwicklungspsychologie", Bern.

Rudinger, G., Chaselon, F., Zimmermann, J., & Henning, H. J. (1985). *Qualitative Daten.* München: Urban & Schwarzenberg.

Runkel, P. J., & McGrath, J. E. (1972). *Research on human behavior.* New York: Holt, Rinehart & Winston.

Schaie, K. W. (1965). A general model for the study of developmental problems. *Psychological Bulletin, 64,* 92–107.

Schaie, K. W. (1977). Quasi-experimental research designs in the psychology of aging. In J. E. Birren & K. W. Schaie (Eds.), *Handbook of the psychology of aging.* New York: Van Nostrand-Reinhold.

Schaie, K. W., & Baltes, P. B. (1975). On sequential strategies in developmental research: Description or explanation? *Human Development, 18,* 384–390.

Shepard, J. L. (1978). A structural analysis of concrete operations. In J. A. Keats, K. F. Collins, & G. S. Halford (Eds.), *Cognitive Development*. Chichester: Wiley.

Singer, B., & Spilerman, S. (1979). Mathematical representations of development theories. In J. R. Nesselroade & P. B. Baltes (Eds.), *Longitudinal research in the study of behavior and development*. New York: Academic Press.

Sterns, H. L., & Alexander, R. A. (1977). Cohort, age, and time of measurement: Biomorphic considerations. In N. Datan & H. W. Reese (Eds.), *Life-span developmental psychology*. New York: Academic Press.

van den Daele, L. D. (1969). Qualitative models in developmental analysis. *Developmental Psychology, 4,* 302–310.

Wittmann, W. W. (1987). Grundlagen erfolgreicher Forschung in der Psychologie: Multimodale Diagnostik, Multiplismus, mutivariate Reliabilitäts- und Validitätstheorie. *Diagnostika, 33,* 209–227.

Wohlwill, J. F. (1973). *The study of behavioral development.* New York: Academic Press.

Wohlwill, J. F. (1980). Cognitive development in childhood. In O. G. Brim, Jr., & J. Kagan (Eds.), *Constancy and change in human development.* Cambridge, MA: Harvard University Press.

Wood, P. K. (in press). Construct validity studies in adult developmental research. In M. Commons, F. Richards & J. Sinnot (Eds.), *Adult intellectual development.* New York: Praeger.

10 Stability of patterns and patterns of stability in personality development

JENS B. ASENDORPF AND FRANZ E. WEINERT

Introduction

What is really meant when it is said that someone grows older but in many respects never ages? What is meant when we have the impression that a child has over the course of a year become less shy yet behaves timidly in social interactions? What is ultimately understood when a child's teacher contends that this student is much less aggressive than before but is still the most aggressive child in the class?

Each of these common statements contains a diagnostic judgment about the development of individuals. Every case poses the same question, What *changes* during a particular time span, and which personal or behavior attributes somehow *remain the same?* The issue, then, is the proportion of stability and change in personality development.

Concepts of stability and change

This issue has attracted much longitudinal research in the last decades. The main interest of these research endeavors is to improve the feasibility of predicting individual behavior (Wohlwill, 1973) and is grounded in the predominant conviction of European and American psychology that invariance in the ontogenesis befits particular meaning for the postulated identity of the individual in his or her life course (Thomae, 1957). Because we are so convinced about our stable individual self, we assume that there must be some stability within developmental change.

Kagan (1980), in an excellent review of the history of ideas about stability and change, pointed to another belief deeply rooted in Western thought – the belief in *connectedness*. Individual development is conceived of as a consequence of different stages that cohere in a causal chain. The developmental theories of Freud and Piaget, for example, try to tell a coherent story about ourselves.

In the case of personality development, connectedness refers to a very broad range of possible continuities in behavioral dispositions. In this context, Kagan (1971) introduced an important distinction between *homotypic* and *heterotypic* continuity. Whereas homotypic continuity refers to the more obvious stabilities of the "same" behavior, heterotypic continuity embraces all kinds of predictive relations between "different" behaviors.

For example, the amount of crying could be longitudinally studied in different individuals. A correlation between the interindividual differences in crying at age 1 and at age 21 (defined by the same behavioral criteria for both ages) would be a measure of homotypic continuity, whereas a correlation between these differences in crying at age 1 and a personality scale tapping impulsivity at age 21 would be a measure of heterotypic continuity. It is very unlikely in this case that homotypic continuity can be expected, because crying among adults and crying among infants seem to be totally different phenomena.

This example illustrates a chronic problem of the longitudinal assessment of personality: the same behavioral disposition (e.g., the tendency to cry often) may have a very different meaning at different ages. This meaning of a certain behavioral disposition at a certain age level cannot be sufficiently captured by studying this disposition in isolation. The meaning is revealed only if we study the disposition in the context of other dispositions, and if we are aware of the fact that in each society social standards exist (and expectations connected with these) that contribute age-specific criteria to the evaluation of dispositions.

Studies on the stability of personality have often disregarded this problem of "sameness" of behavior; instead, researchers have simply defined personality dispositions by a set of behavioral criteria or labels for rating scales independent of the age level. What Wohlwill wrote in 1973 still holds: "With only very few exceptions, work on stability . . . has consisted in the endless proliferation of correlation coefficients, to indicate the degree of relationship between measures of behavior over some given time interval. . . . The result has been that we have learned a little about the 'behavior' of *variables* over age but nothing concerning the behavior of individuals" (p. 359).

Indeed, psychological studies of stability and change have nearly exclusively focused upon interindividual differences in single variables or aggregates of variables, each of which represents a single personality trait. The temporal stability of between-subject differences in single traits is often called the *normative stability* of personality traits (e.g., Kagan, 1980; Moss & Susman, 1980; Rutter, 1987).

However, if we are interested in the study of *personality,* that is, of the "individual organization of behavior" (Allport, 1961), the traditional "variable oriented approach" must be complemented by a "person oriented pattern approach" (Magnusson, 1988) that focuses on the stability and change of individual *patterns* of traits, that is, of within-subject differences between many traits. The temporal stability of these individual patterns is often called the *ipsative stability* of personality (e.g., Kagan, 1980; Moss & Susman, 1980; Rutter, 1987).

Furthermore, the stability and change of these individual patterns should be contrasted with the stability and change of two other types of patterns. First, for each age there exists a characteristic pattern of behavior representing the "age-specific average personality." This pattern can be assessed by the pattern of the sample means of many traits. The structure of this pattern may be studied by factor analysis, and its temporal stability may be assessed by comparing the factor structure across time. This type of stability is often called the *continuity* of personality dimensions (e.g., Emmerich, 1964, 1968; Moss & Susman, 1980).

Second, in each culture stereotypic beliefs prevail about age differences in the behavioral expression of the same trait. For example, children may be assumed to externalize aggression more in terms of physical aggression and less in terms of verbal aggression, whereas the inverse is held true for adults. Thus, for each trait, an age-specific *prototypic pattern* of *assumed* behavioral expressions may be identified and studied for stability and change. Such studies reveal the cultural standards and expectations that provide age-specific criteria for the social evaluation of personality development in different domains. In this way they provide a reference system for interpreting results of the first three approaches (studying normative stability, ipsative stability, and continuity).

One possible way of doing so is to compare the prototypic pattern of a trait with the individual personality patterns found in a sample of subjects. The similarity between the prototypic pattern and the individual pattern of a particular person in the sample constitutes the person's *prototypicality* for the trait. Such a prototypicality score can be obtained simply by correlating a person's individual pattern with the prototypic pattern. The prototypicalities, in turn, constitute a single measure of interindividual differences in the trait. Note, however, that this approach of studying single traits differs from the ordinary assessment of traits.

For example, if we are interested in studying aggressiveness, we may either obtain a traditional measure of aggressiveness (such as self-ratings, peer-ratings, or behavioral observations of aggressive behavior that are sufficiently aggregated to provide a single index of aggressiveness with a high short-term stability), or we may compare each subject's personality pattern with the socially shared prototypic pattern for aggressiveness. For children, aggressive behaviors will score high, and shy behaviors will score low in this prototypic pattern. Children who are both aggressive and shy will obtain a high aggressiveness score on the traditional measures but will receive only a medium prototypicality for aggressiveness, because their high shyness does not fit well with the social stereotype of an aggressive child.

To summarize, there are six possible kinds of stability and change. Three refer to between-subject differences in single variables, aggregates of variables, and prototypicalities, and three others refer to between-variable differences in personality patterns at the level of the individual or at the level of age groups, and to between-variable differences in socially shared prototypic patterns for particular traits (cf. Figure 10.1).

All these types of stability and change could be assessed on the surface level in regard to a rather arbitrary selection of behavioral measures, or on the structural level with indicators for a theoretically based system of constructs. In each of these cases

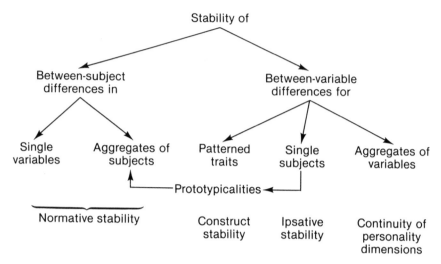

Figure 10.1. Six different kinds of stability.

the analysis remains purely descriptive. Explanations of the empirically observed stability and change by developmental mechanisms require designs other than those applied in conventional longitudinal studies (Nesselroade & Baltes, 1979).

Furthermore, stability findings do not tell us much about specific processes of change. A high long-term stability of between-subject or of between-variable differences indicates that developmental change processes are functionally equivalent across persons or variables but does not reveal anything more specific about these changes. A low long-term stability may be simply due to a short-term instability of the measures obtained. Even if a high short-term stability has been proven, the low long-term stability only indicates that different persons or variables changed in different ways; but the stability data reveal neither the specific nature of these differences nor their similarities that still may exist. Therefore, change is not at all equivalent to nonstability; it is a widespread misunderstanding that stability data would reveal much about developmental change.

In order to obtain information about universal, individual, or differential change, it is essential to reconstruct *developmental functions* (trends or sequences) on empirical bases (cf. Wohlwill, 1973, for the rationale of this approach; Flavell, 1972, for specific classes of changes; and Bryk & Raudenbush, 1987, for a method of studying developmental trends psychometrically). If specific change processes can be empirically reconstructed, this also provides full information about the stability of differences. Thus, studies of change can answer all stability questions, but not vice versa.

The problem with studies of change is, however, that they need more measurement points than do studies of stability in order to study developmental functions with some reliability. Often, at least four measurement points are needed to study change. Also, it depends on the theoretical perspective whether one is more interested in change or in stability. For the developmentalist, it is essential to study change processes in detail, whereas the personologist may be already satisfied with stability data.

In the following, we will address only questions of stability, with a special focus on the stability of individual patterns and on patterns of the stabilities of many variables. We will discuss the desired quality of data that enables reasonable estimates of the various types of stability we have discussed so far. Subsequently, we will illustrate these requirements with data from our ongoing longitudinal study on the development of individual differences in cognitive and social competence.

Desired properties of stability data for personality

What kind of data are needed for assessing the six types of stability depicted in Figure 10.1? We propose that such data should meet at least four requirements.

High short-term stability

Because we are concerned here with the long-term stability of personality and personality traits, this requirement is absolutely necessary. Not every behavioral variable indicates a personality trait; not every individual pattern of variables represents a personality pattern. Instead, they may tap states or patterns of states that change according to a time scale that is quite different from the time scale for developmental changes. In terms of reliability, a high short-term retest reliability is necessary in order to interpret correctly medium or low long-term instabilities as indicators of developmental changes. This applies to the stability of between-subject differences as well as to the stability of between-variable differences.

A high consistency of between-subject or between-variable differences across similar variables (internal consistency) is not sufficient for studies on the stability of personality. It is not sufficient because states and patterns of states may be assessed with a high internal consistency despite a very low short-term stability. Since much confusion has arisen concerning this question, an example may help to clarify what we mean here by short-term and long-term stability.

Adults vary considerably in the short-term stability of their mood: some are very stable, and others show typical cyclic mood changes within a period of some months. The mood variability of a person may be considered to be a rather permanent characteristic of that person; then we might be interested as to whether this personality trait is stable over many years.

In order to do this we must first reliably assess each person's mood variability, for example, by fitting a "cyclicity parameter" to many observations of the person's mood obtained within a period of, say, three months (cf. Larsen, 1987, for such an approach). Whether the person's cyclicity parameter is reliably measured or not obviously cannot be answered by determining the synchrony between many concurrent assessments of the person's mood. Necessary for interpreting the cyclicity parameter as a personality trait is its temporal stability (but obviously not the temporal stability of the mood itself); thus, another three months is needed to assess the retest stability of the parameter. Only when this retest stability is established, a comparison between the cyclicity parameter of the person obtained in the first three months of assessment and the one obtained five years later in another three-month assessment can be interpreted as tapping a developmental phenomenon of personality.

That a high retest reliability must be secured for all measures in studies of personality development is a principle not well respected in many present longitudinal studies. Often, the less costly procedure of proving internal consistency is preferred and defended by the argument that additional retesting intensifies the problems of overtesting and transfer effects that plague most longitudinal studies. But this problem can be easily avoided, because retest reliabilities can be established in a different, parallel sample.

Low retest reliabilities often can be improved very much by aggregating measures and – usually less so – situations over time. Epstein, with a remarkable longitudinal stability, aggregates papers on this simple but very important principle. One-shot measurements such as a single behavioral observation or a single rating of a single observer seldom reach sufficient retest reliability. The study of Moskowitz and Schwarz (1982) nicely demonstrates how the short-term normative stability of behavioral observations and its consistency with ratings of knowledgeable informants can be strongly increased by aggregating the behavior over time and the ratings over different informants.

The retest reliability of patterns of variables may be also somewhat improved by aggregating over similar variables within the pattern. However, a tradeoff between an increasing reliability and a decreasing within-pattern variance exists here; where exactly the optimal balance is reached depends on the research questions to be addressed.

A wide range of variables

Because personality embraces many different domains of psychic functioning, the ipsative stability of personality may be considerably biased if only a small portion of these domains are chosen for analysis. Thus, a wide range of variables should be covered by the assessment procedures. More generally, which results can be obtained and which not strongly depend upon the measures used; measurement is already model building. Whereas this is obvious as a general statement, it can have more subtle consequences in concrete applications that may bias the results in a way that is not easy to detect.

For example, if we are interested in studying aggressiveness by determining children's prototypicalities for a prototypic aggressive pattern construed for a given pool of variables, the stability of interindividual differences in these prototypicalities for aggressiveness partly depends upon the normative stabilities of the variables in the pool used. Different pools of variables that contain the same measures of aggressiveness but differ in other aspects of personality that are related to but not identical with aggressiveness may yield different normative stabilities of the prototypicalities for aggressiveness.

Some redundancy in the pool of variables

Whereas a high between-variable variance is desirable for the reasons pointed out above, it is also useful if the pool of variables contains some redundancy. Similar variables allow the reduction of unsystematic measurement error by aggregating over variables within the pool. Also, for some types of analyses it is necessary to estimate model parameters on the basis of parallel measurements (e.g., LISREL). Because it may be impossible or too costly to obtain a retest for each measurement point in the longitudinal sample, two concurrent, highly consistent measures suffice for this estimation problem.

For example, parallel prototypicalities can be obtained by dividing the pool of variables into halves that allow highly correlated prototypic patterns; the two correlations between each person's individual pattern and the two prototypic patterns are very likely to be also highly correlated over persons, that is, to represent parallel measures of prototypicality.

An ipsative mode of assessment

The assessment procedure for individual or prototypic patterns should be tailored according to this task. Thus, the individual or the construct should be the reference point for assessment, not the mean of a sample or of a population of persons. This requirement is more than just standardizing many variables within subjects a posteriori, which is always possible, of course. The person-oriented approach should be already reflected in the mode of assessment.

For self- or other-ratings, this requirement is easy to meet. Instead of comparing individuals with averages for each of many variables, raters are asked to compare many variables for their saliency for one particular individual (the Q-sort technique, see p. 188). For behavioral observations, measures of time sharing (within-subject percentages of a fixed amount of time spent with certain behaviors) or proportional frequencies (within-subject rates of certain behaviors in a fixed amount of time) are similarly suited. If different behaviors can be scaled on a common intensity scale, within-subject differences in behavioral intensities can also be directly assessed.

All these modes of assessment explicitly contrast different variables within the same individual and generate individual patterns without demanding further standardization. Each component of the pattern can be considered to represent the subject's score on a particular variable; these variables, in turn, can be used for normative analyses. Thus, the ipsative assessment procedures can also be used for normative analyses.

Illustration with data of LOGIC

In order to illustrate these four requirements for the longitudinal study of personality development, we now present some data from the Munich Longitudinal Study on the Genesis of Individual Competencies (LOGIC; cf. Weinert & Schneider, 1986, 1987). In LOGIC, the cognitive, social, and motivational development of a representative sample of more than 220 children from Munich and its vicinity are being systematically investigated. Tests, observational instruments, interview techniques, and rating methods are being applied. Part of the data collection takes place in a psychological laboratory and part under naturalistic conditions in kindergartens. The children were three to four years old at the beginning of the study.

In the meantime, three waves of data collection have been completed, and most of the subjects entered elementary school in the autumn of 1987. Therefore, in the next phase, the study extends to about 50 classrooms, in which many other students are found along with the children from the longitudinal study. In addition, three individual test sessions of about two hours in a psychological laboratory are scheduled every year. The most important goals of LOGIC are the systematic analyses of developmental patterns in various domains, the description of within-subject and between-subject differences in developmental stability and change, and (prospectively) the study of influences of some conditions of schooling (quality of instruction, teacher behavior, peer group interactions) on different aspects of development.

In the remainder of this chapter, we illustrate with some of the data from the LOGIC study how one can study the different kinds of stability discussed in the opening section with an assessment instrument meeting most of the requirements pointed out above. Also, these data help us demonstrate which problems arise if these requirements are not fully met. This assessment instrument is the California Child Q-Sort.

Stabilities of the California Child Q-Sort applied in LOGIC

In the LOGIC study we applied a short version of the California Child Q-Sort (CCQ) in German (cf. Block & Block, 1980, for the original version; Göttert & Asendorpf, 1989, for the German adaptation). This Q-sort consists of 54 items that must be assigned to nine categories of saliency for each child so that six items are assigned to each category. About 200 children were assessed at the age of 3–4, 4–5, and 5–6 years by their teacher in preschool/kindergarten; also, three-week retest data were obtained for 45 children.

The Q-sort method. The Q-sort method (Stephenson, 1953; Block, 1961) is an ipsative procedure for assigning scores on many items to individual subjects. A set of Q-sort-items can be used to describe either an abstract construct or an individual person. Whereas conventional normative rating procedures compare many persons for one particular items, ipsative procedures compare many items for their saliency for one particular person, or construct. The primary advantages of this method are that (a) observers are not required to have detailed knowledge of norms for each item, (b) response biases, such as the tendency to use extreme scores on rating scales, are reduced by requiring items to be sorted into a predetermined number of categories that accord to a fixed distribution, and (c) each item is explicitly evaluated in the context of many other items. Thus, the Q-sort method appears to be particularly valuable for an ipsative assessment of personality by the judgment of knowledgeable informants. Individual patterns, prototypic patterns for various traits, and the prototypicality of individual patterns for such prototypes can be directly computed from the raw data. The most frequently used Q-sort in developmental psychology is the California Child Q-sort.

The California Child Q-sort. This Q-sort was developed by Block and Block (1980) in order to assess the constructs of ego-control and ego-resiliency. Ego-control refers to the tendency of individuals to control their impulses in the service of the ego. A highly controlled person is supposed to exhibit, for example, a high threshold for response, inhibited emotional behavior, an indirect mode of manifesting needs, high delay of gratification, and a highly planned and organized behavior. Ego-resiliency refers to the tendency of individuals to adapt to varying situational circumstances, especially stressful ones. A highly flexible person is assumed to be resourceful in adapting to new situations and in coping with stress.

The items of the original 100-item version of the CCQ were selected to be related to these constructs; this particularly applies to its short version of 54 items (Schiller, 1978, cited in Block & Block, 1980). Because ego-control and ego-resiliency are very broad constructs applying to a wide range of situations and reactions, even the short 54-item version of the CCQ covers a wide range of variables.

Also, the set of 54 items contains enough redundancy for constructing parallel measures of many constructs. However, the CCQ-items are not equally well suited for studying different domains of children's personality. Rather, prototypic sorts for particular constructs can be the better constructed the more closely these constructs correspond to ego-control and ego-resiliency. The set of CCQ-items places clear constraints upon the potential use of this instrument.

The CCQ instruction asks for an equal distribution of the items among the nine categories of saliency. The advantages of this procedure are that the Q-sort is maximally discriminative with regard to within-subject differences and is easy to apply; a slight disadvantage is that the nonnormal distribution does not fit the prerequisites of the correlation as a sufficient measure of statistical dependence (i.e., bivariate normal distribution of scores) if different CCQ-patterns are correlated over items (Q-correlation).

CCQ-prototypes used within LOGIC. Within LOGIC, the CCQ is used mainly for studying children's emerging social and social-cognitive competence (cf. Asendorpf, 1987, 1989a). Six constructs related to this domain of competence are investigated:

Table 10.1. *CCQ prototypes for preschool children.*

Prototype	Definition	Agreement[a]
Desirable child	This is a child you personally would find most desirable in your group.	.96
Aggressive child	This is a child who is often involved in aggressive encounters.	.92
Introverted child	This is a child who appears to be not very interested in other children; the child rarely approaches peers and often plays alone *without* appearing anxious.	.81
Shy child	This is a child who appears to be quite interested in other children but is somewhat anxious and inhibited and hence has problems in establishing contact.	.90

Intercorrelations		DES	ECO	ERE	AGG	INT	SHY
U.S.-Desirability	USD	.87	.10	.87	−.55	.30	−.09
Desirability	DES		.20	.85	−.65	.41	.00
Ego-control	ECO			.13	−.64	.59	.56
Ego-resiliency	ERE				−.51	.37	−.20
Aggressivity	AGG					−.69	−.58
Introversion	INT						.59
Shyness	SHY						

[a]Cronbach-*alpha* of the prototypic sorts of four teachers

ego-control and *ego-resiliency* (as defined by the prototypic sorts provided in Block & Block, 1983), *aggressiveness, introversion, shyness,* and *desirability of personality.* These last four constructs were defined by new prototypic sorts obtained from four preschool teachers of different classes. Table 10.1 contains the definitions of the prototypes presented to the four teachers, their agreement for each prototype, and the intercorrelations of the prototypes as well as the U.S.-prototypes for ego-control, ego-resiliency, and desirability (cf. Waters, Noyes, Vaughn, & Ricks, 1985, for the prototypic CCQ-sort of desirability).

Table 10.1 indicates that the four new prototypes showed a high agreement among the teachers and with the comparable U.S.-sort for a desirable child (it seems as if German teachers tend to prefer more introverted and less aggressive children). The intercorrelations of the prototypes are nearly always substantial; this reflects the fact that the set of CCQ-items "pulls for" ego-control or ego-resiliency. However, the data presented below suggest discriminant validity for each of the six prototypes.

Because the CCQ-prototypicalities reflect teachers' subjective perceptions of the children studied, and because these perceptions had to pass through the filter of the CCQ-items, it is necessary to demonstrate the external validity of the prototypicalities. Table 10.2 provides some of these validity data (for more of these data and for a detailed description of the external variables, see Asendorpf, 1987a,b).

Table 10.2. *Concurrent external validity of the CCQ-prototypicalities obtained for the third wave.*

External criterion	DES	ECO	ERE	AGG	SHY	INT
HAWIK verbal IQ (2nd wave)[a]	.25	.12	.30	−.15	−.09	.23
HAWIK nonverbal IQ (2nd wave)[a]	.29	.28	.29	−.31	.17	.38
Observed % success[b]	.22	−.06	.29	−.05	−.20	.10
Observed % aggression[b]	−.18	−.39	−.13	.34	−.32	−.36
Observed % shyness[b]	−.09	.27	−.16	−.16	.37	.16
Parental rating shy toward peers	−.10	.28	−.13	−.12	.28	.19
Parental rating self-conscious[c]	.13	.34	.05	−.32	.37	.23
Parental rating aggressive	−.16	−.33	−.08	.32	−.40	−.28

Note: Abbreviations of prototypicalities refer to those in Table 10.1.
[a]Hannover-Wechsler-Intelligence Scale for Preschool Children (Eggert, 1978).
[b]In contact initiations with peers during regular free-play in preschool (about 2 hrs. of observation per child).
[c]When in the focus of others' attention.

Table 10.2 demonstrates substantial convergent and discriminant concurrent validity of the CCQ-prototypicalities for both naturalistic observations and parental ratings of children's behavior toward peers. Also, the positive relations to be expected between IQ, desirability, and ego-resiliency were confirmed. The positive correlation between IQ and introversion appeared to be due to the high saliency of attentiveness and concentration, and the low saliency of aggressivity, in the CCQ-prototype for introversion.

Description of CCQ-stabilities as revealed by LOGIC. The longitudinal data obtained for the CCQ within LOGIC were explored for five different types of stability. First, the *stability of interindividual differences in single items* was determined by correlating children's scores in a particular item between two points in time. This type of stability taps the stability of particular traits. Because each child's score in a CCQ-item depends on all other scores of that child, the stabilities of the items are not independent of each other. This dependency reflects the fact that personality is not merely a sum of traits but rather a system of interrelated traits.

Second, the *stability of the item means* was computed by correlating the 54-item means between two points in time. The pattern of item means at a particular point in time reflects the relative saliencies of traits for a certain age, that is, children's "average personality" at that particular age. This pattern may slowly shift over time due to universal developmental trends.

Third, the *stability of individual patterns* was determined for each child by correlating each child's 54 scores between two points in time. This type of stability refers to the stability of each child's personality. Note that these individual stabilities of personality partly depend upon the stability of the pattern of item means: the higher

Table 10.3. *Stability of the CCQ for preschool children.*

Variables	N^a	MEAN	STD	MIN	MAX
Single items					
3-week stability	54	.58	.22	.13	.69
2-year stability	54	.29	.14	.07	.58
Pattern of item means					
3-week stability	1	.91	–	–	–
2-year stability	1	.87	–	–	–
Individual patterns					
3-week stability	45	.64	.28	.28	.86
2-year stability	151	.43	.31	–.44	.88
Individual prototypicalities					
3-week stability	6	.83	.03	.79	.91
2-year stability	6	.59	.02	.44	.66
Stability of one-year stabilities					
single items[b]	1	.77	–	–	–
individual patterns[c]	1	.41	–	–	–

Note: 54 items. Means, standards, and correlations of correlations are based on Fisher's z-transformation. The six prototypicalities were determined for ego-control, ego-resiliency, aggressiveness, introversion, shyness, and desirability.
[a]Number of variables that the mean is based upon.
[b]Correlation between item stabilities.
[c]Correlation between pattern stabilities.

the stability of the average personality, the higher the average stability of individual patterns will be.

Fourth, the *stability of individual prototypicalities with regard to a particular construct* was computed by correlating children's prototypicality for a certain construct between two points in time. The constructs ego-control, ego-resiliency, desirability (German prototype), aggressiveness, introversion, and shyness (cf. Tables 10.1 and 10.2) were used for these analyses.

Finally, it was investigated whether the *stabilities of items or individual patterns were stable* over time. Thus, we correlated the one-year stabilities of the 54 items obtained for wave 1–2 with those obtained for wave 2–3 over items, and the one-year stabilities of the individual patterns obtained for wave 1–2 with those obtained for wave 2–3 over children. These "stabilities of stability" are seldom discussed in the literature. However, the temporal stability of between-variable differences in stability, or of between-subject differences in stability respectively, provides crucial information about the question whether the stability of a trait or a person can be considered to be a permanent characteristic of that trait or person. Table 10.3 contains a summary of the five types of stability discussed so far.

For single items, the mean stability of $r = .29$ over two years is low; the item stabilities ranged from $r = .07$ to $r = .58$. Table 10.3 suggests that the low mean and the high variance of the item stabilities are due to the low mean and the high variance of their retest reliabilities, which ranged from $r = .13$ to $r = .69$. Why was the retest reliability so low for many items? Three possible reasons may play a role here.

First, the low mean retest reliability of the 54 items can partly be attributed to the fact that the items are one-shot measures that are not aggregated (cf. Epstein, 1979, 1980, for the merits of aggregation). Aggregates of the items – for example, the prototypicalities – showed a much higher mean retest reliability of $r = .84$ (cf. Table 10.3). However, this cannot be the full story, because the retest reliabilities showed not only a low mean but also a high variance. The 54 items differed greatly in their retest reliability; the aggregation principle cannot explain these differences. While reliabilities in the upper range of the distribution might be explained by insufficient aggregation, this is not true for retest reliabilities in the lower range; a retest reliability of only $r = .13$ clearly cannot be explained by insufficient aggregation alone.

Second, the very low retest reliabilities of some of the items may reflect a considerable short-term instability of the phenomenon measured. For example, the item with the lowest longitudinal stability of $r = .07$ was "can recoup after stressful experience." This item also showed the lowest retest reliability of all 54 items of $r = .13$. On the other hand, this item showed a respectable correlation of $r = -.47$ with another unstable item, "tends to dramatize mishaps." Both items appear to measure consistently similar, unstable constructs that represent states rather than traits. Therefore, their low retest reliability cannot be explained only by insufficient aggregation. Instead, the items appear to tap unstable coping responses that seem to be so unstable because they are strongly influenced by specific, actual circumstances.

This example nicely illustrates the principle outlined above that a high short-term stability is necessary and a high internal consistency is not sufficient for interpreting low longitudinal stabilities as instances of differential developmental processes.

Third, as was discussed above, the stability of a Q-sort-item partly depends upon the stability of all other items. Thus, the most unstable items also affect the stability of the most stable ones by a kind of snowball effect. Hence, the retest reliability of all items is lowered by those items that tap unstable phenomena.

This effect of the item interdependency was not very strong, however, because clear differences in the stability of the items existed. In the case of long-term stability, these differences were very stable over time, as indicated by a correlation of $r = .77$ between the two one-year stabilities (cf. Table 10.3). Thus, a stable pattern of stability emerged for the single items of the CCQ.

The average stability of the individual CCQ-patterns was higher than the mean stability of the CCQ-items. The very high two-year stability of $r = .87$ obtained for the pattern of item means suggests, however, that the average two-year stabilty of children's personality patterns was due partly to this stereotypic effect. In fact, when the stability of the item means is canceled out by defining individual patterns on the

Table 10.4. *Stable and unstable children: Differences in intelligence.*

Intelligence test	Mean (Std) of IQ				Difference		
	Unstable[a]		Stable[b]		t	df	p
HAWIK[c] verbal, age 3–4	102.2	(9.3)	112.2	(12.6)	3.74	67	.001
HAWIK verbal, age 4–5	108.8	(9.7)	112.8	(7.9)	1.92	70	.06
CMMS[d] nonverbal, age 3–4	103.0	(13.7)	111.3	(11.5)	2.73	67	.01
HAWIK nonverbal, age 4–5	98.7	(12.3)	110.8	(13.8)	3.84	67	.001

[a]Lowest quartile of 2-year stability of individual CCQ-patterns
[b]Highest quartile of 2-year stability of CCQ-patterns
[c]Cf. Table 10.2
[d]Columbia Mental Maturity Scale (Burgemeister, Blum, & Lorge, 1972)

basis of z-scores determined over children separately for each measurement point, the two-year stability drops from .43 to .30.

As Table 10.3 indicates, the one-year stabilities of children's individual patterns were not very stable over time ($r = .41$, for the stability of these stabilities). Thus, the data do not support the notion that the stability of personality is a permanent characteristic of most children at that age. On the other hand, a comparison of the most stable with the most unstable children (as defined by the highest vs. lowest quartile in the two-year stability of the individual patterns) revealed that the stable children had higher scores in all of the IQ-tests applied than the unstable children (cf. Table 10.4). No comparable relations to Piagetian measures of cognitive development of the children were found.

That the children perceived to be more stable by their teachers were somewhat more intelligent on average cannot be attributed to a pure intelligence effect, because children's stabilities between the various IQ-tests of Table 10.4 did not show a clear relation to their intelligence level in these tests (this was analyzed by a new coefficient of individual stability in single variables; see p. 195). Rather, one possible interpretation of the difference between stable and unstable children is that more intelligent chilldren are more visible to their teachers in preschool and are more reliably judged by them, which, in turn, leads to a higher stability in their CCQ-patterns.

A second possible interpretation is that the more stable children were so stable because they had an overall more desirable personality (including high intelligence); thus, their stability would be due to less social pressure exerted upon these children. This interpretation is strongly supported by another result. A correlation of $r = .59$ was found between the initial social desirability of children's personality patterns and the two-year stabilities of these patterns. Thus, the more desirable a child's personality was in the first year of preschool, the more stable this personality remained.

The retest and the longitudinal stabilities of the CCQ-prototypicalities were respectable; the lowest stability was found for ego-resiliency ($r = .44$), a medium one

Table 10.5. *Correlations between prototypicalities of wave one and three and individual stabilities from wave one to three.*

Wave	DES	AGG	ERE	ECO	SHY	INT
1	.29	−.33	.39	.28	−.01	.39
3	.08	−.15	.16	.11	−.08	.21

Note: Abbreviations of prototypicalities refer to those in Table 10.1

for shyness and desirability ($r = .50$), and a rather high one for ego-control, introversion, and aggressiveness (r's between .62 and .66).

These stabilities on the level of aggregates of persons do not preclude substantial interindividual differences in the stability of the prototypicalities, however. We explore these potential differences with a new coefficient of individual stability that is based on the difference between a person's z-scores in the two variables to be compared. The rationale and the statistical properties of this new coefficient are presented in Asendorpf (1989b,c). Here, it may suffice to say that the individual stabilities were approximately normally distributed for each of the six prototypes, with a similar variance.

When the two-year individual stabilities for each prototypicality were correlated with the individual prototypicality scores (e.g., the stability of desirability of a particular child with the child's desirability score at the first assessment), an interesting pattern emerged (see Table 10.5).

The four socially desirable characteristics (cf. Table 10.1) were found to be positively related to their stability. Shyness (which was found to be neutral in respect to social desirability) showed no relation to its stability, and the undesirable trait of aggressivity was negatively related to its stability. Furthermore, this pattern was much clearer for the first assessment than for the assessment two years later. This result may again reflect the effect of socialization toward a socially desirable personality. The less agreeable a child appears, the more social pressure may be exerted upon the child to change in a more desirable direction.

Conclusions

We have shown that the different kinds of stability described in the opening section can be studied with Q-sort data. (We did not assess the stability of prototypic Q-sorts, but this can be done easily by instructing people to generate age-specific prototypic sorts.) The Q-sort data presented met three of the four requirements for stability data outlined in the second section of this chapter. The requirement of a high short-term stability was only partly fulfilled, however. The single items showed a low mean and a high variance of short-term stability that appear to be due not only to an insufficient aggregation of the measures but also to differences among the items in their "trait-likedness," that is, in the degree to which they meet the requirement of a trait. These differences in trait-likedness were found to be very stable over time.

This result helps to clarify some of the confusion that has evolved in the literature around the question of whether interindividual differences are temporally stable or not (e.g., Block, 1977; Epstein, 1979, 1980, 1983; Kagan, 1980; Mischel, 1968; Mischel & Peake, 1982). Obviously, there are as many answers to this question as there are behavioral dimensions and age intervals.

The more interesting question for the psychology of personality is how stable particular traits are over an extended period of time within a certain age range. This question can be answered empirically, but it needs data of a particular quality to be answered correctly. Only variables with a high short-term stability can be used, because this type of stability is a necessary prerequisite for traits.

The temporal stability of traits often is confused with the temporal stability of personality (e.g., Mischel, 1968; Mischel & Peake, 1982). We have shown that the temporal stability of personality can be studied empirically; again, there are as many answers to this question as there are persons and age intervals. And again, a high short-term stability of the individual patterns studied must be demonstrated before answers to these questions can be tried. It simply makes no sense to interpret a low long-term stability of a person's personality pattern as indicating major shifts in this person's personality if this pattern is not stable over a period of a few weeks. Disregarding these necessary prerequisites maintains the stability of confusion about stability issues in personality development.

References

Allport, G. W. (1961). *Pattern and growth in personality.* New York: Holt, Rinehart & Winston.

Asendorpf, J. (1987). Social competence. In F. E. Weinert & W. Schneider (Eds.), *LOGIC – Report No. 2: Documentation of assessment procedures used in waves one to three.* Munich: Max Planck Institute for Psychological Research.

Asendorpf, J. (1989a). *Soziale Gehemmtheit und ihre Entwicklung (Social inhibition and its development).* Berlin: Springer.

Asendorpf, J. (1989b). The measurement of individual consistency. *Methodika, 2.*

Asendorpf, J. (1989c). Individual, differential, and aggregate stability of social competence. In B. H. Schneider, G. Attili, J. Nadel, & R. Weissberg (Eds.), *Social competence in developmental perspective* (pp. 71–86). Dordrecht, Netherlands: Kluwer.

Block, J. (1961). *The Q-sort method in personality assessment and psychiatric research.* Springfield, IL: Charles C. Thomas.

Block, J. (1977). Advancing the psychology of personality: Paradigmatic shift or improving the quality of research. In D. Magnusson & N. S. Endler (Eds.), *Personality at the crossroads: Current issues in interactional psychology* (pp. 37–63). Hillsdale, NJ: Erlbaum.

Block, J. H., & Block, J. (1980). The role of ego-control and ego-resiliency in the organization of behavior. In W. A. Collins (Ed.), *Minnesota Symposium on Child Psychology* (Vol. 13, pp. 39–101). Hillsdale, NJ: Erlbaum.

Block, J. H., & Block, J. (1983). *Rationale and procedure for developing indices of ego-control and ego-resiliency.* Unpublished manuscript. Berkeley: University of California.

Bryk, A. S., & Raudenbush, S. W. (1987). Application of hierarchical linear models to assessing change. *Psychological Bulletin, 101,* 147–158.

Burgemeister, B., Blum, L., & Lorge, J. (1972). *Columbia Mental Maturity Scale.* New York: Harcourt Brace Jovanovich.

Eggert, D. (1978). *Hannover Wechsler Intelligenztest für das Vorschulalter (HAWIVA).* Bern: Huber.

Emmerich, W. (1964). Continuity and stability in early social development. *Child Development, 35,* 311–332.

Emmerich, W. (1968). Personality development and concepts of structure. *Child Development, 39,* 671–690.

Epstein, S. (1979). The stability of behavior: I. On predicting most of the people much of the time. *Journal of Personality and Social Psychology, 37,* 1097–1126.

Epstein, S. (1980). The stability of behavior: II. Implications for psychological research. *American Psychologist, 35,* 790–806.

Epstein, S. (1983). The stability of confusion: A reply to Mischel and Peake. *Psychological Review, 90,* 170–184.

Flavell, J. H. (1972). An analysis of cognitive developmental sequences. *Genetic Psychology Monographs, 86,* 279–350.

Göttert, R., & Asendorpf, J. (1989). Eine deutsche Version des California-Child-Q-Sort, Kurzform (German version of the California-Child-Q-Sort, short version). *Zeitschrift für Entwicklungspsychologie und Pädagogische Psychologie, 27,* 70–82.

Kagan, J. (1971). *Change and continuity in infancy.* New York: Wiley.

Kagan, J. (1980). Perspectives on continuity. In O. G. Brim, Jr., & J. Kagan (Eds.), *Constancy and change in human development* (pp. 26–74). Cambridge, MA: Harvard University Press.

Larsen, R. J. (1987). The stability of mood variability: A spectral analytic approach to daily mood assessments. *Journal of Personality and Social Psychology, 52,* 1195–1204.

Magnusson, D. (1988). *Individual development from an interactional perspective: A longitudinal study.* Hillsdale, NJ: Erlbaum.

Mischel, W. (1968). *Personality and assessment.* New York: Wiley.

Mischel, W., & Peake, P. K. (1982). Beyond déjà vu in the search for cross-situational consistency. *Psychological Review, 89,* 730–755.

Moskowitz, D. S., & Schwarz, J. C. (1982). Validity comparison of behavior counts and ratings by knowledgeable informants. *Journal of Personality and Social Psychology, 42,* 518–528.

Moss, H. A., & Susman, E. J. (1980). Longitudinal study of personality development. In O. G. Brim, Jr., & J. Kagan (Eds.), *Constancy and change in human development* (pp. 530–95). Cambridge, MA: Harvard University Press.

Nesselroade, J. R., & Baltes, P. B. (Eds.) (1979). *Longitudinal research in the study of behavior and development.* New York: Academic Press.

Rutter, M. (1987). Continuities and discontinuities from infancy. In J. D. Osofsky (Ed.), *Handbook of infant development* (Vol. 2, pp. 1256–1296). New York: Wiley.

Stephenson, W. (1953). *The study of behavior.* Chicago: University of Chicago Press.

Thomae, H. (1957). Problems of character change. In H. F. David & H. v. Bracken (Eds.), *Perspectives in personality theory* (pp. 242–254). New York: Basic Books.

Waters, E., Noyes, D. M., Vaughn, B. E., & Ricks, M. (1985). Q-sort definitions of social competence and self-esteem: Discriminant validity of related constructs in theory and data. *Developmental Psychology, 21,* 508–522.

Weinert, F. E., & Schneider, W. (Eds.) (1986). *First report on the Munich Longitudinal Study on the Genesis of Individual Competencies (LOGIC)* (Technical Report). Munich: Max Planck Institute for Psychological Research.

Weinert, F. E., & Schneider, W. (Eds.) (1987). *LOGIC – Report No.2: Documentation of assessment procedures used in waves one to three* (Technical Report). Munich: Max Planck Institute for Psychological Research.

Wohlwill, J. F. (1973). *The study of behavioral development.* New York: Academic Press.

11 Beyond correlations: From group data analyses to single case studies

FINI SCHULSINGER

Introduction

The pretentious title of this chapter does not represent any special affectation or ambitiousness. On the contrary, this chapter is a modest attempt to provoke a discussion of ways to solve some elementary problems that have arisen as a natural consequence of a special, but not uncommon, type of longitudinal research. The collection of experiential and behavioral data through personal contacts over many years from a specific population may leave the researchers with at least two classes of data: (1) relatively simple (reduced) variables that naturally lend themselves to all kinds of multivariate statistics, and (2) other variables that have been recorded during unstructured parts of the regular interviews and that reflect positive and negative life experiences or events.

At the conclusion of such a longitudinal study, the first kind of data on various subgroups of the research sample will be analyzed statistically in traditional correlational ways with the purpose of testing the original hypotheses behind the study. Also, assumptions that have appeared during the intermediate waves of the group data analyses will be tested this way at the conclusion of the study.

But the second kind of data, which are not collected systematically because they were not hypothetical predictors of outcome and which are not always reduced variables, are still left untreated. In consideration of the enormous historical utility of such "qualitative" data, even in "$n = 1$ studies," the research group behind this project has asked me to show how this class of data can be utilized in a meaningful way.

The body of literature on qualitative data analysis is very large. However, very little of it pertains to the actual situation within our own longitudinal project. For that reason, I expect that a specific discussion of our problems among a number of longitudinal researchers may bring about solutions that meet our needs. This chapter is meant as an opening of this discussion.

The project

In 1962 Sarnoff Mednick and the author began a prospective, longitudinal study of children of severely schizophrenic mothers (Mednick & Schulsinger, 1965). It was

Table 11.1. *List of experimental measures: 1962 high-risk assessment.*

Psychophysiology
   Conditioning-extinction-generalization
   Response to mild & loud sounds
Wechsler Intelligence Scale for Children (Danish adaptation)
Personality inventory
Word association test
Continuous association test
   30 words
   1 minute of associating to each word
Adjective checklist used by examiners to describe subjects
Psychiatric interview
Interview with parent or rearing agent
School report from teacher
Midwife's report on subject's pregnancy & delivery

the first prospective study in the field of psychiatry of a population at special high risk. It was designed to test Mednick's (1958) theory on schizophrenia as a learned thought disorder in individuals with a physiological disposition towards avoidance learning. When such individuals during their childhood were exposed to repeated or chronic anxiety-provoking situations, they learned, in order to avoid the anxiety, to think in a disordered (tangential) way.

Because it was a major effort to collect and examine the sample of 207 high-risk subjects and their 104 matched low-risk controls – a total of 311 subjects – more comprehensive variables than those absolutely necessary for testing the initial hypothesis were collected, for example, the midwives' reports.

These variables appear in Table 11.1. The 311 subjects were examined between December 1962 and March 1964. They were between 10 and 20 years old (15.1 average), and none of them were clinically mentally deviant.

The idea was to follow these children through the major part of the risk period for schizophrenia, which at that time was considered to be from 15–45 years of age. Eventually, we would be able to determine which of the original variables discriminated those children who became schizophrenic from those with other outcomes. Variables with such predictive power might then be considered as potential targets for preventive intervention.

As the project was the first prospective longitudinal study in the mental health area, we really did not know the ideal length of the intervals between the reassessments of the sample. We wanted, of course, to get as much prospective data collection as possible. On the other hand, we were afraid of making the study just another therapeutic facility for adolescents and young adults, and thus influence the natural history of schizophrenia. These problems, however, solved themselves by the scarcity of funds available at that time for such an adventurous undertaking as a study whose

Table 11.2. *Years of assessments.*

1962	1967	1972–74	1980
Initial assessment	5-year follow-up	10-year diagnostic inter-view follow-up	Subsample follow-up
Children of schizo-phrenic mothers ($n =$ 207)	Social worker interview		Diagnostic reexamina-tion
			CAT-scan examination
Children of nonschizo-phrenic mothers ($n =$ 104) age 15.1 years	Preliminary comparison of "sick," "well," and control groups		
Psychological examina-tion			1980–83 Diagnostic in-terview study of the children's fathers
Psychiatric examination			
Rearing environment			
Parent interview			
Psychophysiological ex-amination			
Perinatal history			
School behavior			

Table 11.3. *Characteristics distinguishing "sick" from "well" and control groups: 1967 follow-up.*

Lost mother to psychiatric hospitalization relatively early in life
Teacher reports of disturbing, aggressive behavior in school
Evidence of associative drift
Psychophysiological anomalies (skin conductance)
   Marked fast latency of response
   Response latency evidenced no signs of habituation
   Resistance to experimental extinction of conditioned skin conductance response
   Remarkably fast rate of recovery following response peak
Sick group (70%) suffered serious pregnancy/birth complications

results first could be expected about 25 years later. Table 11.2 shows the years of reassessments.

At the 1967 reassessments none of the subjects could be designated as schizo-phrenic or psychotic, but 20 of the high-risk subjects were having severe behavioral problems of various kinds. Table 11.3 shows the statistically significant differences between this "sick" group and a matched "well" high-risk group, and also a demo-

Table 11.4. *Diagnoses at 10-year follow-up.*

	Interviewer		CAPPS-DIAGNO II		CATEGO (PSE + SCL + AS)		"Consensus" diagnoses	
Schizophrenia[a]	13	(1)	30	(6)	10	(1)	15	(1)
Borderline states (including schizoid and paranoid personality disorders)[b]	71	(5)	20	(1)	35	(3)	55	(4)
Psychopathy	5	(4)	2	(1)	4	(4)	5	(4)
Other personality disorders	26	(10)	3	(2)	22	(9)	22	(9)
Neuroses (symptoms & character)	34	(44)	31	(16)	43	(38)	30	(33)
Nonspecific conditions	0	(0)	43	(17)	24	(17)	13	(11)
No mental disorder	23	(27)	44	(47)	15	(17)	25	(27)
Other conditions (including affective & paranoid psychoses)	1	(0)	0	(1)	20	(2)	1	(0)
Disagreement among the 3 diagnoses							7	(2)
Total	173	(91)	173	(91)	173	(91)	173	(91)

[a]Two additional schizophrenics had died before the 1972–74 assessment, but hospital charts clearly indicated the presence of schizophrenia.
[b]These 71 individuals comprise 29 borderline schizophrenics (SPD), 29 schizoid personality disorders, and 13 paranoid personality disorders.

graphically matched low-risk control group. Further details may be found in Mednick and Schulsinger (1968).

At the next folllow-up, which took place from 1972 to 1974, the sample had reached an age at which some severe psychopathological outcomes could already be expected. For this reason the assessment included an extremely thorough clinical evaluation (H. Schulsinger, 1976) of which the main results appear in Table 11.4.

Apart from a traditional clinical interview based on an eclectic psychiatric frame of reference, two standardized interviews were applied simultaneously: the CAPPS (predecessor of SADS-L) and the PSE, ninth edition (PSE eighth edition was used in the WHO International Pilot Study of Schizophrenia). These standardized interviews yielded computer-derived diagnoses. They differed from each other and also from the clinical interview. Based on face validation, supported by the "middle way view" advocated by Gottesman and Shields (1972), we have used the clinician's own (ICD-8) diagnoses in subsequent data analyses. Also, the incidence of schizophrenia was in accordance with what could be expected from numerous classical pedigree studies, after age had been corrected using the abridged Weinberg method and Strömgren's method.

Based on this 1972–1974 assessment, a number of correlational data analyses were carried out using different paradigms (Mednick et al., 1978). Our first approach was to use multivariate analyses in the form of the path-finding analysis program LISREL (Jöreskog & van Thello, 1972). See Figure 11.1. In principle, this method is a natural choice in longitudinal projects insofar as one of its potentials is to find which

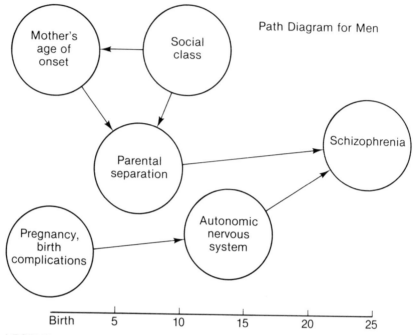

Figure 11.1. Example of path diagram for male high-risk subjects.

indicators of unmeasured variables (constructs) lead to a certain outcome and how much of the variance they were responsible for.

On the other hand, the parameters are factor analysis derived, and therefore the overall results are reduced to such an extent that they are not immediately understandable. Certainly, they are far from being of a causal nature. But the method may be extremely powerful with regard to creating the background for new hypotheses.

A later approach was to analyze the data with psychopathological (diagnostic) outcome and genetic risk as the independent variables, and hypothesize contributing etiological factors as the dependent variables, one at a time. This turned out to be a very fruitful paradigm for data analyses and gave some evidence for the following conclusions:

1. Pregnancy and birth complications (PBC) were the worst for schizophrenics, best for schizotypal personality disorders, and intermediate for the psychopathologically healthy high-risk subjects (Parnas et al., 1982).

2. Institutional rearing during the first years of life was most frequently associated with a schizophrenic outcome. It was second to most, with a schizotypal personality

disorder outcome, and was least associated with a no-mental illness outcome in the high-risk subjects (Parnas, Teasdale & Schulsinger, 1985).

3. Cerebral ventricular atrophy (in the 1979/80 subsample) was most prominent in schizophrenics, least prominent in the schizotypals, and in an intermediate position in the healthy high-risk subjects. This was a distribution comparable to the distribution of pregnancy and birth complications. There was a significant but not very high correlation between the PBCs and the ventricular size, which indicates that other factors affecting the brain might be contributing towards the manifestation of schizophrenia (Schulsinger et al., 1984). Mednick, Machon, Huttunen, and Bonnet (1988) produced evidence for neurotoxic viral infections as such factors.

Presently, the final follow-up of the high-risk and low-risk subjects is going on. Results from the multivariate statistical analyses using the same paradigm as above will be out during 1990. The final follow-up comprises a thorough social and psychopathological interview, CT-scans of the brain, and the examination of smooth pursuit eye movements (SPEM), by many considered the most promising hypothetical trait marker for schizophrenia at the present (Holzman et al., 1974).

Of the original 311 subjects, 12 have died, most of them due to suicide. Some have emigrated, and a few will refuse to participate in the final follow-up, especially in the medical parts of it (the social home interview is accepted by most). The multivariate statistical analyses will of course yield a substantial amount of results on possible predictors and constellations of predictors that may be used to establish new projects on the possibilities of primary prevention of a number of cases of schizophrenia. If the present results will be replicated in the final follow-up, it means that the schizotypal personality disorder subjects are close to being expressors of the genotype for schizophrenia. If such subjects in utero or during childhood (or even later) are exposed to various biological and psychosocial stressors, they may manifest schizophrenia. Results of that nature will, of course, be of great interest. They are, however, not results that document *causal* relationships.

Possibilities for establishing causal relationships

We estimate that 250–270 of the original 311 subjects from 1962 will participate in the final follow-up study. Presently, approximately half of this number have participated in this examination.

We will, from this and from earlier assessments, have a substantial number of data that do not fit into the multivariate statistical analyses. Either they have not been collected systematically, and therefore will not be present for every subject, or they will be unreduced and therefore unsuitable for ordinary statistical procedures. Many of these data will consist of subjects' accounts of experiences or of the examiners' accounts of their impressions. This raises the following problems:

1. Is it meaningful to try to take advantage of such unsystematic, "qualitative," or humanistic and unreduced data?

2. If so, how should one proceed to take advantage, considering the size of the sample (approximately 250 subjects)?

These two problems will now be dealt with.

As indicated, we will end up with 250–270 files, each consisting of a large amount of structured and systematically collected data on the subject. In addition, each file will also contain thorough systematic information on the psychopathology of the fathers, collected through personal interviews (Parnas et al., 1985). Furthermore, each file will be supplemented with an extremely thorough and structured set of data on the mothers' schizophrenia, collected from the mothers' complete hospital charts up to date (Jørgensen et al., 1987). As a whole, these files may be considered as 250–270 single case stories, of which a certain preplanned part will enter the multivariate statistical analyses.

An immediate solution would be to subject all these single case files to some kind of qualitative analysis, that is, to try to *understand* them. Much has been achieved in behavioral science through understanding just a few cases or even one single case. From Shipley (1961) a few of these studies will be mentioned:

> Jean Piaget, *The language and thought of the child.*
> August Aichhorn, "The meaning of the reality principle in social behavior" (ch. 9 in *Wayward Youth*).
> Josef Breuer and Sigmund Freud, *Studies on hysteria.*
> Julius Wagner von Jauregg, *The effect of malaria on progressive paralysis* (9 cases).
> Eugen Bleuler, *Dementia Praecox, or the group of schizophrenias* (ch. 1 on "The fundamental symptoms").

Bleuler's book was based on many patients, but his conclusions were of the "understanding nature," not statistically derived. He was contemporary with Kraepelin, who coined the "Dementia Praecox" concept, and did it on a true quantitative empiristic basis. Whereas Bleuler's mode of understanding dynamic aspects of his patients' experiences and behavior had a positive influence on therapeutic attitudes, it seems now that Kraepelin's statistically derived concept is in close accordance with today's biologically oriented theories on schizophrenia.

A newer example of qualitative research is the 800-page book by Wallerstein (1986) on the psychoanalytic therapies of 42 patients. It is a most impressive and inspiring exercise, full of well-documented messages on therapy and on method. However, even if our own 250–270 case files are not as long and detailed as the Menninger Foundation therapy cases in Wallerstein's book, we judge it absolutely impossible to study them in a purely qualitative way. In order to profit from such a study, more than one researcher would have to read the cases. It will simply be too much for a group of "judges" to keep so many cases separate from each other mentally in a meaningful way.

Compromises

Qualitative research of human behavior is not in itself a compromise due to lack of sufficiently structured and reduced data. It may be the only way to understand complexities of human life and behavior, and it is not "less scientific" than empiristically carried out research. It is just a different strategy for data analysis. Various studies of long-term outcome in drug addiction have yielded highly interesting results on prognosis. But personal accounts from sociologists who have lived for some time in drug-addict environments with, say, one or two addicts teach us much more about the phenomenon of drug addiction and drug culture than the big surveys.

But how can we learn from 250–270 cases apart from the empiristic collection of data? The answer is: By compromising. The first compromise in our study will be to reduce the number of cases that will be studied qualitatively. We are interested in outcomes, and our basic statistical analyses will use Schizophrenia, Schizotypal Personality Disorder, Other Psychiatric Outcomes, and No Mental Illness as four dichotomous dependent outcome variables against which we will analyze independent potential predictor variables. Logically, we would then have to select a representative subsample of subjects from four outcome groups – 30–50 cases.

Now, qualitative research is based on understanding. Is it also based on objectivity, or compulsive avoidance of any bias? Is it possible to *understand* without knowledge of the case stories, and can bias be avoided when knowledge is needed? Of course not. We therefore intend to maximize knowledge and postpone the problem of bias for a little while. The qualitative analysis is proposed to be carried out by four investigators, each of whom has his or her own separate and very personal experience of the whole sample (see Table 11.2):

1. The 1962–64 interviewer
2. The 1972–74 interviewer
3. The present final follow-up interviewer
4. The 1967, 1972–74, 1979–80, and present final follow-up social worker

We are going to read the 30–50 cases, one at a time, and then meet to discuss them one case at a time. But how will it be possible to learn something from this? Our intention is to try to agree on a causal hypothesis for each case. In order not to get too many hypotheses, two compromises must be adopted:

One is to agree, before the exercises start, upon a common frame of reference for our hypotheses. That may not be so difficult. As a consequence of the results from our earlier assessments, we all adhere to a diathesis-stress concept of schizophrenia. This means that we believe that schizophrenia is a result of an interaction between certain hereditary liabilities on the one hand and a variety of experiential factors on the other. Some of the experiential factors are included in the planned data collection as bricks in our general scientific hypotheses. The other experiential factors may be any kind of life experience related to the working life, the love life, the parental obligations and ties, illnesses, accidents, crime, encounters with the mental health care delivery system, successes, defeats, and so forth. Our common frame of reference then will be to adhere to the diathesis-stress concept and to include all those events and grade them according to a preconceived system before we include them in our causal explanations for each of the 30–50 subjects.

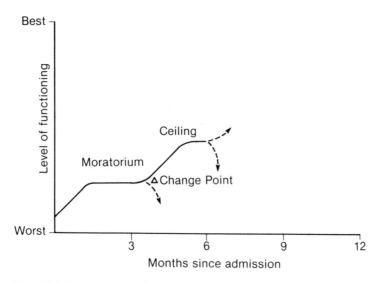

Figure 11.2. Common pattern of the course of psychiatric disorder in 28 patients.

The second compromise is to agree on the application of a pattern recognition technique. This is one of the several approaches to single cases studies as, for example, described in Yin (1984). Unfortunately, this technique has not been widely used in psychopathology research. The only examples known to the present author are described by Strauss, Hafez, Lieberman, and Harding (1985). They studied 28 patients hospitalized for functional psychiatric disorder in an attempt to explore systematically the course of psychiatric disorder over a 2-year period. Their variables were, apart from outcome, personality characteristics, work experiences, family and other network experiences, and so forth. They recognized through a qualitative approach a common pattern composed of what they named "longitudinal principles." This pattern appears Figure 11.2.

Moratoriums are periods of stability in symptoms and functioning, but with relatively "hidden" silent changes such as reconstitution of identity, strengthening of skills in subtle ways, and so forth.

Change points involve considerable shifts in functioning and symbols over a brief period, for example, changing to a more exciting job.

Ceilings are defined as the highest level of functioning reached in the given period of time.

Strauss et al. (1985) describe a number of longitudinal principles, for example, "nonlinearity" of the course. They also describe periods of "decay of vulnerability" and "phases of environmental response" such as convalescence and backlashes.

It is difficult to predict where these patterns and longitudinal principles will be recognized in our sample, which consists of a population with a highly diversified outcome – from no mental illness, over a spectrum of almost any mental disorder, to schizophrenia. Strauss et al.'s sample consists of patients who all had the same diagnosis. But the approach described makes a great deal of sense, and it will be tried out in our attempts to describe and understand what are beyond the correlations.

How to proceed from the qualitative analysis

We imagine that it will be possible to achieve consensus between the four qualitative researchers about a few causal models pertaining to most or all of the 30–50 cases. However, it may take some time to solve initial disagreements. Causal models in this context should be understood as interpretations of a combination of the main results from the analyses of the earlier assessments and from the statistical analyses of this final assessment, plus the patterns recognized and agreed upon during the described qualitative exercise.

It will be necessary to express this combination of old results and new patterns in a way that the causal models can be subject to statistical analyses with the purpose of testing their validity within the total sample. Nobody expects a 100% validity. There will be a number of cases for which the causal models are not appropriate. It is hoped that this number will not be too large. We will then try another qualitative exercise with the purpose of understanding why the models did not fit in these cases.

When we feel that our qualitative powers are exhausted, it may be possible to ascertain statistically the types and number of items that characterize the cases in which none of the causal models fit.

Conclusions

What has been described is a tentative procedure with the purpose of utilizing longitudinal data that do not fit into multivariate statistical programs. The procedure is presented in order to discuss this kind of problem, which most likely is unavoidable in a longitudinal prospective study of the length described (25 years), with relatively rare reassessments, and in a field where the phenomenon under study, that is, schizophrenia, is extremely complex. Furthermore, during the 25 years new knowledge about the etiology of schizophrenia has been found in different areas – from genetics, to obstetrical complications, cognitive functioning, psychophysiology, rearing conditions, and even course and prognosis – not to mention treatment strategies. When we began selecting children of schizophrenic mothers in 1962, the reason was to get a higher than average population risk for a schizophrenic outcome. But at that time this risk was considered as psychologically caused in wide academic circles. Only several years later it became evident that the high-risk mainly could be ascribed to hereditary liabilities. Since the project began in 1962, brain imaging has become an important research tool. The etiological assumptions with the best face validity presently describe schizophrenia as a result of a genetic liability, which may in part be manifest as a fetal, possibly genetic, defect of the cyto-architecture in parahippocampal and entorhinal areas of the brain. It is assumed that this cerebral defect may show itself later in life as subtle, or less subtle, neuro-integrative defects. If children with such a disposition are exposed to certain stressors, for example, neurotoxic viral infections in utero, obstetrical complications (asphyxia), stressful childhood rearing, serious psychosocial defeats, and so forth, clinical schizophrenia may then be the result.

The more factors involved in etiology and pathogenesis, the more complicated is data analysis. On the other hand, the chance of finding factors that can be prevented is larger. The complexity, however, makes it impossible to design a longitudinal prospective study in which all useful variables can be selected premorbidly. Therefore, it is necessary to operate with the possibility of ending up with a larger number of data that can be utilized only after a qualitative procedure.

As already stated, this is not seen as an obstacle for a good quality of research. On the contrary. To limit a longitudinal study of a complex phenomenon as schizophrenia to variables only of a kind that can be predicted from the beginning, and also can be reduced sufficiently for quantitative analyses, is a much stronger guarantee for research of disputable quality or importance. In this context it should be noted that many of the most serious and most common human illnesses − mental as well as physical − most likely fit the same type of diathesis-stress concept as does schizophrenia.

The quality of qualitative research is difficult to determine from the outset. As already stated, guidelines for the present field of research are scarce. Considering, however, the high quality of much research in literature, history, and anthropology, one should not despair. Gregory Bateson (1941), whose contributions towards an understanding of schizophrenia are much disputed, was otherwise an outstanding and highly recognized anthropologist of his time. In a charming paper read at the Seventh Conference on Methods in Philosophy and the Sciences in 1940, he described in some detail his approach to understanding new phenomena and coherences. He writes:

So far I have spoken of my own personal experiences with *strict* and *loose* thinking, but I think actually the story which I have narrated is typical of the whole fluctuating business of the advance of science. In my case, which is a small one and comparatively insignificant in the whole advance of science, you can see both elements of the alternating process − *first the loose thinking* and the building up of a structure on unsound foundations and *then the correction of stricter thinking* and the substitution of a new underpinning beneath the already constructed mass. And that, I believe, is a pretty fair picture of how science advances, with this exception, that usually the edifice is larger and the individuals who finallly contribute the new underpinning are different people from those who did the initial loose thinking. . . .

And if you ask me for a recipe for speeding up this process, I would say first that we ought to accept and enjoy this dual nature of scientific thought and be willing to value the way in which the two processes work together to give us advances in the understanding of the world.

Appendix

The discussion of the paper upon which this chapter is based was introduced with a paper prepared by Wolfgang Edelstein. In spite of certain initial remarks, Edelstein contributed in a constructive way to solving problems raised in the paper. Based on his own background in developmental psychology, he emphasized the importance of studying patterns of change. He proposed giving up the distinction of qualitative and quantitative research. It is now possible to deal with categorical–qualitative data in similarly sophisticated ways as it is possible to deal with continuous variables. There are now methods available for assessing typologies as well as pattern hypotheses. Edelstein illustrated his points with examples from his own Piagetian research, which showed ways of quantitative analyses of various categorical patterns. In his detailed discussion he did not forget to emphasize the necessity of understanding of the theoretical nature of the patterns observed. The discussion became very constructive, for which reason Edelstein's references are appended to the references of this chapter.

References

Bateson, G. (1941). Experiments in thinking about observed ethnological material. *Philosophy of Science, 8,* 53–68.

Gottesman, I. I., & Shields, J. (1972). *Schizophrenia and genetics* (p. 415). New York: Academic Press.

Holzman, P. S., Proctor, L. R., Levy, D. L., Yassilo, N. J., Meltzer, N. Y., & Hurt, S. W. (1974). Eyetracking dysfunctions in schizophrenic patients and their relatives. *Archives of General Psychiatry, 31,* 143–151.

Jöreskog, K. G., & van Thello, M. (1972). LISREL-A: General computer program for estimating a linear standard equation system involving multiple indicators of unmeasured variables. *Research Bulletin: 56–72.* Princeton, NJ: Educational Testing Service.

Jørgensen, A., Teasdale, T. W., Parnas, J., Schulsinger, F., Schulsinger, H., & Mednick, S. A. (1987). The Copenhagen high risk project: The diagnosis of maternal schizophrenia and its relation to offspring diagnosis. *British Journal of Psychiatry, 151,* 753–757.

Mednick, S. A. (1958). A learning theory approach to research in schizophrenia. *Physiological Bulletin, 55,* 316–327.

Mednick, S. A., Machon, R., Huttunen, M. O., & Bonnet, D. (1988). Fetal viral infection and adult schizophrenia. *Archives of General Psychiatry* (in press).

Mednick, S. A., & Schulsinger, F. (1965). A longitudinal study of children with a high-risk for schizophrenia: A preliminary report. In S. Vanderberg (Ed.), *Methods and goals in human behavior genetics* (pp. 255–296). New York: Academic Press.

Mednick, S. A., & Schulsinger, F. (1968). Some premorbid characteristics related to breakdown in children with schizophrenic mothers. In D. Rosenthal & S. S. Kety (Eds.), *The transmission of schizophrenia* (pp. 267–291). New York: Pergamon Press.

Mednick, S. A., Schulsinger, F., Teasdale, T. W., Schulsinger, H., Venables, P. H., & Rock, D. R. (1978). Schizophrenia in high-risk children: Sex differences in predisposing factors. In G. Serban (Ed.), *Cognitive defects in the development of mental illness* (pp. 169–197). New York: Brunner/Mazel.

Parnas, J., Schulsinger, F., Teasdale, T. W., Schulsinger, H., Feldman, P. M., & Mednick, S. A. (1982). Perinatal complications and clinical outcome in children of schizophrenic mothers. *British Journal of Psychiatry, 140,* 416–420.

Parnas, J., Teasdale, T. W., & Schulsinger, H. (1985). Institutional rearing and diagnostic outcome in children of schizophrenic mothers. *Archives of General Psychiatry, 42,* 762–769.

Schulsinger, F., Parnas, J., Petersen, E. T., Schulsinger, H., Teasdale, T. W., Mednick, S. A., Moller, L., & Silverton, L. (1984). Cerebral ventricular size in the offspring of schizophrenic mothers. *Archives of General Psychiatry, 41,* 602–606.

Schulsinger, H. (1976). A ten year follow-up of children of schizophrenic mothers: A clinical assessment. *Acta Psychiatrica Scandinavica, 53,* 371–386.

Shipley, T. (Ed.) (1961). *Classics in psychology* (p. 1342). New York: Philosophical Library.

Strauss, J. S., Hafez, H., Lieberman, P., & Harding, C. M. (1985). The course of psychiatric disorder. III: Longitudinal Principles. *American Journal of Psychiatry, 142*(3), 289–296.

Wallerstein, R. S. (1986). *Forty two lives in treatment* (p. 784). New York: Guilford Press.

Yin, R. K. (1984). *Case study research: Design and methods.* Applied Social Research Methods Series (Vol. 5, p. 160). Beverly Hills, London, New Delhi: Sage.

The following references are from Wolfgang Edelstein's discussion paper:

Dayton, C. M., & MacReady, G. B. (1976). A probabilistic model for validation of behavioral hierarchies. *Psychometrika, 42,* 189–204.

Hildebrand, D. K., Laing, J. D., & Rosenthal, H. (1977). *Prediction analysis of cross classifications.* New York.

Lazarsfeld, P. F. (1972). *Qualitative analysis: Historical and critical essays.* Boston.

Lazarsfeld, P. F., & Barton, A. H. (1951). Qualitative measurement in the social sciences: Classification, typologies, and indices. In ? Lerner & ? Laswell, *The political sciences* (pp. 155–192). Stanford, CA: Stanford University Press.

Lazarsfeld, P. F., & Robinson, W. S. (1940). The quantification of case studies. *Journal of Applied Psychology, 24,* 817–825.

Rudinger, G., Chaselon, F., Zimmermann, H. J., & Henning, H. J. (1985). *Qualitative Daten: Neue Wege sozialwissenschaftlicher Methodik.* München, Wien, Baltimore.

12 Age, period, and cohort in the study of the life course: A comparison of classical A-P-C-analysis with event history analysis or Farewell to Lexis?

KARL ULRICH MAYER AND JOHANNES HUININK

Introduction

The story of the past

In all of the relevant disciplines – psychology, sociology, political science, and demography – the impact of the effects of age, period, and cohort (or of what these indicators stand for) were in the past primarily treated in accordance with the logic of Lazarsfeld's scheme of testing for spurious correlation. However, the major dimension of interest – and correspondingly what was considered of minor substantive interest and was to be controlled for – tended to be quite different for the various disciplines. Therefore, the term *cohort analysis* denotes something technically very similar but substantively very dissimilar. To avoid confusion, it is worthwhile to elaborate on these distinctions within the social sciences.

In sociology, initially, the units of analysis tended to be total societies identical with nation-states. The substantive focus concentrated on their overall change (often assumed to be a trend as in the logic of modernization, secularization, and the like). Thus, time series of representative cross sections were first to be scrutinized for age variation and later for cohort variation in order to corroborate true period changes of action patterns, values, or attitudes.

In a following step, age variations became of interest as a quasi-universal functional feature of society. Conceptually, this was developed most fully in Riley's model of normative age grading and age stratification (Riley, Johnson, & Foner, 1972). Following the work of Linton (1939) and Eisenstadt (1956), use of the concepts of age roles and age groups as units of social structure opened the way for the idea of corresponding and *causally connected* life stages (for a critique, see Mayer & Müller, 1985). Again, one and only one of the A-P-C-dimensions was of substantive interest, and the others were just to be controlled for.

As a continuous undercurrent, the Janus-faced concept of "generation" as borrowed from Mannheim (1952), that is, as both a universal of the human population process and as specific sociohistorical cohorts, was present in sociology. But it was hardly ever dealt with within the quantitative A-P-C framework. Only recently in theory (Ryder, 1965) and in empirical analysis (Müller, 1978; Mayer, 1977) has cohort been reintroduced in sociology as a means to study societal change, (i.e., as something historically specific, rather than an expression of the universal metabolism of any society), as it is still treated in the age stratification model of Riley.

However, with few exceptions within sociology, all three aspects – age, period, and cohort – basically had the character of accounting proxies without specific substantive interpretations of *particular* age groups, *particular* birth cohorts, or *particular* historical periods. The general model, then, in sociology tended to be one either of primordial cross-sectional structures (Mayer, 1986) or of secular and global societal change, thought of most frequently in a trend-like fashion.

In contrast, within psychology the general model is focused entirely on age-dependent ontogenetic development or maturation. The paradigmatic introduction of cohort sequential models (Schaie, 1965; Baltes, 1968; Schaie & Baltes, 1975) had the sole purpose of guarding against the fallacy of drawing developmental conclusions where cohort or period effects might exist. Despite various efforts of interpretation (Nesselroade & Baltes, 1984; Schaie, 1986) neither period nor cohort effects have any substantive meanings within psychology; they are residual control variables. Where "period" might interest psychologists, it would refer to phylogenetic development or evolution and thus falls far outside the scope of any empirical longitudinal observations (Featherman, 1985; Grossmann & Grossmann, 1986).

In demography, cohort is the primary notion, because cohort size at time of birth and cohort attrition are major elements of the demographic accounting system and because only within a cohort-analytic frame of reference are aggregate computations and forecasts of fertility and mortality feasible (Ryder, 1965).

It is only in political science – a discipline without its own theoretical core – that all three A-P-C-dimensions were treated in a substantive manner with equal weight (Beck, 1976; Jennings & Niemi, 1981). Age related to the hypothesis of growing conservatism over the life course, cohort to long-term effects of early political socialization or times of political mobilization, and periods to election events or duration of specific political regimes. Beck even succeeded in bringing all three dimensions into one coherent theory of political party alignment and realignment.

However, the relevance of the cohort approach is far greater in sociology than in demography and developmental psychology, because it does not simply relate to the empirical problem of decomposing variance. It relates to the crucial problem of mediating processes between different levels of social organization. Already in 1965 Ryder demonstrated impressively the potential of cohort analytical designs in the social science beyond the more strategic intentions of demography and psychology (Ryder, 1965). This is even more true if one thinks of an integration of life course analysis into this conceptual context.

Let us argue this claim more fully: Classical cohort analysis, especially in the form of "A-P-C-analysis," was originally introduced as a method for exploring aggregated demographic data. Information about the members of cohorts is broken down only by age and historical year. These variables – together with the discrete indicators of age, period, and cohort – indicate, above all, macro-sociological settings that change over time. But in terms of theory we have to deal with a typical multilevel problem: the characteristics of a cohort are aggregated outcomes of the individual behavior of cohort members in the societal context, indicated crudely by calendar time. The analysis of the dynamics of social change therefore needs refinements in the data basis in two ways.

First, we need to obtain more information on the heterogeneity of individual life courses within different cohorts. This is the central aim of life course research. On such a basis it becomes immediately apparent that the life course is an integration of many different time scales on the individual level. Technically, each life event might be taken as the starting point of a new duration of time, changing the configuration of statuses and experiences in these statuses.

Social change, that is, the development of the institutional, cultural, and social conditions of individual life courses, defines the time scales on the societal level. Thus, the second refinement is that we need more differentiated knowledge of historical events and processes that make up the dimensions of the macro-scales of time.

The cohort analytical design structures the model of the multilevel relation between the individual (life course) and societal (social change) processes in a specific way. The impact of the societal process is conceptualized in its historical (cohort effects) and actual (period effects) dimension. Both act on the individual level in structuring the individual life courses by providing time-dependent opportunity structures and age-grading norms. The differential exposure of the cohorts to social conditions is the source of changing cohort composition, which in turn is a vehicle for social change again. Ryder and others try to construct this multilevel relation exclusively via the relation of physical age and calendar time. However, one needs a multiple net of relations of time scales on the individual and societal level. For example, it is not just "youth" that is the carrier of societal change. More specifically, one might ask when people left school, married, had children, and what the relations between these events are. One might further ask how opportunity structures in the environment develop across the life course.

In this chapter we will discuss these issues of the study of the life course in the context of traditional age–period–cohort models and in the recently developed context of stochastic event history models. First we will introduce the concepts of classical cohort analysis and life course analysis. Then we will discuss the specific advantages of both. We will focus in particular on the differential treatment of cohort influences in the two approaches. Finally, we will discuss some methodological strategies and practical issues of data design in life course studies as event histories.

Classical cohort analysis: The A-P-C-model

We define a cohort as a set of social units (in the following, individuals) who experienced a certain event (cohort-defining event) at a certain time (origin of the cohort), measured usually in calendar time. A prominent cohort-defining event is the birth of an individual, producing a birth cohort. But cohorts may likewise be defined by marriage, school exit, or first entry into the labor force. Although these cohort-defining events are events in the individual life course, one may also think of cohorts defined by historical events such as war or an exposure to innovations like the pill. (For an alternative taxonomy of cohort definers, see Baltes, Cornelius, & Nesselroade, 1979.) In principle, one could in this manner distinguish between cohort-defining events that occur at a specific time in the individual life course and those that stem from general historical events. There are two interconnected time scales along which a cohort may be observed: the duration of time since the origin of the cohort (age of the cohort) and the calendar time in terms of historical years (period). Birth cohorts are especially convenient because their age is equal to the physical age of the cohort members. In other cases one will obtain duration times, such as the duration since the first marriage or the first entry into the labor force, as the age of the respective cohorts. These duration times usually are not simply linear transformations of physical age, because the cohort-defining events will not occur at the same age for each individual. But with this definition we have a linear dependency of the origin of the cohort, the cohort age, and the period.

The empirical basis of classical cohort analyses follows the centuries-old conventions of demographic, highly aggregated data collection, differentiated by age (A), period (P), and consequently by cohort (C). These dimensions are measured on the micro-level, that is, the occurrence of a marriage, an entry into the labor force, the birth of the first child. Consequently, the dependent variables in this type of analysis are based on counts of the observed events (birth of a child, marriage, etc.) for the cohorts in single years, and yield, for example, the percentages of cohort members who experienced a given event during a single year. Thus, we may obtain, for example, age-specific marriage or birth rates for women by calendar year.

The starting point of cohort analysis, then, is an Age × Period matrix of rates; this design is equivalent to the Lexis-diagram. It can easily be rearranged as a Cohort × Period or Age × Cohort matrix. The condition for this reorganization is the exact correspondence of the measurement of age, period, and cohort. Again, age has to be understood as the age of the cohort and not necessarily as the chronological age of individuals. The statistical properties of the classical cohort analytical design are essentially identical, whether the data used come from census tables, from prospective developmental studies, or from retrospective surveys on life courses. The analysis of data of this type, with the simultaneous inclusion of all three factors – age, period, cohort – is called A-P-C-analysis.

These factors may be understood as proxies for more complex constructs of processes, such as maturation, accumulation of resources, networks, or experience. However, confusion of age as proxy and age as substantive variable occurs frequently.

One way to explain the variance of the dependent variable by cohort membership, age, and period is the approach of a linear A-P-C-model. It is well known that multiple classification analysis in cohort analysis leads to an identification problem that in many instances cannot be solved in a satisfactory manner (Mason, Mason, Winsborough, & Poole, 1973; Pullum, 1980; Rodgers, 1982; Jagodzinski, 1984; Kupper, Janis, Salama, Yoshizawa, & Greenberg, 1983; Fienberg & Mason, 1979; Mason & Fienberg, 1985). However, one may obtain unique estimates of the second order differences of the parameters for the cohort, age, and period indicators (Huinink, 1989). This is not possible for the first order differences without exogenous restrictions (Pullum, 1980). The second order differences provide information about the acceleration of the change, that is, the change in velocity of the variation in the dependent variable across cohorts, ages, and periods.

An additional problem with the linear A-P-C-model lies in its assumption of additivity. It might well be the case that certain period-specific events have an impact only on the behavior of a certain cluster of cohorts in a certain age phase. For example, oral contraceptives were not immediately available for all women after they had been introduced in the early sixties. In the case of Germany, it is possible to demonstrate by a cohort analysis on birth rates that oral contraceptives spread from the older to the younger women over time, namely, cohorts. In other words, there may be interaction effects that cannot be handled satisfactorily in traditional A-P-C-analysis.

A more intuitive, explorative method to demonstrate A-P-C effects on a semigraphical basis has been proposed by Huinink (1988, 1989). This method takes the second order differences into account and tries to locate patterns of interactions. Suppose that one has a complete Age × Period table. For each age, then, one may calculate the rate of change in the variable scores of adjacent periods (cohorts), and one gets a new table with these rates of change, where the additive effects of age are partialed out (time-lag rates of change). If one follows the same procedure for single cohorts or for the periods, one obtains additional tables with rates controlled for the additive cohort; or period effects (longitudinal vs. cross-sectional rates of change) (Palmore, 1978). In a two-step procedure one may also calculate rates controlling for two of the three factors. Each of these tables can be used to identify dominant effects of one of the three factors. Take the table where age is being controlled for, and color in the regions with similar rates; for example, rates lying above, below, and in an arbitrary interval around zero. The structure of the colored regions now informs directly about cohort and period effects as well as about interactions of cohort and period with age. Diagonal boundaries between arrays of different colors indicate cohort effects, sometimes only for special age intervals (interaction effect). Vertical boundaries indicate period effects. Horizontal boundaries indicate the dominance of an interaction between age and period, namely, cohorts.

This strategy provides a straightforward but still powerful way to identify cohort, period, and age effects, even if interactions between these three factors do exist (Huinink, 1988).

Figure 12.1 gives an application of this comparative method to fertility. Take the age-specific birth rates for women in the Federal Republic of Germany in the historical years between 1963 and 1982. The Age × Period matrix of time-lagged

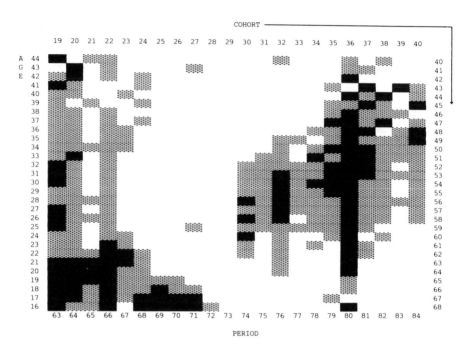

Figure 12.1. Colored Lexis-diagram of the time-lag rates of age-specific birth rates for the FRG 1963–1984. Black areas: rates above +0.02, gray areas: rates between −0.02 and 0.02, white areas: other.

rates of change in the birth rates is given in Table 12.1. In Figure 12.1 we show only a colored Lexis-diagram. Black areas indicate rates of change larger than 0.02, gray areas indicate rates between −0.02 and +0.02, and the white areas show negative rates smaller than −0.02.

Coming back to our remarks on the diffusion of oral contraceptives, we are now able to verify our hypothesis. Note the "dark" regions in the young age interval until 1972. In Germany during the sixties social norms on premarital sexual relations relaxed, but the younger women did not yet have easy access to the pill. Thus, the number of unplanned births increased for these ages. We also know from the German Life History Study (GLHS) data that especially women with complete vocational training, mostly having their children at later ages, show a higher rate of premarital conceptions when they experience an early birth.

Furthermore, by this method one can discover cohort differentials causing postponed births (again based on an interaction effect) as well as period effects in the years 1979/80 (most likely brought about by the introduction of maternity leave for employed women in the middle of 1979). By means of a purely additive model we would not have been able to identify these phenomena.

Classical cohort analysis possesses many virtues. Even though it is purely descrip-

Table 12.1. Lexis-diagram of the time-lag rates of age-specific birth rates for the FRG 1963–1984 (for period p the table shows the rate of change from period p − 1 to period p).

AGE	63	64	65	66	67	68	69	70	71	72	73	74	75	76	77	78	79	80	81	82	83	84
44	0.08	0.07	0.00	0.00	-0.04	-0.04	-0.08	-0.11	-0.03	-0.16	-0.06	-0.10	-0.11	0.00	-0.17	-0.25	-0.13	0.00	-0.08	0.00	-0.11	-0.07
43	-0.09	0.08	-0.06	-0.02	-0.05	-0.05	-0.05	-0.07	-0.01	-0.13	-0.12	-0.08	-0.13	-0.10	-0.16	-0.16	-0.15	0.00	0.00	-0.09	-0.04	-0.07
42	0.00	0.03	-0.05	-0.02	-0.11	0.01	-0.04	-0.06	-0.06	-0.14	-0.09	-0.08	-0.11	-0.17	-0.15	-0.11	-0.13	0.03	-0.03	-0.03	-0.05	-0.04
41	0.04	-0.01	-0.03	-0.08	-0.03	-0.02	-0.05	-0.07	-0.04	-0.12	-0.12	-0.11	-0.16	-0.12	-0.14	-0.14	-0.02	-0.06	0.04	-0.08	-0.04	-0.01
40	0.02	-0.01	-0.05	-0.04	-0.02	-0.03	-0.07	-0.06	-0.05	-0.10	-0.12	-0.14	-0.16	-0.10	-0.09	-0.10	-0.06	0.03	0.00	0.03	-0.06	-0.02
39	0.01	-0.03	-0.02	-0.03	-0.04	-0.02	-0.06	-0.08	-0.04	-0.11	-0.15	-0.16	-0.10	-0.07	-0.12	-0.10	-0.01	-0.01	0.06	-0.01	-0.05	-0.05
38	0.00	0.01	-0.04	-0.02	-0.04	-0.03	-0.03	-0.08	-0.08	-0.16	-0.16	-0.10	-0.12	-0.04	-0.11	-0.06	-0.02	0.11	-0.02	0.01	0.01	-0.03
37	0.01	0.01	-0.05	-0.01	-0.04	-0.01	-0.05	-0.08	-0.10	-0.15	-0.13	-0.10	-0.10	-0.07	-0.06	-0.07	0.05	0.06	0.01	0.04	-0.03	0.00
36	0.02	0.00	-0.03	-0.01	-0.02	-0.03	-0.06	-0.12	-0.09	-0.14	-0.12	-0.09	-0.08	-0.05	-0.07	-0.02	0.00	0.08	0.05	-0.03	-0.01	0.04
35	0.01	0.01	-0.04	0.00	-0.01	-0.03	-0.07	-0.13	-0.08	-0.13	-0.11	-0.08	-0.07	-0.02	0.00	-0.03	0.01	0.12	0.01	0.01	-0.02	0.03
34	0.02	0.01	-0.02	-0.01	-0.02	-0.06	-0.08	-0.12	-0.07	-0.12	-0.12	-0.06	-0.05	0.02	-0.04	-0.02	0.07	0.05	0.03	0.00	-0.01	-0.02
33	0.01	0.03	-0.03	0.00	-0.05	-0.07	-0.05	-0.13	-0.06	-0.12	-0.14	-0.04	0.00	0.00	-0.05	0.05	0.01	0.07	0.04	0.00	0.00	-0.01
32	0.05	0.01	-0.03	-0.02	-0.04	-0.05	-0.06	-0.12	-0.08	-0.11	-0.11	-0.02	-0.02	0.02	-0.01	0.02	0.04	0.09	0.04	0.00	-0.04	0.02
31	0.03	0.01	-0.04	-0.01	-0.03	-0.05	-0.07	-0.12	-0.08	-0.11	-0.09	-0.01	-0.02	0.03	0.01	0.01	0.05	0.06	0.03	-0.01	-0.02	0.02
30	0.03	0.00	-0.03	-0.01	-0.03	-0.05	-0.07	-0.13	-0.06	-0.10	-0.08	-0.02	0.02	0.03	0.00	0.04	0.04	0.06	0.00	0.02	-0.04	-0.01
29	0.02	0.00	-0.03	0.01	-0.03	-0.05	-0.09	-0.12	-0.06	-0.08	-0.10	0.01	0.01	0.06	0.00	0.02	0.03	0.04	0.02	-0.01	-0.04	0.02
28	0.01	0.00	-0.02	0.00	-0.04	-0.06	-0.10	-0.11	-0.04	-0.10	-0.08	0.04	0.00	0.04	0.00	0.02	0.01	0.05	-0.01	0.00	-0.02	-0.02
27	0.03	0.01	-0.02	0.00	-0.04	-0.06	-0.10	-0.10	-0.05	-0.08	-0.05	0.02	0.00	0.05	-0.02	-0.02	0.02	0.05	-0.01	0.01	-0.04	-0.01
26	0.03	0.00	-0.02	-0.01	-0.01	-0.06	-0.10	-0.11	-0.03	-0.07	-0.06	0.03	0.01	0.03	-0.03	0.00	0.00	0.05	0.00	-0.01	-0.04	-0.02
25	0.04	0.00	-0.03	0.00	-0.04	-0.06	-0.09	-0.10	0.01	-0.09	-0.06	0.02	0.00	-0.01	-0.02	-0.01	0.00	0.05	-0.01	-0.08	-0.04	-0.03
24	0.02	0.01	-0.04	0.00	-0.02	-0.06	-0.11	-0.08	-0.03	-0.08	-0.08	0.03	-0.05	0.02	-0.04	-0.03	0.00	0.03	-0.03	-0.01	-0.05	-0.06
23	0.02	0.00	-0.03	0.03	0.00	-0.04	-0.07	-0.09	-0.04	-0.09	-0.08	-0.02	-0.04	0.00	-0.07	0.00	-0.03	0.03	-0.02	-0.03	-0.06	-0.09
22	0.02	0.01	0.01	0.04	0.03	-0.01	-0.10	-0.09	-0.04	-0.12	-0.12	-0.02	-0.04	-0.02	-0.03	-0.04	-0.05	0.04	-0.01	-0.04	-0.11	-0.10
21	0.04	0.03	0.04	0.07	0.06	-0.02	-0.08	-0.08	-0.06	-0.14	-0.13	-0.03	-0.09	0.02	-0.06	-0.07	-0.04	0.05	-0.04	-0.08	-0.12	-0.13
20	0.05	0.07	0.07	0.10	0.01	-0.04	-0.10	-0.07	-0.16	-0.14	-0.15	-0.05	-0.06	-0.02	-0.09	-0.05	-0.04	0.03	-0.08	-0.07	-0.16	-0.12
19	0.11	0.12	0.04	0.06	0.10	0.00	-0.02	-0.01	-0.06	-0.13	-0.16	-0.05	-0.11	-0.04	-0.09	-0.07	-0.05	-0.02	-0.07	-0.13	-0.16	-0.12
18	0.17	0.07	0.02	0.03	0.01	0.01	0.05	0.00	0.02	-0.12	-0.12	-0.09	-0.16	-0.09	-0.10	-0.05	-0.14	0.02	-0.11	-0.10	-0.21	-0.15
17	0.07	0.03	-0.01	0.07	-0.02	0.01	0.07	0.07	0.07	-0.04	-0.15	-0.09	-0.19	-0.09	-0.10	-0.17	0.00	-0.07	-0.12	-0.14	-0.19	-0.12
16	0.04	0.00	0.02	0.04	-0.04	-0.07	-0.07	0.15	0.15	0.00	-0.08	-0.10	-0.14	-0.11	-0.18	-0.12	-0.06	0.06	-0.14	-0.13	-0.20	-0.04
	63	64	65	66	67	68	69	70	71	72	73	74	75	76	77	78	79	80	81	82	83	84

PERIOD

tive, it is able to provide qualitative information about the relevance of cohort membership, age, and current situation for the processes under investigation. This is an important first step in the exploration of data.

Because of the relatively simple type of observations required, it is easier to collect data for continuous follow ups of cohorts and periods. The standard example is aggregate tables from yearly censuses. In this way one may get a rough but complete picture of a small piece of history.

On the surface it appears as if the significance of the A-P-C scheme resided in its nature as an easy-to-handle methodological tool, that is, in its potential for data exploration and analysis. Its limitations were therefore almost exclusively expressed in methodological terms (identification, operationalization, estimation). Much more is at stake, however. It now becomes clear that the major significance and appeal of the traditional A-P-C-model as well as its limitations must rather be seen in the fact that it constituted a highly parsimonious, self-contained scheme with a high degree of suggestive congruence between the levels of theoretical, explanatory categories and empirical indicators. It suggested that all the important dependent variables and all the important independent variables were part of the scheme and that most of the problems could be solved if only one could obtain sufficient data and fill the cells of the Lexis-diagram. In particular, the A-P-C-model flourished because it is isomorphous both with the "general developmental model" in psychology and the "age stratification model" in sociology.

Using data on birth cohorts from the census and surveys to assess the impacts of the Second World War on the life course (Mayer, 1988)

In the following we want to exemplify the use of A-P-C-analysis for the study of the life course. How did World War II affect the military experience, working life, educational opportunities, and initial occupational status of the various birth cohorts living through it? The main question in our context is whether war effects were mainly period effects, spreading fairly evenly across a number of cohorts, or whether such effects operated differently on cohorts located at different points in the life course during the war years.

Military recruitment and prisoners of war

The first wave of data from the Socio-Economic Panel Study reveal that military mobilization reached its peak in 1944 when for all men 16 years and older 50–97% of given cohorts were enlisted (Table 12.2). The cohorts that "lost" the largest number of active years in the war and in imprisonment were those born between 1914 and 1919. Similarly, the cohorts born between 1920 and 1925 were called up almost completely during the war years.

The figures for 1945 and later indicate the degree to which men became prisoners

Table 12.2. *Proportion of men in military service or imprisonment during and after World War II, by year and birth cohort.*

Birth cohort	Year												
	1938	1939	1940	1941	1942	1943	1944	1945	1946	1947	1948	1949	1950
1902–1904	12	21	35	37	49	52	55	51	37	29	24	12	5
1905–1907	6	20	34	40	39	46	49	45	29	29	22	25	11
1908–1910	8	24	41	47	51	54	58	54	33	21	13	5	2
1911–1913	17	39	57	66	72	75	78	75	41	26	16	7	4
1914–1916	56	67	75	76	76	78	78	68	32	17	11	2	3
1917–1919	49	73	83	87	90	91	89	78	47	28	17	8	1
1920–1922	4	20	49	79	88	89	90	84	42	20	10	6	4
1923–1925	2	1	6	23	65	92	97	92	60	40	27	12	7
1926–1928	–	–	–	2	9	25	61	71	33	18	13	4	–
1929–1931	–	–	–	–	–	–	8	8	4	3	1	1	1

Source: Socio-Economic Panel (1984).

of war. In 1946, 60% of those born in the 1923–1925 period were in prison camps, decreasing to 40%, 27%, and 12% in the ensuing years. Relatively long prison terms are also characteristic of the men born between 1902 and 1907. These figures show that certain cohorts were drawn into the war almost entirely and that their members often lost 6–9 years in their occupational careers.

This evidence supports the utility of using birth cohorts as collectivities to assess the effects of World War II. It also gives rise to the hypothesis that the war had the greatest effects on the later life course of those cohorts who served as soldiers in the greatest proportions and for the longest time (i.e., the cohorts born between 1915 and 1925).

Occupational placement of men

What were the effects of war (i.e., military service, imprisonment, decreased educational opportunities) on the occupational placement and early careers of West German men? The crucial issue that the data at hand can illuminate is who were most disadvantaged? Those male cohorts whose working lives were interrupted by military service and imprisonment or those cohorts entering the labor market in the turmoil of the postwar period?

From a supplementary survey for the 1971 micro-census, occupational information is available on men for the years 1939, 1950, 1960, and 1971. Thus, we must be careful not to confound cohort and career stage differences.

For present purposes the proportion of manual workers in the cohort- or age-specific labor force will serve as an indicator of (lower) occupational status (Tables 12.3 and 12.4). Of the 20- to 30-year-old men in 1939, 67–54% were manual workers. After the war, in the same age band the corresponding proportions ranged from 81% for the youngest to 57% for the oldest men. In 1960 the corresponding proportions (i.e., 77% and 65%) still exceeded the figures for 1939. Judged against prewar conditions, cohorts born between 1926 and 1930 had approximately 15% more manual workers.

In contrast, the cohort born in 1920, the occupational careers of whose members were severely disrupted by the war, does not exhibit a markedly higher proportion of manual workers when compared to their age peers before the war (Mayer, 1977). The data on occupational distribution appear to indicate that the war affected those cohorts most adversely whose members had to enter the labor market for the first time toward the end of and after the war rather than those whose members served in the military in high proportions and for long periods.

Impacts on the later life course

So far, only the immediate consequences of World War II and its aftermath on the life conditions of different birth cohorts were examined. It was established that wartime events affected the life course most adversely if they coincided with the formative years, especially those periods when crucial educational and occupational choices are

Table 12.3. *Size of occupational categories of men by cohorts (in percent).*

| Year of birth | Manual workers in labor force | | | |
	1939	1950	1960	1971
1931–1932	–	81	65	53
1929–1930	–	76	60	51
1927–1928	–	70	56	49
1925–1926	60	63	52	46
1923–1924	64	60	51	46
1921–1922	70	57	49	45
1919–1920	67	55	49	44

Source: Microcensus-Supplementary Survey "Berufliche und soziale Umschichtung der Bevölkerung" (1971).

Table 12.4. *Size of occupational categories of men by age.*

| Age | Proportion of manual workers in labor force (in percent) | | | |
	1939	1950	1960	1971
19–20	67	81	77	63
21–22	62	76	70	48
23–24	55	70	68	57
25–26	54	63	69	56
27–28	55	60	67	50
29–30	54	57	65	50
31–32	54	55	60	52
33–34	–	54	56	51
35–36	–	51	52	53
37–38	–	49	51	54
39–40	–	50	49	53
41–42	–	52	49	51

Source: Microcensus-Supplementary Survey "Berufliche und soziale Umschichtung der Bevölkerung" (1971).

made. But how lasting were these disadvantages? Were they not compensated for in the boom years of economic reconstruction, the so-called Wirtschaftswunder of 1948 to 1965?

Occupational attainment

Table 12.3 presents data on the occupational achievements of aggregate cohorts of men at several points between 1939 and 1971. For the purpose of this discussion, one can compare the careers of cohorts born in 1919/20 and those born in 1931/32.

As noted above, the occupational lives of those in the earlier cohorts were severely disrupted by years of military service and imprisonment, whereas the younger men suffered particularly bad conditions at occupational entry. For the earlier cohorts the proportion employed in manual occupations declined from 67% in 1939 to 49% in 1960 when they were about 40 years old. Among the more recent cohorts, the proportion in manual work was 81% in 1950, declining to 53% in 1971 at age 40. Comparing these two sets of cohorts at age 30, the relative proportion of manual workers was 55% for the earlier one and 65% for the later one.

Thus, in 1960 the more recent cohorts were still markedly disadvantaged when compared to the earlier ones at about the same chronological age, even though the general economic conditions were much better in 1960 than in 1950. Ten years later the more recent cohorts were still more heavily concentrated in manual work than the earlier ones, though the discrepancy has decreased.

These findings support the hypothesis that wartime experiences affected the whole life course, because initial disadvantages were not fully compensated for in later career stages, despite highly favorable economic conditions. This finding is particularly significant, because Germany's postwar boom gave rise to a marked shift in the occupational structure, including an expansion of the white collar sector.

The life course as an event history

In an event history model of the life course we assume that, given a well-defined population at risk, the rate $r(t)$ of instantaneous change of a discrete variable in continuous time (such as changing a job, migrating, marrying, becoming pregnant, voting for a party, reaching a developmental stage) depends on:

1. The individual *process (exposure, waiting) time* (such as duration from legal marriage age to marriage).

Further, it may depend on:

2. A set of *time independent covariates,* for example, attributes of the person, such as status of social origin;
3. Membership in a given *cohort,* such as birth cohorts, marriage cohorts, labor market entry cohorts;
4. *Specific attributes of given cohorts,* such as labor market conditions at time of occupational entry or educational opportunities at time of transition to secondary school;
5. *Age* (if process time is different from age);
6. A set of *time-dependent covariates* of the individual in addition to age, such as marriage or employment status, income, amount of training, tenure status;
7. *Continuous period effects of the environment,* such as the supply of open jobs, public spending, the housing market;
8. *Discrete period effects of the environment,* such as periods of political regimes.

Let us now consider the differences and contrasts to the A-P-C-model.

First, it is important to recognize that models comprising all or many of the parameters listed above can indeed be estimated. Therefore, the above distinctions are not purely analytical and conceptual, but they can be modeled and tested. The identification problem that has for a long time preoccupied researchers in this area does not exist anymore. Here one should take note that new problems arise. It may be difficult to decide whether time dependencies of transition rates are in fact due to unobserved heterogeneity. Contrary to the identification problem in cohort analysis, this problem can be solved by extending the information basis.

There must be above all a conscious theoretical decision about the process time. When does exposure to risk of an event, such as attaining a Piaget level of cognitive ability, reaching a Kohlberg-moral stage, or mastering a certain memory level, start? As all the available evidence from life course applications of event history shows, duration is usually more important than age. Thus, process time is probably only rarely identical with age or historical time per se. Correspondingly, the observation points must relate to all the points in time where changes did or will occur.

Within process time (duration at risk) the functional form of time dependency should and often can be theoretically predicted and directly tested. Thus, there is a transition from the inductive mode of empirical accounting in A-P-C-analysis to a much more precise deductive mode of theory testing. In the current literature on job shifts, for instance, the competition between explanatory theories does not simply relate to overall age- or working-life dependency, but rather to the particular shapes of time dependency.

The dimensions of time multiply with corresponding theoretical choices. To give just a few examples from our own studies, there are age, time after World War II, labor market experience, job duration, membership in a firm, lifetime of a firm, duration in a given socioeconomic class, duration of upward occupational mobility, duration until father's status is reached, duration from legal to actual age at marriage, first conception to marriage and vice versa, spacing between children, and leaving the parental home after school-leaving age.

Once age is only one among many "life times," it very quickly can be shown that duration in a state (like marriage, employment, etc.) is generally a far more powerful predictor of rates of change than age. Chronological age becomes less and less important, and institutional membership (social age) becomes more so. It is most likely that something similar would characterize hitherto assumed age dependencies of psychological development.

Period can be defined both as an extended period of time, like government of the Social-Liberal coalition 1969–1981, or as ongoing changes of the environment as measured in monthly or quarterly time series, like consumer demand, job vacancies, Dow-Jones Index. More than one definition of cohort can be introduced simultaneously, such as birth and labor market entry or marriage cohorts.

Models can be used for prediction because the formal processes are well-defined.

Event history analysis allows one to make explicit empirical distinctions between membership in a given cohort as a contextual property, and cohort characteristics such as exposure to external events, as an individual property. Multivariate analysis is matched by explicit theorems of substantive multilevel analysis, for example, for the level of the individual, the primary group, the cohort, the region, and the overall society.

It should further be noted that the observation plan of event histories is in some respects much less restrictive than in A-P-C-analysis. Because it is a true individual level design, both age and cohort can, in principle, vary freely among individuals. It is only if cohorts or age groups are introduced as categorical variables that for any single one a sufficient fraction of the sample must fall into any category.

Analysis is not confined to panel designs of few observation points with equal intervals. Individual cases can have varying lengths of observation. Subjects who dropped out of the study can reenter, because populations at risk are continuously adjusted. Because maximum likelihood estimation techniques allow for right-censored data, processes can be observed at any point in time and not only after they have been completed for all subjects.

Career opportunities: A dynamic approach to the study of the life course, cohort, and generation effects (Blossfeld, 1986).

To illustrate the use of event history analysis as an alternative to A-P-C-analysis we will draw on an analysis based on the German Life History Study by Hans-Peter Blossfeld (1986). The main topic of his analysis is to explain occupational career opportunities by characteristics of the individual, characteristics of the career trajectory as an institutional pathway, and characteristics of the changing labor market. Cohort effects are assumed to operate in the beginning of careers in the sense that historical conditions have differential impacts on birth or labor market entry cohorts, whereas period effects are those of the economic cycle affecting all members of the labor force in a similar manner, speeding up or impeding their careers.

It is a well-established fact that careers (i.e., the rate of job shifts of various types) are highly time dependent. According to human capital theory, not age but past and expected remaining time in the labor force are the decisive time scales, because past time in the labor force is supposed to measure amount of acquired human capital and because expected remaining time in the labor force reduces the likelihood of new training (due to lower expectations of returns the smaller the remaining working life), and thus consequent gains in attainment.

According to vacancy chain theory, a similar time dependency related to labor force experience should be observed, but for very different reasons. For a given level of educational resources, opportunities for better jobs decline as the level of attainment already achieved increases. This reflects a decreasing gap between actual and expected rewards, and not an increase in personal ability. In addition, careers develop according to general trend-like shifts in the composition of the occupational structure and according to cyclical changes of the economy that affect the labor demand.

These considerations generate 10 time scales where 7 time scales are entered into the analyses simultaneously. The three dependent variables are defined as waiting time distributions: (a) duration until an upward job shift occurs, (b) duration until there is a lateral move, (c) duration until there is a downward job shift.

The independent variables constitute 7 interrelated time scales: (d) time in the labor force, (e) education as time varying covariate measured at beginning of given job spell, (f) relative social status of given job, (g) level of economic development at time of entry into the labor force, (h) labor market conditions at time of entry into the labor force, (i) level of general economic and social development at time *t*, (j) labor market conditions at time *t*.

All individual attributes have been measured on a monthly basis within the survey. The statistics on variables *g* to *j* are based on quarter-year time series of 17 socioeconomic indicators that were transformed into two constructs by factor analysis.

The model estimated can be written as

$$r(t/\mathbf{X}(t); \tau_i, i = 1, \ldots, n) = \exp(\beta'\mathbf{X}(t)) \cdot \sum_{i=1}^{n} f_i(\tau_i)$$

where $\mathbf{X}(t)$ is the vector of the time-dependent exogenous variables, and τ_i are duration times on the different time scales, such as time in the labor force, time in the actual job, and so forth. The number of time scales included in the model is represented by *n*. An identification problem does not arise, because the measures on cohort and period conditions are not taken from the survey data set but from external sources. But even if they would have to be taken from the survey data, the identification problem could be avoided, because duration in labor force is not identical with age, and the equation $A = P - C$ does not hold. This is also true for entry into the labor force, which defines cohort independently of year of birth (see Figure 12.2a–c).

The empirical results show strong independent effects of career duration, cohort as historical time of entry into the labor force, and actual historical time at any month of employment (see Figures 12.3 and 12.4). Moreover, it is clearly shown that career opportunities depend only in part on purely individual attributes, even if those are taken as dynamic variables changing over time.

Some methodological strategies and practical issues of life course studies as event histories

Strategies for the construction of a data base

Information on life courses of single individuals should be collected in retrospective or prospective surveys on cohort-specific representative samples. Data may be collected by interviewers using questionnaires in the field or computer-assisted telephone interviews. Both methods are costly in time and money and impose severe constraints on the sample size. For cohort analysis, however, one needs stable esti-

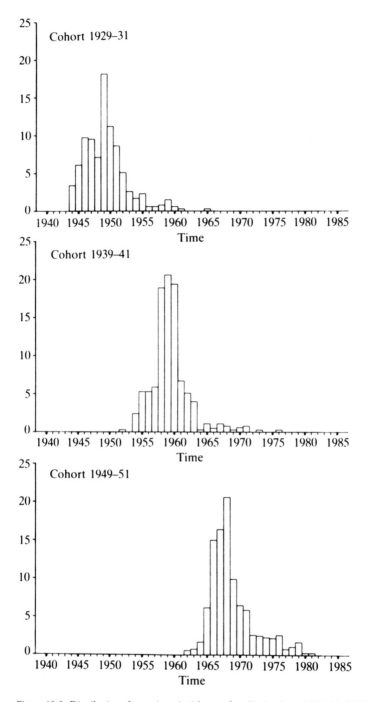

Figure 12.2. Distribution of entry into the labor market (Birth cohorts 1929–31, 1939–41, 1949–51). Source: Blossfeld (1986).

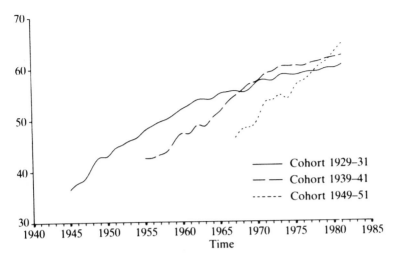

Figure 12.3. Development of prestige scores for men in historical time (Birth cohorts 1929–31, 1939–41, 1949–51)
Source: Blossfeld (1986).

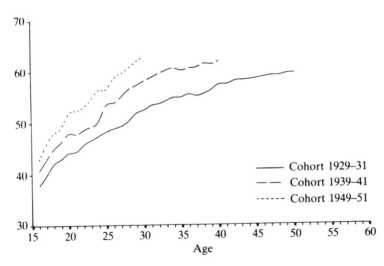

Figure 12.4. Development of prestige scores for men over the life course (Birth cohorts 1929–31, 1939–41, 1949–51)
Source: Blossfeld (1986).

mates of structural parameters in each cohort to be able to compare between cohorts or to conduct intracohort analysis, such as event history modeling.

Several decisions must be made before data collection: Which type of cohorts should be included? How many cohorts should be included? How large should be the size of cohort-specific subsamples? The latter problem is important due to the constraint of overall sample size. As a consequence one will usually be able to include only a few cohorts. In contrast to classical cohort analysis, based on demographic data, a continuous succession of cohorts will rarely be available. There is then an unavoidable tradeoff between the number of cohorts and the degree of richness of intracohort, life-course data. However, effects of cohort membership as such or other indicators of it could be tested in a parametric model (such as the one proposed above) even without a cohort-specific stratified sample. We do think, however, that by abandoning the opportunity of powerful intracohort life course analysis one also forgoes the advantages of an effective analysis of the interactions of individual and historical processes.

Therefore, the selection of specific cohorts becomes a strategic and far-reaching decision. Methods of classical cohort analysis are well suited for that purpose. In the case of the German Life History Study, data on single-year cohorts from the 1% micro-census of 1971 formed the selection base. The 1929–1931 cohort was chosen because – as we have shown above – it occupies an extremely disadvantaged position, and the cohort 1939–1941 was chosen because it comprised the birth cohorts largest in absolute size. As another illustration, one could study period and cohort effects on the change of age-specific birth rates on the basis of data of the official statistics. Our own research experience shows that on that basis both cohort- and period-specific turning points in the trends concerning age patterns and levels of birth rates can be detected. This might be supplemented by an analysis of marriage rates, marriage duration–specific birth rates, age-specific rates of illegitimate births, employment rates, and so forth. Based on such kinds of results and a theoretical background, cohorts can be selected that play a key role in, for example, the process of changes in family formation. One only has to be aware of the fact that the information derives from aggregated data.

As a consequence, effects of changing group composition might remain undetected for two reasons. First, one may have no information about changes of the population in the composition of the critical sociostructural variable. Second, precise information about the relevance of this sociostructural attribute for the studied phenomena may be lacking, because cohort analyses cannot be applied separately for different subgroups. In many cases this would be possibly only on the basis of continuous event history data.

Conventional cohort analysis can also be employed in an inductive manner to form reasonable clusters of adjacent cohorts of single-birth years to reduce sampling costs.

Retrospective data and recall error

Within the field of psychology of memory there is a large literature on biases and errors of recall. The conclusions drawn from studies on the recall differences between "episodic" and "semantic" memory would suggest that retrospective life history data should not be used for collecting event histories.

Retrospective data do not suffer from the more serious problems of panel data, such as mortality and changing measurement conditions (Featherman, 1979). However, they are potentially subject to errors of recall, and for this reason, in the German Life History Study (GLHS) special precautions were taken to ensure the quality of the data. Prior to data collection at the national level, a pilot study was conducted in 1979 to compare retrospective data with data on residential, familial, and occupational changes collected 10 years earlier from the same individuals (Tölke, 1989; Papastefanou, 1980). The findings corroborated the feasibility of retrospective questions on objective life events and trajectories, given appropriate instruments. These findings were used to develop interview schedules and field procedures that generated the most accurate responses. After the national data were collected, the life history protocols were checked thoroughly. Over 4,000 working hours (and as much money as for actual interviewing) were spent reviewing the internal consistency of the interview information and soliciting initially missing data. In this task, about 15% of the respondents were contacted again by phone or letter.

Our confidence in the quality of our own retrospective data from the GLHS on objective life events such as job change, marriage, and migration is based on a fairly large and systematic amount of circumstantial evidence: statistical comparison of the GLHS-data with comparable data drawn from the 1971 and 1982 micro-census (Blossfeld, 1987), census data on fertility (Tuma & Huinink, 1989), official data on cohort-specific marriages (Papastefanou, 1987), methodological studies of our migration data (Wagner, 1989), comparisons of job-shift and class-shift processes (Mayer & Carroll, 1987), and cross-national comparisons of German and Norwegian life history data (Mayer, Featherman, Selbee, & Colbjørnsen, 1989).

Different strategies of testing for the quality of the retrospective data were applied. Blossfeld assessed the representativeness of the GLHS data at the time of interview and retrospectively 10 years earlier, using the micro-census of 1982 and 1971. He concentrated on main sociostructural variables of the respondents, such as age (cohort), level of education, occupational position, and place of residence. The results provide a good fit of the sample distribution of these variables to those that people usually obtain from official statistics. Major differences concerning education and occupation are due to different definitions of categories. To assess the quality of retrospective data in particular, one can compare the goodness of fit obtained for 1982 and 1971. Again the results are very encouraging.

Huinink compared age-specific birth rates for the first, second, and third child, estimated from the GLHS data, to those from official statistics. The difference in the age-specific percentages of women with no or fewer than two, or three children never exceeds 4%. A similar good fit Papastefanou found for age-specific marriage rates. The congruence of age distributions of marriage or child birth (as for other life events), respectively, of survival and rate functions supports the quality of the retrospective information in a particular way.

Wagner discussed the quality of the retrospective data on migration. He analyzed the proportion of respondents who had been contacted to correct dates of their migration history because of inconsistent reports in the interview (correction rate). He found a percentage of identified incorrect reports larger than 20% when the move took place early in age. For migrations at ages older than 20 the correction rate is mainly near 10%. It did not differ substantially from cohort to cohort.

Given this evidence, we believe that the retrospective life history data can be at least as good – and is most likely better – than the conventional concurrent measurements in social science surveys. More important than the absolute measurement quality of the data, however, are questions of possible systematic recall error that might confound empirical findings (Jabine, Straf, Tanur, & Tourangeau, 1984). The most plausible hypotheses of this sort are (1) that events closer to the time of the interview will be better recalled, thus monotonically confounding recall with age or cohort, and (2) that episodes of longer duration will be remembered better than those of shorter duration, again causing interference with age or cohort variables. We cannot, in some instances on the basis of the available data, definitively rule out either hypothesis. On the other hand, it is shown by Tuma and Hannan that these kinds of biases have almost no effect on estimates of effects of covariates (Tuma & Hannan, 1984).

References

Baltes, P. B. (1968). Longitudinal and cross-sectional sequences in the study of age and generation effects. *Human Development, 11*(3), 145–171.
Baltes, P. B., Cornelius, S. W., & Nesselroade, J. R. (1979). Cohort effects in developmental psychology. In J. R. Nesselroade & P. B. Baltes (Eds.), *Longitudinal research in the study of behavior and development* (pp. 61–87). New York: Academic Press.
Beck, P. A. (1976). A socialization theory of partisan realignment. In R. G. Niemi & H. F. Weisberg (Eds.), *Controversies in American voting behavior.* San Francisco: Freeman.
Blossfeld, H.-P. (1986). Career opportunities in the Federal Republic of Germany: A dynamic approach to the study of life-course, cohort, and period effects. *European Sociological Review, 2,* 208–225.
Blossfeld, H.-P. (1987). Zur Repräsentativität der Sfb-3-Lebensverlaufsstudie: Ein Vergleich mit Daten aus der amtlichen Statistik. *Allgemeines Statistisches Archiv, 71,* 126–144.
Eisenstadt, S. N. (1956). *From generation to generation.* New York: Free Press of Glencoe.
Featherman, D. L. (1979). Retrospective longitudinal research: Methodological considerations. *Journal of Economics and Business, 32*(1), 152–169.
Featherman, D. L. (1985). Individual development and aging as a population process. In J. R. Nesselroade & A. von Eye (Eds.), *Individual development and social change: Explanatory analysis* (pp. 213–241). New York: Academic Press.
Fienberg, S. E., & Mason, W. M. (1979). Identification and estimation of age-period-cohort models in the analysis of discrete archival data. *Sociological Methodology, 10* 1–67.
Grossmann, K. E., & Grossmann, K. (1986). Phylogenetische und ontogenetische Aspekte der Entwicklung der Eltern-Kind-Bindung und der kindlichen Sachkompetenz. *Zeitschrift für Entwicklungspsychologie und Pädagogische Psychologie 18,* 287–313.
Huinink, J. (1988). Methoden der explorativen Kohortenanalyse. In *Zeitschrift für Bevölkerungswissenschaft, 14,* 69–87.
Huinink, J. (1989). Kohortenanalyse der Geburtenentwicklung in der Bundesrepublik

Deutschland. In A. Herlth & K. P. Strohmeier. *Lebenslauf und Familienentwicklung.* Leverkusen: Leske und Budrich.

Jabine, T. B., Straf, M. L., Tanur, J. M., & Tourangeau, R. (Eds.). (1984). *Cognitive aspects of survey methodology: Building a bridge between disciplines.* Washington, DC: National Academy Press.

Jagodzinski, W. (1984). Identification of parameters in cohort models. *Sociological Methods and Research, 12*(4), 375–398.

Jennings, M. K., & Niemi, R. G. (1981). *Generations and politics: A panel study of young adults and their parents.* Princeton: Princeton Press.

Kupper, L. L., Janis, J. M., Salama, I. A., Yoshizawa, C. N., & Greenberg, B. G. (1983). Age-period-cohort analysis: An illustration of the problems in assessing interaction in one observation per cell data. *Communications in Statistics, 12,* 2779–2807.

Linton, R. (1939). A neglected aspect of social organization. *American Journal of Sociology, 45* 870–886.

Mannheim, K. (1952). The Sociological Problem of Generations. In P. Kecskemeti (Ed.), *Essays on the sociology of knowledge* (pp. 276–322). New York: Routledge and Paul.

Mason, K. O., Mason, W. M., Winsborough, H. H., & Poole, W. K. (1973). Some methodological issues in cohort analysis of archival data. *American Sociological Review, 38,* 242–258.

Mason, W. M., & Fienberg, S. E. (Eds.). (1985). *Cohort analysis in social research: Beyond the identification problem.* New York: Springer.

Mayer, K. U. (1977). *Recent developments in the opportunity structure of (West)German society 1935–1971* (SPES-Arbeitspapier Nr. 67). Mannheim/Frankfurt: Sozialpolitische Arbeitsgruppe.

Mayer, K. U. (1986). Structural constraints on the life course. *Human Development, 29,* 163–170.

Mayer, K. U. (1988). German survivors of World War II: The impact on the life course of the collective experience of birth cohorts. In M. W. Riley (Ed.), *Social structures and human lives. Social change and the life course* (pp. 229–246). Newbury Park et al.: Sage.

Mayer, K. U., & Carroll, G. R. (1987). Jobs and classes: Structural constraints on career mobility. *European Sociological Review, 3,* 14–38.

Mayer, K. U., Featherman, D. L., Selbee, L. K. & Colbjørnsen, T. (1989). Class mobility during the working life: A comparison of Germany and Norway. In M. L. Kohn (Ed.), *cross-national research in sociology* (pp. 218–239). Newbury Park et al.: Sage.

Mayer, K. U., & Müller, W. (1985). The state and the structure of the life course. In A. B. Sørensen, F. E. Weinert, & L. Sherrod (Eds.), *Human development and the life course.* Hillsdale, NJ: Erlbaum.

Müller, W. (1978). Der Lebenslauf von Geburtskohorten. In M. Kohli (Ed.), *Lebensverlauf und Biographie.* Neuwied: Luchterhand.

Nesselroade, J. R., & Baltes, P. B. (1984). Sequential strategies and the role of cohort effects in behavioral development: Adolescent personality (1970–72) as a sample case. In S. A. Mednick, M. Harway, & K. M. Finello (Eds.), *Handbook of longitudinal research* (Vol. 1, pp. 55–87). New York: Praeger.

Palmore, E. (1978). When can age, period, and cohort be separated? *Social Forces, 57,* 282–295.

Papastefanou, G. (1980). *Zur Güte von retrospektiven Daten: Eine Anwendung gedächtnis-psychologischer Theorie und Ergebnisse einer Nachbefragung* (Sfb 3-Arbeitspapier Nr. 29). Frankfurt/Mannheim: Sonderforschungsbereich 3.

Papastefanou, G. (1987). Gender differences in family formation: Modelling the life course specificity of social differentiation. In K. U. Mayer & N. B. Tuma (Eds.), *Applications of event history analysis in life course research* (Materialien aus der Bildungsforschung Nr. 30) (pp. 327–403). Berlin: Max-Planck-Institut für Bildungsforschung.

Pullum, T. W. (1980). Separating age, period, and cohort effects in white U.S. fertility, 1920–1970. *Social Science Research, 9,* 225–244.

Riley, M. W., Johnson, M., & Foner, A. (1972). *Aging and society. III: A sociology of age stratification.* New York: Sage.

Rodgers, W. L. (1982). Estimable functions of age, period, and cohort effects. *American Sociological Review, 47,* (774–787).

Ryder, N. B. (1965). The cohort as a concept in the study of social change. *American Sociological Review, 30,* 843–861.

Schaie, K. W. (1965). A general model for the study of developmental problems. *Psychological Bulletin, 64*(2), 92–107.

Schaie, K. W. (1986). Beyond calendar definitions of age, time, and cohort: The general developmental model revisited. *Developmental Review, 6,* 252–277.

Schaie, K. W., & Baltes, P. B. (1975). On sequential strategies in developmental research: Description or explanation. *Human Development, 18,* 384–390.

Tölke, A. (1989). Möglichkeiten und Grenzen einer Edition bei retrospektiven Verlaufsdaten. In K. U. Mayer & E. Brückner (Eds.), *Lebensverläufe und Wohlfahrtsentwicklung.* (Materialien aus der Bildungsforschung Nr. 35) (pp. 173–225). Berlin: Max-Planck-Institut für Bildungsforschung.

Tuma, N. B., & Hannan, M. T. (1984). *Social dynamics: Models and methods.* Orlando: Academic Press.

Tuma, N. B. & Huinink, J. (1989). Postwar fertility patterns in the Federal Republic of Germany. In K. U. Mayer & N. B. Tuma (Eds.), *Event histories in life course research.* Madison, WI: University of Wisconsin Press (in print).

Wagner, M. (1989). *Räumliche Mobilität im Lebensverlauf.* Stuttgart: Enke.

13 New possibilities for longitudinal studies of intergenerational factors in child health and development

JOHN FOX AND KEN FOGELMAN

Introduction

Background

Primary prevention of psychosocial disorders has derived much from studies of continuities over the span of human development and of behavioral variation (Mednick & Baert, 1981). As well as focusing on the processes underlying developmental stabilities or transitions, the new field of developmental psychopathology is concerned with questions about individual differences and about heterogeneity in the developmental process and in behavioral outcomes (Rutter & Garmezy, 1983). Longitudinal studies have contributed to this field, because they can provide increased precision in timing and measurement, heterogeneity of outcome, timing by age of onset, observation of intraindividual change, and potential for analyzing causal chains (Rutter, 1987). Recent interest in how health and development are affected by the family, school, and locality in which children are brought up (Rutter, 1985; Maughan, 1987) has been accompanied by the development of new statistical methods for handling data at different levels of aggregation (Aitken & Longford, 1986; Goldstein, 1987). Each of these contemporary developments suggests that the time is ripe for the collection of data that will allow us to investigate simultaneously the influences of inter- and intragenerational, individual, and aggregate factors.

The National Child Development Study (NCDS) is one of three major British birth cohort studies. It covers approximately 17,000 children born in one week in March 1958. In addition to information about the cohort, it has collected a limited range of characteristics of the cohort's parents, the schools the cohort attended, and the neighborhoods they lived in.

We now see an opportunity to use the experiences of the past few decades to strengthen NCDS. This takes up and extends suggestions from Gruenberg and Le Resche (1981), who commented:

The next follow-up wave of the survey should enrich the data base along a whole new dimension by providing information on the children of the original cohort. These possibilities make the National Child Development Study an invaluable resource for medicine and social science.

Here we describe how we plan to include others in the cohort members' families, to build on the wide use that is currently being made of data collected over a period of more than 20 years, and to make full use of the interdisciplinary strengths of those researchers who will be most involved in the analysis of further data collected in the study.

Although Mednick and Baert (1981) describe a large number of longitudinal studies in different countries, the possibilities for direct international comparisons have been limited. There is much to be gained when planning data collection from a review of similar studies in other countries. In the case of NCDS, this review has given us ideas about topics to cover and has highlighted similarities between our study and others, particularly two longitudinal surveys being conducted by the National Opinion Research Center (NORC) at Chicago University in the United States. These are the National Longitudinal Survey of Youth (NLS/Y) and the National Educational Longitudinal Survey (NELS). NORC has already collected information on the children of the female members of the NLS/Y cohort. Consequently, we decided to incorporate ideas about comparative analysis between longitudinal studies on parents and children into our plans.

In the first part of this chapter we describe NCDS and our objectives for the future of this study. We then outline the design that we believe will best meet those objectives. Finally, we illustrate how the broader scope of the study may lead to a greater understanding of intergenerational antecedents and consequences of problems in child health and development.

National Child Development Study

Blaxter (1986) describes in some detail the range of British longitudinal studies, the type and sources of information they contain, and the main uses that have been made of them. The National Child Development Study (NCDS) began as a perinatal mortality survey designed to examine social and obstetric factors associated with early death or abnormality among the 17,000 children born in England, Scotland, and Wales in the week of March 3–9, 1958. The National Children's Bureau subsequently collected information about the children, their families, and their environment in 1965 when the subjects were seven, in 1969 when they were 11, in 1974 when they were 16, and in 1981 when they were 23. These phases are referred to as NCDS1, NCDS2, NCDS3, and NCDS4. From NCDS1–3 the birth cohort was augmented with immigrant children born in the sampling week. In addition, details of public examination entry and performance were obtained from schools, sixth-form colleges, and colleges of further education in 1978.

Figure 13.1 summarizes the timing of these phases and indicates how in each phase information was obtained from a variety of sources. In the initial birth survey, data were obtained from the mother and from the midwife's medical records. In the first three follow-up surveys, data were gathered from parents by health visitors, from head teachers and class teachers by questionnaire, from medical examinations

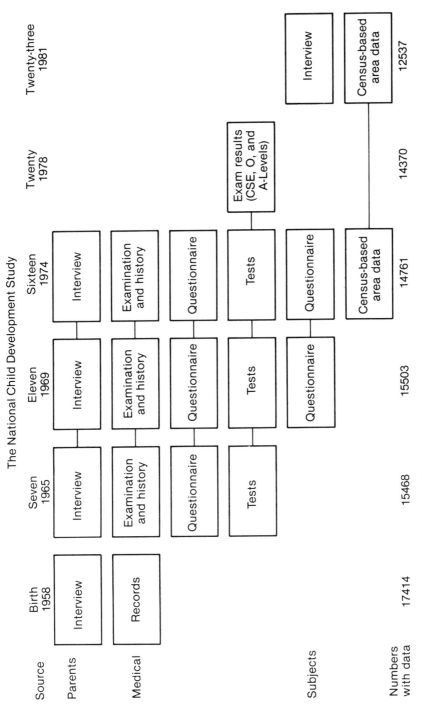

The National Child Development Study

Source	Birth 1958	Seven 1965	Eleven 1969	Sixteen 1974	Twenty 1978	Twenty-three 1981
Parents	Interview	Interview	Interview	Interview		Interview
Medical	Records	Examination and history	Examination and history	Examination and history		
		Questionnaire	Questionnaire	Questionnaire		
		Tests	Tests	Tests	Exam results (CSE, O, and A-Levels)	
			Questionnaire	Questionnaire		
				Census-based area data		Census-based area data
Subjects						
Numbers with data	17414	15468	15503	14761	14370	12537

Figure 13.1. NCDS1–4 timing of surveys, sources of information, and responses.

235

carried out by the school health service, and from tests of ability and questionnaires completed by the subjects themselves. In NCDS4, data were obtained from the subjects themselves by professional survey research interviewers, and the data were supplemented by small area statistics based on the 1971 and 1981 national censuses.

The study is best known for work on child health and development (Davie, Butler, & Goldstein, 1972; Fogelman, 1983). It has also given rise to a number of books and articles dealing with subgroups, such as adopted children (Seglow, Pringle, & Wedge, 1972), children in one-parent families (Ferri, 1976), and children from disadvantaged backgrounds (Wedge & Essen, 1982).

About 12,500 cohort members were successfully traced at age 23 and interviewed about many aspects of their lives, including family formation and dissolution; employment history, earnings, and experiences; postschool education, training, and apprenticeships; housing history; and health.

High response rates were achieved in each phase (Figure 13.1). Attrition arises from death, emigration, and failure to trace, as well as refusal. The decline in numbers interviewed in 1981 mainly reflects difficulties in tracing members of the cohort after they had left compulsory schooling. The majority of the cohort had not yet settled down by age 23 but would be expected to have done so by 1989/90 when we plan next to interview them. Since 1981, contact has been maintained with the sample by sending them a birthday card each year to let them know what is happening to the study and what research is being undertaken, and to ask them one or two questions, including their new addresses if they have changed.

Analysis of nonresponse to the main stages indicates only small biases overall, though with some tendency for disadvantaged children to be underrepresented. The one more important bias is an underrepresentation of ethnic minority children. Repetition of some of the analyses of data collected in the earlier phases of the study suggests that the relationships found are, however, reasonably robust to nonresponse bias (see Appendix in Fogelman, 1983).

NCDS5

Objectives for NCDS5

When we started to plan the next phase, we decided to build on the unique information that has been collected in NCDS in the following ways:

1. To enhance it as a national longitudinal data set for studying changes in health, socioeconomic, and demographic circumstances, and their interrelationships within and between generations;
2. To increase the use of the data set, including the collection of new ad hoc specialized data, in the detailed study of particular subgroups of the cohort;
3. To develop further the accessibility of these data to the research community and also to administrators and policymakers; and
4. To facilitate and encourage more wide-ranging and systematic comparisons between the three British birth cohort studies.

There is increasing emphasis on childhood and early adult experiences in studies of health and socioeconomic circumstances in middle and old age (Marmot, Shipley, & Rose, 1984; Barker, Osmond, Golding, Kuhn, & Wadsworth, 1987; and Medical Research Council, 1987). From the outset we insisted that researchers, advising us about what information to collect, recognize the value of investing in information that will be useful in the medium and longer term, even at the expense of information that, although highly topical, is likely to become dated and irrelevant as the cohort ages.

The first objective is central to the topic of this paper, because it indicates the importance of design as a way of increasing the usefulness of the study to those wishing to address a variety of different questions. We hoped to emphasize the need to build upon issues already addressed by the study that would be better understood if we had more data on "change," both in circumstances and in status. We also wished to point to many questions that in recent years had been asked about intergenerational continuities and discontinuities (Rutter & Madge, 1976; Brown & Madge, 1982; Blaxter & Paterson, 1982; Atkinson, Maynard, & Trinder, 1983; Rutter, 1985).

The limitations of a large study such as NCDS are to be found when one wants to consider particular aspects of people's lives and circumstances in more depth, and to observe changes over a shorter time period. However, NCDS can be used to identify reasonable numbers of people with particular characteristics, and, as in earlier phases, these people can be the subject of more intensive investigation. Similarly, we felt that our work to encourage new users of the data set had identified clear demand for the sort of data we were able to offer, and we felt that demand would grow as more and more people began to appreciate the strengths of the study.

The final objective has since been extended to incorporate a wish to compare *between countries* for the same generation. When we first started to think about the next phase, we thought this was highly unlikely, if not impossible, and we wished to encourage comparisons drawing on the two other British birth cohort studies. However, discussions we have been having with NORC have indicated that two studies for which they are responsible offer considerable potential for comparative work and complementary analysis. NORC and the NCDS User Support Group are considering how to maximize collaboration, but recognize that each study will need to maintain its own integrity and to achieve its own objectives.

NCDS5 and the research community

The NCDS User Support Group established by City University with initial support from the Economic and Social Research Council has in the past few years established a wide network of users and potential users of data collected in NCDS1–4. There are more than 50 projects currently based on NCDS data in institutions in the United Kingdom and the United States. These include projects looking at postschool education and training; at transition in young adulthood; at health education and social mobility among young adults; at depression among young adults; at factors influencing alcohol consumption among young adults; and at respiratory disease among young adults.

Regular contact is maintained with researchers so that we can find out what they are discovering from the study and tell others about the work that is going on. Two mechanisms publicize work using NCDS. These are NCDS Working Papers, which are prepublication draft reports, and NCDS NEWS, a newletter that contains brief descriptions of work in progress and lists recent publications based on the study.

This network has provided an important strength in the development of ideas for the next round. It meant that there was a sizeable group of researchers with different disciplinary perspectives – many international experts in their own fields, yet all with a common interest in the cohort and its development through early adult life.

Themes for NCDS5

It was natural that we would seek to collect further information about family and social networks; occupation and income dynamics; housing and environment; health continuities; mental health; health behavior, beliefs, and education; reproductive performance; and child rearing, health, and education. These areas all build upon information already collected in the study to age 23.

Parenting is just one theme that crosses most of these different areas and that emphasizes our interest in relationships between the three generations covered by our study. In order to coordinate the interests of potential users of NCDS we have established a network of collaborators and group coordinators (Table 13.1). Collaborators have interests in individual projects, and group coordinators represent those interests at meetings where we make the main decisions about the design and balance of the next round. The extent to which the areas are interrelated is clear from the number of people who are involved in the development of more than one aspect of the study.

Group coordinators also help us keep collaborators informed about progress in their areas and will help us coordinate the main applications for funding. Although our central focus is parenting, applications will highlight a number of "problems" that the new data will be used to address. These will include the antecedents and consequences of teenage pregnancy, illegitimacy, and divorce; adult sequelae of serious educational difficulties in childhood; intergenerational continuities and discontinuities in child health and development; intergenerational factors in reproductive performance; influences of characteristics and experiences of cohort members in childhood on the mental health of their children; and continuities and discontinuities between child and adult psychopatholoogy.

NCDS5 design

In 1981, when the cohort was last contacted, information was obtained in the main from a single interview with cohort members. This was supplemented with informa-

Table 13.1. *NCDS5 network of researchers.*

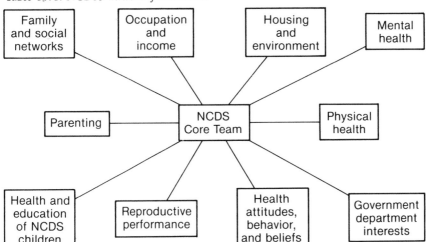

Theme	Coordinator	Institution
Overall planning	Bynner and Fox	City University
Family and social networks	Kiernan	City University
Parenting and U.S.A. interests	Michael/Willis	NORC, Chicago
Occupation and income	Dalton	Bristol University
Housing and environment	Holmans	Dept. of Environ.
Reproductive performance	Alberman	London Hospital
Child health and education	Fogelman	City University
Mental health	Rutter	Inst. Psychiatry
Physical health	Joffe	St. Mary's, London
Health attitudes, behavior, and beliefs	Calnan	Kent University
Government department interests	Marsh	City University
NCDS User Support Group	Shepherd	City University

tion about the locality in which they lived based on small area statistics from the two most recent national censuses. If we are to obtain the information necessary to address the wide range of issues highlighted above, we will need to use a more diverse strategy to data collection, more along the lines of earlier contacts with the sample in which other people, such as parents and teachers, were also contacted. Our current plans include two main interview surveys and a series of self-completion tests and questionnaires (Table 13.2).

In the first interview, which is expected to last for up to two hours, we expect to collect from the cohort member information about family and household formation; labor market histories; housing and migration histories; physical and mental health; use of health and social services; health beliefs and attitudes; and parents' health, well-being, and whereabouts. We may also interview the cohort member's current partner about his or her social and family background, physical and mental health,

Table 13.2. *Elements and content of NCDS5.*

Survey	Element	Respondent	Content	Average time needed	Approx. sample size
Preliminary	Self-completion	Cohort member & any part-ner	Economic history Marital history Family history Housing history		16,000
Main	Interview	Cohort member	Family & household forma-tion Labor market histories Housing & migration histo-ries Physical & mental health Use of health & social services Health beliefs & attitudes Parents' health, well-being, & whereabouts	90	16,000
	Measure 1	Cohort member	Height	15	16,000
	Measure 2	Cohort member	Weight	15	16,000
	Interview	Partner	Social and family background Occupation and income Health	30	10,000
	Measure 1	Partner	Height	15	10,000
	Measure 2	Partner	Weight	15	10,000
Supplementary	Interview	Mothers	Reproductive histories Health & development of their children (including Rutter A scale) Attitudes & child care behav-ior (including use of ser-vices)	30	10,000[a]
	Test 1	Children	Intellectual & language devel-opment		
	Test 2	Children	Mathematical ability		
	Test 3	Children	Reading ability	60	17,000[b]
	Test 4	Children	Health & physical develop-ment		
	Test 5	Children	Temperament Scale (if < 8 years)? SAICA (if 8–16 years)		
	Postal	Teachers	School Child		17,000

Table 13.2. *(cont.)*

Survey	Element	Respondent	Content	Average time needed	Approx. sample size
Emigrants	Postal	Cohort members living ex-G.B.	Economic history Marital history Family history Housing history Health history		400

[a]10K–c6K female cohort members & c4K female partners
[b]Tests will be age specific.

and educational abilities and achievements. We will probably also need to obtain similar information for parents of cohort members' children who are no longer living with the cohort member.

In the second interview, lasting about 90 minutes and conducted two or three weeks after the first, we would interview mothers and all the children of the cohort members. Mothers would be asked about their reproductive histories; about the health and development of their children; about their attitudes and child care behavior; and about schooling and use of services. The children would be tested for intellectual and language development; mathematical and reading ability; and health and physical development.

The proposed design is ambitious, and we will need to mount field tests to convince ourselves that it is practicable. To a limited extent we will build on the experiences of the NORC studies. We are now starting to investigate how best to collect the information we require and how to cope with competition for limited interview time. As in earlier rounds, we will want to assess the quality of information collected by building in checks for consistency within the interview, with information collected earlier, and where possible with other records.

Studies in child health and development

Studying the third generation

By 1989 the NCDS cohort will have had approximately 17,000 children. Although at this stage we are only planning the first contact with these children, it is clear that to achieve many of our objectives we will need to observe their health and development longitudinally. NORC is contacting the children of female members of the NLS/Y cohort at three-year intervals.

NCDS and similar longitudinal studies based on representative samples of children have shed light on the influences on the health and development of children of a broad range of experiences and characteristics of parents *during the period of parenthood* and on the sequelae in the early adult experiences of the cohort member. While extending our observations on the careers and experiences of this particular cohort into their early thirties, we wish to add into NCDS information on the children, partners, and parents of the original NCDS cohort in order to open up three new dimensions: first, and most important, to study relationships between the *childhood* experiences, characteristics, and behavior of the cohort and those of their children; second, to investigate in more detail than previously the influence of experiences and characteristics of the parents in *early adulthood before the child was born;* and third, to observe the influences of both these and current circumstances on the development of *more than one child in the same family.* It will also be possible to identify period effects by comparing the relationships found for the children of the cohort with those found a generation earlier when the cohort were children. However, this must be seen as a by-product rather than an objective of the new design. We amplify on the potential gains in the next five sections. These sections refer to outlines of topics of interest given in Fox and Fogelman (1987). These topics include changes in family situation and their effects on children; parenting – fathering; school choice; continuities and discontinuities in material disadvantage; poverty, unemployment, and child health; intergenerational continuities in health; development delay; parental depression; and deviant behavior.

Contemporary circumstances

In the three British birth cohort studies, at each contact during childhood the cohort member provided the primary focus of questioning and testing. Information about the child's contemporary home environment was obtained from his or her parents, but questions were generally directed around the child, and when questions were asked about the parents they tended to be limited in scope and depth. NCDS, for example, collected factual information about educational background, socioeconomic circumstances, and family history of the cohort members' parents, and supplemented this with limited information about their parenting behavior and their aspirations and expectations for the child's future education and employment.

We expect the descriptions of the circumstances in which the children of the cohort members are being brought up to be substantially richer than those of the NCDS cohort member's childhood. Because the NCDS cohort member will continue to be the principal focus of the investigation, the next round should provide a more detailed and accurate account of factors that have previously been found important in child-development studies. At the same time the emphasis on the cohort member's own situation should enable us to investigate the influences of new factors that have not previously been included in a systematic way in nationally representative longitudinal studies. The information we are seeking on the cohort members and their partner's own lives and their physical and mental health as well as about their children's health and development illustrates the ways in which we hope to strengthen our description of the home environment. In this way we hope to provide a clearer view of the situations in which children thrive and those that increase the risk of problems.

There are a number of questions that can only be addressed if better data are collected on the contemporary circumstances in which children are brought up. For example, Fox and Fogelman suggest how this type of data could be used to investigate the role of parental depression in children's behavior problems and early cognitive and language problems associated with family breakdown, single parenthood, and unemployment, and how it would contribute to studies of developmental delay, deviant behavior, and school choice.

Intergenerational relationships between childhood experiences, characteristics, and development

The main reason for wanting to test and examine the children of the cohort is the potential NCDS would then offer for addressing questions about intergenerational relationships between childhood experiences, characteristics, and development in a population sample. There are three main types of issues of interest: continuities and discontinuities between generations; problems in children that are related to different problems in their parents' childhoods; and indirect consequences to children of their parents' childhoods.

Under the first heading we would include studies of, for example, growth, development delay, and particular medical conditions such as asthma, eczema, or epilepsy, in which the researcher was concerned with the extent to which problems are inherited from one generation to the next and the circumstances in which they are not.

Under the second heading we would include those studies that were attempting to identify a broader range of childhood characteristics or problems that may be inherited but whose origins may be apparent in different symptoms in the childhood of the parent. It will be of interest, for example, to see whether the children of those cohort members who had eczema as children were at increased risk of developing asthma or epilepsy.

The third heading is concerned with indirect relationships and their consequences for children. For example, how is the cohort members' parenting behavior related to their childhood relationships with their own parents, and what are the consequences for their children? Fox and Fogelman also highlight examples of questions on continuities and discontinuities in material disadvantage and on poverty, unemployment, and child health and development that would be included under this heading.

NCDS provides a promising base for such a series of studies of children, because substantial data have been systematically collected throughout the childhood and early adulthood of one of their parents (i.e., the cohort member). Also, much data were collected on one set of grandparents (i.e., the cohort member's parents) and on the relationships between those grandparents and the relevant parent during the parent's childhood.

For the intergenerational studies proposed in this section we need information on the second parent, his or her background, health, and development, and on the second set of grandparents. We will be able to make use of the fact that for a little over half the sample the second parent will be the father, and for a little under half it will be the mother. However, NCDS will be greatly strengthened if we are able to interview partners about the most important aspects of their background, childhood, and development, as well as about their parents, and to give them tests similar to those being given to the cohort member.

Early adult careers and successful parenting

Because the British birth cohort studies began their data collection around the time of the birth of the children, little information was collected about the early adult experiences and circumstances of the parents. The primary objective was to describe the contemporary circumstances and events during the life of the child.

NCDS already contains substantial detail about the early adult careers and experiences of the cohort to age 23, including information about partnership and family formation, further education, and entry to and experiences of the labor market. A study of the cohort's children would therefore be able to draw on this information. It would allow one to ask whether cohort members' transition to adulthood was predictive of successful parenting and to identify particular situations or experiences that were likely to lead to problems.

At the same time it would enable us to investigate further variables, such as the age of each parent, that are found to be so important in child-development studies.

Data on early adult careers would be of interest in projects on change in family situation and its effect on children, on parenting, and on continuities and discontinuities in material disadvantage.

Within family differences in child development

Few studies have collected information systematically on siblings, and those that have have generally focused on twins (Loehlin & Nichols, 1976) or adopted children (Scarr, Webber, Weinberg, & Wittig, 1981). The proposed interviewing of all of the NCDS cohort's children is intended to allow us to look at within-family variation for a national population sample. We are interested in the extent to which problems cluster in families and in understanding how competition between siblings and the ways in which they support each other influence their development. An initial question concerns the significance of the sex composition of the family, the spacing between children, and their respective attainments.

Period comparisons

We are not putting forward a study of NCDS cohort members' children as equivalent to a new longitudinal study of a more recent generation of children. In 1989 our sample of children will vary in age from the newly born to teenagers. As children with a parent born in March 1958, those who are older will have young parents who will be more likely to have minimum education, to have manual rather than nonmanual occupations or to have no jobs, and who will have experienced a variety of problems during their childhood and early adulthood as compared with older parents of children of the same age. In contrast, children from more affluence and privileged sections of society will be overrepresented among the young children. The children would therefore not be representative of their age group. However, they are a sample of children growing up in the 1980s and 1990s, and as a result they will provide a basis for comparisons of findings with previous generations.

There have been many changes in family life over the past thirty years (Kiernan, 1988). We described earlier an interest in teenage pregnancy, illegitimacy, and divorce, each of which has been found to be of major importance in terms of the health and development of children. The frequency of and the responses to each have changed dramatically in recent years. Little is known, however, as to how the significance of each to children varies with changes in social mores. Comparisons of the significance of these factors between generations can shed useful light on the mechanisms underlying the relationships, albeit somewhat crudely. They can suggest whether the apparent consequences of these factors are intrinsic to the situation implied (e.g., a very young or a single parent) or more related to the behavior of people in particular situations (e.g., the way such parents cope with their children). The argument would be similar, for example, to those used by Rutter (1985) when asking whether relationships between divorce and conduct disorder reflect the loss of a partner or discord and conflict between partners.

A number of authors (Kiernan, 1987; Joshi, 1985; Golding, 1987) have been using data from the three cohort studies to make comparisons between successive generations. Although there are compelling arguments for mounting a new study based on a representative sample of children born in the late 1970s or early 1980s, the proposals put forward here would meet many of the requirements of such a study.

Conclusions

As with all longitudinal studies, the reasons for continuing NCDS and the primary focus of the study change as the cohort ages and passes through different life stages. The NCDS cohort of children born in one week in March 1958 has been followed in great detail through childhood and early adulthood. We now want to focus on the cohort as parents. In drawing up our plans for the next stages of data collection, we have tried to build upon the strong links the study has established with a growing community of users of the data we have already collected. We have also tried to ensure that we maximize the value of data that we have already collected. To do this we believe that we should collect more information about the cohort's immediate family, their partners, their children, and their parents. We have only now started to identify all the practical problems of such a design and have not yet secured the necessary funding. However, we believe that the arguments for such a strategy are very persuasive.

Appendix

Preliminary thoughts on projects on change in family situation and its effects on children

It is now widely recognized that family patterns are becoming more and more diverse (Kiernan, 1983, 1988). Teenage pregnancy is increasing and more often than previously is giving rise to a child who in the early period of his or her life at least is being brought up by the natural mother (Werner, 1986). More and more young people are cohabiting and are starting to have families outside marriage (Brown & Kiernan, 1981; Werner, 1982). Although the numbers eventually marrying remain high, breakdown of marriage through separation or divorce is on the increase, as is remarriage among those who are divorced (Kiernan, 1988; Haskey, 1983). There is therefore considerable interest in comparing the partner and family formation experiences of cohort members from different family backgrounds, in assessing whether differences can be explained by some of the known consequences of family backgrounds, and in asking how these changes might be affecting children.

Many studies have described the family circumstances of different cohorts of children and their effects on attainment and behavior during childhood, and on partnership and family formation during early adulthood. The principal references using NCDS can be found in Fogelman (1983) and Kiernan (1987).

By collecting information on cohort members' children, researchers would be able to investigate longer-term effects of these experiences on cohort members and their children. They would wish to ask whether and how they lead to "successful" or "unsuccessful" parenting. This would require an assessment of how far choices and experiences in early family careers were influenced by family backgrounds and experiences, how far they reflected consequences of low educational attainment and behavioral problems apparent during the childhood of the cohort member, and how far they reflected their, and their partners', achievements and difficulties during early adulthood.

Although much is known about the consequences of family problems, the change in pattern of family formation and dissolution calls into question many of the well-known consequences. Are the experiences of divorce, of being brought up in a single-parent family, or of step-families more or less traumatic for children now that these are more common experiences and more is known about the potential adverse consequences? How important is the socioeconomic climate in which these changes are taking place? Are people more or less likely to experience multiple problems? How do the responses of children depend on their ages at the time the family problems occur? What does this tell us about the "formative years," as referred to in the child-development literature? Such questions would be addressed by comparing the consequences to the children of the cohort who experienced these particular family situations between Great Britain and the United States, and contrasting them with the consequences to the cohort members who experienced similar situations a generation earlier.

Family size has always been a particularly important variable in explaining child health and development. The reasons for this will be better understood once we can examine whether such relationships are stable across generations and cultures, and once we can compare the development of different children within the same family. We need to consider how the frequency and type of problem associated with increased family size is related to the spacing of births and the position of the individual child in the family, and whether there are patterns of problems within families and how these relate to the circumstances and experiences of families. In addition to studying parent-child relationships, we will need to assess the ways in which children in the same family help and compete with each other.

References

Aitken, M., & Longford, N. (1986). Statistical modelling issues in school effectiveness studies. *Journal of Royal Statistical Society (A) 149*, 1–26.

Atkinson, A. B., Maynard, A. K., & Trinder, C. G. (1983). *parents and children: incomes in two generations*. London: Heinemann.

Barker, D. J. P., Osmond, C., Golding, J., Kuhn, D., & Wadsworth, M. E. J. (1989). Growth in utero, blood pressure in childhood and adult life, and mortality from cardiovascular disease. *British Medical Journal, 298*, 564–567.

Blaxter, M. (1986). Longitudinal studies in Britain relevant to inequalities in health. In R. Wilkinson (Ed.), *Class and health: Research and longitudinal data*. London: Tavistock.

Blaxter, M., & Paterson, E. (1982). *Mothers and daughters: A three-generational study of health attitudes and behaviour*. London: Heinemann.

Brown, A., & Kiernan, K. E. (1981). Cohabitation in Great Britain: Evidence from the General Household Survey. *Population Trends, 25*, 4–10.

Brown, M., & Madge, N. (1982). *Despite the welfare state*. London: Heinemann.

Davie, R., Butler, N., & Goldstein, H. (1972). *From birth to seven*. London: Longman.

Ferri, E. (1976). *Growing up in a one-parent family*. Windsor: NFER.

Fogelman, K. (1983). *Growing up in Great Britain: Collected papers from the National Child Development Study*. London: Macmillan.

Fox, A. J., & Fogelman, K. (1987). *New possibilities for longitudinal studies of intergenerational factors in child health and development*. NCDS Working Paper No. 26, Social Statistics Research Unit, City University, London.

Golding, J. (1987). *Plus ca change: Predictors of birthweight in two national birth surveys*. Paper presented to meeting of the British Society of Population Studies, June 26, 1987.

Goldstein, H. (1987). *Multi-level models in education and social research*. London: Griffin.

Gruenberg, E. M., & Le Resche, L. (1981). Reaction: The future of longitudinal studies. In S. A. Mednick & A. E. Baert (Eds.), *Prospective longitudinal research: An empirical basis for the primary prevention of psychosocial disorders* (pp. 319–325). Oxford: Oxford Medical Publications.

Haskey, J. (1983). Children of divorcing couples. *Population Trends, 31*, 20–26.

Joshi, H. (1985). Motherhood and employment: Change and continuity in post-war Britain. In British Society for Population Studies, *Measuring socio-demographic change*. OPCS Occasional Paper No. 34.

Kiernan, K. (1983). The structure of families today: Continuity or change? In British Society for Population Studies, *The family*. OPCS Occasional Paper No. 31.

Kiernan, K. (1987). Transitions on young adulthood. In J. N. Hobcraft & M. Murphy (Eds.), *Population research in Britain*. Oxford: Oxford University Press.

Kiernan, K. (1988). The British family: Contemporary trends and issues. *Journal of Family Issues, 9*(3), 298–316.

Loehlin, J. C., & Nichols, R. C. (1976). *Heredity, environment and personality: A study of 850 sets of twins*. Austin: University of Texas Press.

Marmot, M., Shipley, M. J., & Rose, G. (1984). Inequalities in death: Specific explanations of a general pattern. *Lancet*, 1003–1006.

Maughan, B. (1987). *School experiences as risk/protective factors*. To be published by European Science Foundation.

Medical Research Council. (1987). Childhood health and adult diseases. *MRC News*, Autumn 1987, 9–10.

Mednick, S. A., & Baert, A. E. (1981). Prospective longitudinal research: An empirical basis for the primary prevention of psychosocial disorders. Oxford: Oxford Medical Publications.

Rutter, M. (1985). Family and school influences oon behavioural development. *Journal of Child Psychology and Psychiatry, 26*, 349–368.

Rutter, M. (1987). *Longitudinal data in the study of causal processes: Some uses and some pitfalls*. To be published by European Science Foundation.

Rutter, M., & Garmezy, N. (1983). Developmental psychopathology. In E. M. Hetherington (Ed.), *Socialization, personality and social development* (Vol. 4 of *Handbook of child psychology*, 4th ed.), pp. 775–911. New York: Wiley.

Rutter, M., & Madge, N. 91976). *Cycles of disadvantage*. London: Heinemann.

Scarr, S., Webber, P. L., Weinberg, R. A., & Wittig, M. A. (1981). Personality resemblance among adolescents and their parents in biologically related and adoptive families. *Journal of Personality and Social Psychology, 40*, 885–898.

Seglow, J., Pringle, M. K., & Wedge, P. (1972). *Growing up adopted*. Windsor: NFER.

Wedge, P., & Essen, J. (1982). *Children in adversity* New York: Pantheon Books.

Werner, B. (1982). Recent trends in illegitimate birth and extra-marital conceptions. *Population Trends, 30*, 9–13.

Werner, B. (1986). Family building intentions of different generations of women: Results from the General Household Survey, 1979–1983. *Population Trends, 44*, 17–23.

14   Archiving longitudinal data

ANNE COLBY AND ERIN PHELPS

Advantages of sharing data

Sharing of research data is a critical part of the scientific method. Sharing data reinforces open scientific inquiry, allows for verification, refutation, and refinement of original findings, and ensures more efficient use of financial and other research resources. Although open access to all kinds of social and behavioral science data is important, sharing data from longitudinal studies is especially valuable. Because carrying out long-term longitudinal research requires such a major investment of time and money, only a few such studies are conducted. And yet, longitudinal data are necessary for addressing many research questions. The special value of longitudinal data is generally recognized as deriving from their unique ability to preserve information about the nature of individual development. Sequences of events and patterns of change that occur within the individual, the family, or some other unit can be studied most effectively through the use of longitudinal data. Alternative methods such as retrospective or cross-sectional studies are subject to serious error that can be reduced by using longitudinal designs. Clearly, research questions about lifelong and intergeneration causal relationships are best answered by following respondents in real time, rather than retrospectively.

Very long-term longitudinal data are difficult for researchers to collect during their own lifetimes, however. Few individual investigators are able to make the kind of time investment that is required and still meet their career goals. Consequently, there are only a relatively small number of investigators who are collecting longitudinal data at any given time. By making the data available and accessible to others, data sharing makes it possible for individuals to conduct longitudinal studies in a few years that would otherwise require a prohibitive time commitment.

There are several reasons that a researcher may want to analyze someone else's data. One is a desire to check on the accuracy of another's results, either by directly replicating the analyses or by using somewhat different analytic techniques that may, for example, statistically control for a confounding variable not accounted for in the original analyses. Lee, Brooks-Gunns, and Schnur (1988), for example, reanalyzed data on an early education intervention program in the United States called Head Start. Earlier reports on the effectiveness of this preschool program for economically disadvantaged children had not controlled for initial differences between Head Start and comparison groups. When these differences were taken into account, the Head Start children could be seen to have gained significantly more on the outcome measures than the comparison groups. The new analyses reverse previous findings, with important policy implications for the Head Start program. Sharing data for this kind of reanalysis is required by scientific conventions that promote objectivity in research.

Another reason for using existing data is to address original research questions without collecting new data. Often this involves analyzing data that were collected but never analyzed by the original investigators. The economics of doing research are improved in this case, both for the original investigator, because information is not wasted, and for the secondary analyst, because the costs of data collection are decreased or avoided.

Finally, and perhaps of most importance, a researcher may have questions that are very difficult to answer adequately without using existing data. These questions include the effects of social change or historical events on the lives of the people who experience them, the relations between very early development and outcomes in middle and late adulthood, and the early causal factors that explain the development of rare outcomes, such as alcoholism or extraordinary achievement in adulthood. Some examples may clarify the unique value of using archival longitudinal data for this kind of research.

Elder (1974) examined the effects of the economic Depression in the United States in the 1930s on the subjective situation and experiences of families and individuals, and the implications of drastic socioeconomic change for family and intergenerational relations. Archival data from the Oakland Growth and the Berkeley Guidance Studies (Institute of Human Development, University of California, Berkeley) were used to investigate the social and psychological effects of differential economic loss. For the Oakland subjects who were entering adolescence, Elder found that the transition into adolescence during the crisis was more punishing for girls than boys, especially in families that suffered greater economic loss. This disadvantage disappeared in adulthood, in that the experience of economic deprivation was not related to lower adult accomplishments or poorer health. However, different findings were obtained with the Berkeley cohort of subjects who were young children at the start of the Depression. In the younger Berkeley cohort, hardship clearly impaired the development and psychological functioning of boys, and this disadvantage persisted through adulthood. Elder attributes these cohort differences, in part, to the length of time spent in economic hardship and the length of time spent in dependence upon others during these hard times. Prior to this work, only historical and retrospective accounts had been used to describe the effects of this historical event on the lives of the people who lived through it.

A second example of the value of using existing archival data comes from Block (1971), who studied personality formation and change in subjects from early adolescence through their thirties, a period of almost 30 years. He also used data obtained from the Oakland Growth and the Berkeley Guidance Studies. Such an enterprise would take at least 35 years, if time spent designing the study, obtaining funding, and collecting and analyzing the data are included. This would require most of an investigator's career. By using archival data, the time required to carry out the project was reduced to 8 years. In this work, a major achievement was the creative way in which information in the subjects' files was transformed into personality data. Disparate and incomplete quantitative data had to be synthesized. Naturalistic, open-ended, and uncoded data needed to be incorporated to enrich the evaluations of the subjects. In order to do this, case assemblies were constructed for each subject. These included ratings and interviews by staff members, intelligence tests, Rorschach and Thematic Apperception Test protocols, teacher ratings and interviews, peer ratings, measures of attitudes and likes/dislikes, news clippings – in short, any available information about the subject as presented by him- or herself, by teachers, or by institute staff. This material was evaluated by 27 trained clinicians and rating according to the California Q-sort as a way of obtaining personality ratings. These ratings were then used to develop a personality typology that provided the basis for a study of personality development over time. Through the use of large amounts of data collected by other investigators, Block was able to make a major contribution to the study of personality in the book *Lives Through Time* without devoting his entire career to this one study.

Another example of a study that benefited greatly from the use of existing data is a 17-year follow-up of a sample of adolescent mothers (the Baltimore Longitudinal Study) conducted by Furstenberg, Brooks-Gunn, and Morgan (1987). The follow-up allowed the investigators to link the life choices of the mothers with the developmental trajectories of their children, who were adolescents themselves at the time of the follow-up. The investigators also compared their data with national sample survey data in order to assess the generalizability of their findings.

A third type of study that can benefit greatly by reanalyzing already-collected data is research that looks at the growth of individuals who develop pathologies, unusual talents, or other statistically rare characteristics. Vaillant (1983) reanalyzed data from 660 men that were gathered from adolescence into late mid-life in order to study the course of alcoholism over the life span. At the time of this work, most studies of alcoholism had been cross-sectional, and no study had followed alcoholics for more than five years. Yet, this disorder develops in otherwise normal individuals and changes over many years. Thus, a complete understanding requires information that is collected over such a time span. Further, in order to understand its development, alcoholism needs to be studied in a normal population, starting before the onset of the problem. Because, as is true of most medical research, only a relatively small percentage of the normal population will ever develop the disorder (3–10% in the case of alcoholism), a large initial sample is required to guarantee a sufficient sample of individuals who will eventually manifest the problem. Therefore, unless existing data were used, Vaillant would have had to collect data on 660 people for 40 years and then throw away at least 80% of it in order to carry out this project.

Obstacles to using existing data

Although it is fairly easy to make a case for the benefits of using others' data, the research literature in human development contains relatively few examples. Researchers in other fields are more likely to analyze and report on secondary data. For example, two American studies in the field of education (the National Longitudinal Study of the Class of 1972 [National Center for Education Statistics, 1972] and the High School and Beyond study [National Center for Education Statistics, 1980]) have provided a wealth of data for educational researchers and have been used to answer a wide variety of important theoretical and policy questions, such as the effects of different kinds of secondary school experiences on later life choices and achievement. Economists and sociologists have long had access to and used national survey data, such as the Panel Study of Income Dynamics (Duncan & Morgan, 1980) and the National Longitudinal Surveys (Parnes, 1983). The use of archival data in studies of human development is much less widespread and lacks the extensive history of secondary analysis in these other fields.

One factor in this reluctance to analyze existing data involves a perception that relevant data are not easily accessible. This is true to some extent. There are more computerized survey data available than the kinds of data that are likely to interest developmental researchers. However, data archives are more numerous than most researchers realize, and individual data sharing is becoming more common. Some archives house data from a few related studies, such as the Institute of Human Development at the University of California, Berkeley, which oversees data collection, organization, and analysis of information from the Berkeley and Oakland longitudinal studies. Other archives obtain data from a large number of individual investigators in order to make them available to other researchers. Representative of this group are ICPSR, the Inter-university Consortium for Political and Social Research at the University of Michigan, which provides computer data from hundreds of studies to consortium members, and the Henry A. Murray Research Center of Radcliffe College, which focuses on longitudinal or panel data and archives original records as well as machine-readable information.

Even with the increasing availability of others' data, a more important problem remains – that of finding the right kind of information. The original investigator may not have collected some information that the new analyst needs. Except through linking records from several sources or obtaining data retrospectively, there is little that can be done to remedy this situation. Just as likely as the omission of a variable is the categorization of it that makes it impossible to retrieve the original form. For example, one researcher might collect data in terms of broad age groups, whereas another might need subjects' exact age in years. This kind of impasse can be avoided in the future if investigators collect data in their most basic form and preserve the data in the form in which they were collected.

Perhaps the best solution to the problem of availability of the specific information that is needed is the preservation of original subject records. This allows the researcher to recode original interviews or projective test responses, audiotapes of interviews or group interactions, and videotapes of group interactions. Whereas some of these media raise difficult confidentiality issues, if they can be overcome the data become extremely valuable. They can then be recorded and reinterpreted by the secondary researcher in order to yield the information necessary for addressing his or her own research questions.

In addition, creative and innovative uses of data can be used to overcome deficiencies in the available data. As described earlier, Block's *Lives Through Time* provides an excellent model of synthesizing disparate data obtained from the Institute of Human Development (IHD) through the use of the Q-sort technique, in a way that allowed him to create uniform variables and perform the analyses of interest. Similarly, Elder (in press) worked extensively with the IHD archives, until he devised a method of constructing a life trajectory for each family. This radical restructuring of the data allowed him to investigate the interacting effects of history and family situation on family and individual development. As these examples show, original records can provide an unparalleled source of reusable data.

Another obstacle that may prevent more widespread use of secondary analysis is the perception that reanalyses involve simple recombinations of existing information and so are atheoretical and uncreative. Some secondary analyses fit this stereotype, and these studies contribute little. Exemplary reanalyses, such as those described here, are very creative and require that the researcher radically restructure the existing data according to the research questions they bring to the data.

This misperception, that secondary analysis involves a simple-minded recombination of variables, arises in part because researchers in human development are not provided training in the analysis of existing data. We would argue that training for pre- and postdoctoral students should include practice in conducting sophisticated reanalyses. Courses could be designed around the analysis of a major data set, especially one that includes original records. A course emphasizing in-depth analysis by students who are guided by a skilled researcher would certainly augment most graduate and postdoctoral programs.

High quality training in the use of archival data should help students in conducting both primary and secondary research later in their careers. A critical step in any research project is the development of a research question that is well grounded in theory and that is operationalized well. This is especially true for effective uses of archival data. Otherwise, the researcher is likely to become mired in the details of the data or to give the available data too much power in framing the questions. The studies cited as examples here all began with a research question, which in turn guided the search for data.

Because many graduate departments discourage secondary analyses for doctoral dissertations, the potential for experience in this area is further minimized. Clearly, students need to learn the skills of instrument selection or development and data collection, but these skills can be obtained through course work or participation in other research projects. Another aspect of the reluctance may be due to a belief that secondary analyses do not provide the students with experience in formulating their own research questions. As we have argued above, this belief derives from a misunderstanding of secondary analysis.

For established researchers, start-up costs (in time as well as money) and funding issues may be the greatest deterrent to ambitious reanalyses. When first encountering an archive, the investigator must immerse him- or herself in the data. The "start" costs, in terms of learning the details of the data set, are sufficiently demanding that they frequently discourage all but the most committed. Moving past this stage to the formulation of a plan of action is a critical challenge that will be encountered (Elder, in press). Obtaining funding for reanalysis of existing data is another obstacle. Success depends on having knowledgeable and sympathetic reviewers. Because so few people are experienced in using existing data, research proposals are often judged by reviewers who are not knowledgeable about or sympathetic toward seondary analysis. This situation does not seem likely to change until secondary analysis is included as a part of every researcher's training.

The value of data archives

The two primary ways that data can be made available for secondary analysis are (1) that the original investigators may give others direct access to their records, and (2) the investigators may contribute a copy of the data to an archive, which then makes the data available to interested researchers. There are some advantages to the first alternative. The main advantage to the primary investigators is that they retain control of the data, giving access only to researchers they trust to perform competent reanalyses and analyses that will complement but not conflict with their own. The advantage to the secondary analysts is that they are likely to have access to the primary investigators for valuable consultation on how the study was originally conceptualized and how the data were collected and coded. This interchange between primary and secondary researchers may contribute to the quality of the reanalyses. This kind of data sharing is fairly widespread, especially in the case of long-term longitudinal studies. At relatively early stages of the study, it may be the only practical approach to sharing data.

The second approach to sharing data, the use of centralized data archives, has advantages as well, and in many cases these may outweigh the advantages associated with the first approach. The first advantage concerns the costs to the original investigators of making data available to other researchers. The burdens of putting the data into a form that is accessible to others and educating others about the nature of the data can be great, especially in the case of large and complex data sets. When data are contributed to an archive, there is an initial period during which the investigators must provide documentation about the data set, but after the data are documented and prepared for use, the archive takes over the burdens of providing access to and assistance in using the data. The report of the American National Academy of Sciences Committee on National Statistics (Fienberg, Martin, & Straf, 1985) recommended that open sharing of data be adopted as a regular practice and that plans for sharing data be an integral part of the research plan whenever this is feasible. The report notes, however, that investigators are often reluctant to make their data available, partly because they lack the funds and staff time to do so. If these costs are assumed by archives, a major obstacle to sharing data is greatly reduced.

A second, and perhaps even more important, advantage to the research community of data archives is that they can bring together a relatively large number of data sets in one place and use a consistent form of documentation and data preparation across the data sets that they hold. The most critical obstacle to using existing data is the interested investigators' inability to locate data sets that meet their complex research needs, with respect to the substantive issues addressed, samples, instrumentation, and so on. For some research questions, the investigator may even need to find two or more data sets with comparable procedures that can be combined to create a multicohort study or a study that allows cross-national comparisons. This problem of finding just the right data sets is sometimes insurmountable. At other times, however, it only appears to be insurmountable as a result of lack of information about the availability of appropriate data sets. Clearly, the more data sets that are available and easy to locate, the more likely it is that researchers looking for data with particular characteristics will be able to find what they need. The creation of centralized data archives is one way to make this possible.

Another advantage of using archives as a mechanism of sharing data is more controversial and involves the issue of quality control. As Elder has pointed out (in press), it is very difficult to assess the value of a data set for secondary analysis independent of the research questions that the new investigator brings to the data. To the extent that this is true, selection by archives should probably err by being overly inclusive rather than very exclusive. Even so, it is possible for archives to exert some quality control by excluding studies that are clearly deficient in sampling procedures, sample maintenance (in the case of longitudinal studies), or instrumentation.

With some selectiveness on the part of the archive and the new investigator, some of the well-known problems of longitudinal research can be avoided by the secondary analyst. The often-cited difficulties of longitudinal research include the great investment of time and money required for data collection, the problem of subject attrition, the use of measures in the early waves that become dated by the time of the later waves, and design problems, such as the confounding of individual and social change in single cohort longitudinal studies. Clearly, the investment of time and money involved in conducting longitudinal research can be greatly reduced through the use of archival data. The problems of subject attrition and dated measures can also be mitigated to a large degree through selection of those studies that in hindsight can be seen to have succeeded in finding robust measures and maintaining a high response rate. The confounding of individual development and social change can be addressed by adding a new cohort to an existing single cohort study or by integrating two or more data sets into a single multicohort study, as Elder has done so well in his reanalyses of the Oakland and Berkeley longitudinal studies.

In spite of the many advantages of centralized archives, their feasibility and usefulness may vary considerably from one country to another. For example, in Sweden, due to laws concerning open access to public records, archives may encounter special difficulties protecting the confidentiality of study participants. Although it is possible and often very useful to archive data outside the country of origin, or to share data across national boundaries, this kind of exchange may also raise special problems under some circumstances. In general, one must take the legal and political realities of the research site into account in determining the best approach to sharing data.

What archives should be doing

In order for data archives to be most effective, they have to offer a wide range of data sets, with effective mechanisms for locating suitable data. They must offer data that are well suited to the research needs of their constituencies, including original subject records in some cases. And they must adopt policies and procedures that allow the data contributors the proper amount of control over their data, protect the privacy of the study participants, and offer appropriate acknowledgment of both the primary and secondary researchers' contributions to studies based on the data.

Data availability

If researchers seeking to use existing data are to find material suited to their research questions, they must have access to as wide a range of data sets as possible. Clearly, no single archive can possibly make available every data set that may be useful for further analysis. Archives vary in the content area in which they specialize, in the types of data they make available, and in the procedures they follow in making data available. Some archives concentrate on a specialized topic such as adolescent pregnancy (Data Archive on Adolescent Pregnancy and Pregnancy Prevention in Los Altos, California) or public opinion regarding political and social issues (e.g., the Roper Center at the University of Connecticut). Others focus on areas as broad as social and political research and include subdepartments on specific topics (e.g., the Inter-university Consortium for Political and Social Research at the University of Michigan). The types of data made available by archives include census data, survey data, voting records, institutional records, and qualitative material such as video-taped observations and responses to open-ended interviews and projective tests. Policies and procedures differ across archives, but generally computer data are made available on magnetic tapes (sometimes on disks), and raw data (original subject records) are usually made available on microfilm or paper. Most archives make their data and services available for cost.

In light of the specialization of archives, it will be important eventually to develop an information retrieval system that will allow researchers to search all relevant

variables. Collection of unprocessed behavioral data rather than precategorized encodings of behavior has been especially useful, for example, when changes have been made in accepted criteria of psychiatric diagnoses. In some cases this may be too cumbersome to be feasible. In other cases, however, it may simply mean running a tape recorder during an interview while also taking notes. If preferred, coding can be based on the notes. Even if not used by the original investigator, the tapes provide a valuable record of the complete interview. In long-term longitudinal studies, diagnostic categories, theoretical constructs, and variables of interest often change over the years of the study. When this happens, the original investigators may themselves want to go back to the data in an unprocessed form to recover needed information.

Third, investigators who expect to share their data should at some point ask the consent of their subjects to make the data available. Conditions under which data would be released to others should be specified in the consent form: for example, whether names and other identifiers would be removed; whether the data would be released for use by other researchers through the original investigator or through an archive; if the data are to be given to an archive, who would have access; and so on. It is obviously preferable, in many cases even necessary, to remove names from raw data before allowing access by anyone outside the immediate research team. For taped interviews that are to be transcribed, it is advisable to have typists substitute code names or numbers for real names at the transcribing stage in order to avoid many hours of deidentification later. For ease of storage and manipulation, it is very useful to transcribe interviews directly onto a computer.

Conclusions

Because large-scale long-term studies are so valuable and so rare, we believe it is critical to make full use of them through data sharing. In order for this to happen effectively, on a larger scale than it has until now, several changes need to occur.

First, the research community needs to develop a set of shared expectations or conventions with respect to the use of data by researchers outside the original team. These conventions should address:

1. Whether, when, and how the principal investigator will give others access to the data;
2. How to deal with consent and confidentiality issues;
3. How to assign credit to both the original investigators and the researchers who are reanalyzing the data; and
4. How much control over the use of data the original investigators should retain.

Second, investigators conducting longitudinal studies should collect and preserve data in their most basic or unprocessed form. They should also document the data collection and processing as completely as possible.

Third, data archives and others offering access to data need to provide the best information possible on how to find appropriate data sets. This will involve developing more and better methods for searching available sources for data sets with characteristics that match the requirements of the investigator.

Fourth, excellent training programs must be developed. In order to do this, the most creative and effective reanalyses need to be highlighted because, as with any research, secondary analysis can be done poorly or well. Then such examples can be used as models for teaching both graduate students and researchers how they may be able to use existing data profitably to answer their own research questions.

References

Block, J. (1971). *Lives through time.* Berkeley, CA: Bancroft Books.

Clubb, J. M., Austin, E. W., Geda, C. S., & Traugott, M. (1985). Sharing research data in the social sciences. In S. Fienberg, M. Martin, & M. Straf (Eds.), *Sharing research data.* Washington, DC: National Academy Press.

Duncan, G. J., & Morgan, J. N. (1980). *Panel study of income dynamics: Waves I–XII* (Machine-readable data file). Ann Arbor: University of Michigan, Institute for Social Research (Producer). Ann Arbor: Inter-university Consortium for Political and Social Research (Distributor).

Elder, Jr., G. H. (1974). *Children of the great depression.* Chicago: University of Chicago Press.

Elder, Jr., G. H. (in press). Studying women's lives: Research questions, strategies, and lessons. In S. I. Powers (Ed.), *Studying women's lives: The use of archival data.* New Haven, CT: Yale University Press.

Fienberg, S., Martin, M., & Straf, M. (Eds.) (1985). *Sharing research data.* Washington, DC: National Academy Press.

Furstenberg, F. F., Jr., Brooks-Gunn, J., & Morgan, P. (1987). *Adolescent mothers in later life.* New York: Cambridge University Press.

Lee, V. E., Brooks-Gunn, J., & Schnur, E. (1988). Does Head Start Work? A one-year follow-up comparison of disadvantaged children attending Head Start, no preschool, and other preschool programs. *Developmental Psychology, 24,* 2.

Migdal, S., Abeles, R. P., & Sherrod, L. R. (1981). *An inventory of longitudinal studies of middle and old age.* New York: Social Science Research Council.

National Center for Education Statistics. (1972). *National Longitudinal Study of the Class of 1972* (Machine-readable data file). Washington DC: National Center for Education Statistics (Producer, Distributor).

National Center for Education Statistics. (1980). *High School and Beyond* (Machine-readable data file). Washington DC: National Center for Education Statistics (Producer, Distributor).

Parnes, H. S. (1983). *The National Longitudinal Surveys 1966–1982* (Machine-readable data file). Washington DC: U.S. Department of Labor, Office of Manpower Policy, Evaluation, and Research (Producer). Columbus, OH: Ohio State University, Center for Human Resource Research (Distributor).

Vaillant, G. E. (1983). *The natural history of alcoholism.* Cambridge, MA: Harvard University Press.

Verdonik, F., & Sherrod, L. R. (1984). *An inventory of longitudinal research on childhood and adolescence.* New York: Social Science Research Council.

Author index

Subject index

271